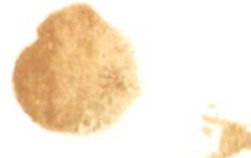

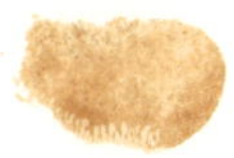

5781693400

AF443347

57 PN 8169340 0

WITHDRAWN
WITHDRAWN

Nutritional Toxicology

VOLUME II

NUTRITION: BASIC AND APPLIED SCIENCE
A SERIES OF MONOGRAPHS

WILLIAM J. DARBY, Editor
Professor of Biochemistry (Nutrition)
Vanderbilt University School of Medicine
Nashville, Tennessee

Anthony W. Norman. *Vitamin D: The Calcium Homeostatic Steroid Hormone*, 1979.

Donald S. McLaren (Editor). *Nutritional Ophthalmology*, 1980.

John N. Hathcock (Editor). *Nutritional Toxicology*, Volume I, 1982. Volume II, 1987.

J. Christopher Bauernfeind (Editor). *Vitamin A Deficiency and Its Control*, 1986.

Nutritional Toxicology

VOLUME II

Edited by

JOHN N. HATHCOCK

Experimental Nutrition Branch
Food and Drug Administration
Washington, D.C.

1987

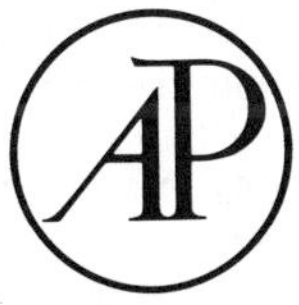

ACADEMIC PRESS, INC.

Harcourt Brace Jovanovich, Publishers

Orlando   San Diego   New York   Austin
Boston   London   Sydney   Tokyo   Toronto

LIBRARY AND INFORMATION SERVICE
POLYTECHNIC OF NORTH LONDON
HOLLOWAY ROAD
LONDON N7 8DB

POLYTECHNIC OF NORTH LONDON

Control No.	615.954 NuT
Class No.	616.399 NuT
Accession No.	5781693400

COPYRIGHT © 1987 BY ACADEMIC PRESS. INC.
ALL RIGHTS RESERVED.
NO PART OF THIS PUBLICATION MAY BE REPRODUCED OR
TRANSMITTED IN ANY FORM OR BY ANY MEANS. ELECTRONIC
OR MECHANICAL. INCLUDING PHOTOCOPY. RECORDING. OR
ANY INFORMATION STORAGE AND RETRIEVAL SYSTEM. WITHOUT
PERMISSION IN WRITING FROM THE PUBLISHER.

ACADEMIC PRESS, INC.
Orlando, Florida 32887

United Kingdom Edition published by
ACADEMIC PRESS INC. (LONDON) LTD.
24–28 Oval Road, London NW1 7DX

Library of Congress Cataloging in Publication Data
(Revised for vol. II)

Nutritional toxicology.

   (Nutrition, basic and applied science)
   Includes bibliographies and index.
   1. Nutritionally induced diseases—Collected works.
2. Nutrition—Collected works. I. Hathcock, John N.
II. Series. [DNLM: 1. Food contamination. 2. Food
additives—Adverse effects. 3. Food poisoning.
WA 701 N976]
RC622.N894   1982   616.3'99   82-4036
ISBN 0–12–332602–8 (v. 2 : alk. paper)

PRINTED IN THE UNITED STATES OF AMERICA

87 88 89 90   9 8 7 6 5 4 3 2 1

Contents

3 Metabolic and Nutritional Effects of Ethanol

Helmut K. Seitz and Ulrich A. Simanowski

4 Effects of Malnutrition on Drug Metabolism and Toxicity in Humans

Kamala Krishnaswamy

5 Nutritional Influences on Chromatin: Toxicological Implications

C. Elizabeth Castro

6 Mutagens in Cooked Foods

Walter A. Hargraves

10 Toxicology of Pesticide Residues in Foods

Joel R. Coats

11 Nutritional Importance of Pesticides

S. Berger and K. Cwiek

Contributors

Numbers in parentheses indicate the pages on which the authors' contributions begin.

Steven A. Belinsky[1] (41), Department of Pharmacology, University of North Carolina, Chapel Hill, North Carolina 27514

S. Berger (281), Institute of Human Nutrition, Warsaw Agricultural University, Warsaw, Poland

Jack Bergman (199), Harvard Medical School, Boston, Massachusetts 02115

C. Elizabeth Castro (129), Helicon Foundation, San Diego, California 92109

Joel R. Coats (249), Department of Entomology, Iowa State University, Ames, Iowa 50011

K. Cwiek (281), Department of Food Research, National Institute of Hygiene, Warsaw, Poland

P. B. Dews (199), New England Regional Primate Research Center, Southborough, Massachusetts 01772

Janet L. Greger (223), Nutritional Sciences Department, University of Wisconsin, Madison, Wisconsin 53706

Walter A. Hargraves (157), ABC Research Corporation, Gainesville, Florida 32607

Frederick C. Kauffman (41), Department of Pharmacology, University of Maryland, Baltimore, Maryland 21201

Kamala Krishnaswamy (105), National Institute of Nutrition, Hyderabad, India

Helen W. Lane (223), Department of Nutrition and Foods, Auburn University, Auburn, Alabama 36830

[1]Present address: S.A.B. National Institute of Environmental Health Sciences, P.O. Box 12233, Research Triangle Park, North Carolina 27709.

Mohsen Meydani (1), USDA Human Nutrition Research Center on Aging at Tufts University, Boston, Massachusetts 02111

Helmut K. Seitz (63), Alcohol Research Laboratory, Department of Medicine, University of Heidelberg, Heidelberg, Federal Republic of Germany

Ulrich A. Simanowski (63), Alcohol Research Laboratory, Department of Medicine, University of Heidelberg, Heidelberg, Federal Republic of Germany

Steve L. Taylor (173), Food Research Institute, University of Wisconsin, Madison, Wisconsin 53706

Ronald G. Thurman (41), Department of Pharmacology, University of North Carolina, Chapel Hill, North Carolina 27514

During the past few years nutritional toxicology has become increasingly recognized as an important new discipline with unique value as a scientific viewpoint. This perspective that nutrition and toxicology are fundamentally linked has led and continues to lead to a new and deeper understanding of each discipline. The intensity and diversity of interactions between nutritional phenomena and toxicologic processes and end points require extensive specification of experimental conditions for results to be predictable. Nutrients modify toxic responses and toxicants modify nutritional requirements and responses.

The purpose of this book is to expand on the topics covered in Volume I of Nutritional Toxicology. More specifically, it addresses particular subjects that have become substantially more important through the development of new knowledge, significant increases in knowledge, or increased awareness of potential effects on human health and well-being. The implications of such knowledge have impact on basic research, toxicity testing, public health, food and agriculture programs, and food safety regulation.

John N. Hathcock

Contents of Volume I

Index

Nutritional Toxicology

VOLUME II

1

Dietary Effects on Detoxification Processes

Mohsen Meydani

I. INTRODUCTION

Humans and animals are continuously exposed to wide varieties of chemical compounds which have some deleterious effects on well-being. The requirement of riboflavin for reduction of carcinogenic azo dye 4-methylaminobenzene by liver homogenates was the stimulating observation of Mueller and Miller (1950), which attracted a broad spectrum of scientists to investigate the role of nutrients on the metabolism and detoxification of foreign compounds. Chemical compounds foreign to the body, such as natural food products, food additives, pesticides, and industrial products, by-products, and pollutants are collectively named xenobiotics. Xenobiotics, after entry into the body, undergo metabolic changes whereby lipid-soluble compounds are converted into polar, water-soluble products and excreted from the body.

Several groups of enzymes participate in the biotransformation and detoxification of xenobiotics as well as in the metabolism of the endogenous substances such as fatty acids, prostaglandins, cholesterol, steroids, and vitamins. Some of the biotransformation process may take place in one tissue such as the liver and

1

Copyright © 1987 by Academic Press, Inc.
All rights of reproduction in any form reserved.

then be further processed in another tissue like the kidney. Some of the enzymes involved in the biotransformation process are localized in the membrane and some in soluble fractions of cytoplasm. The biotransformation and detoxification of chemical compounds take place in two major phases: (1) functionalization (phase I) processes, where foreign compounds are converted to more potent or less potent compounds than the parent compounds to render them ready for the next stage of processing, and (2) conjugation (phase II) processes, whereby metabolites produced in phase I processes are combined with endogenous molecules and become less toxic and harmful and more water-soluble and readily excretable. In the phase I processes, compounds may undergo either oxidation, reduction, or hydrolysis and become functionalized and sequestered for subsequent biotransformation. Mixed-function oxidases (MFO) or "monooxygenases" are the general terms used for the enzyme systems involved in oxidative reactions. The system has an absolute requirement for reducing equivalents of NADPH or NADH, and molecular oxygen and a reducing agent. Central for the MFO system are cytochrome P-450s, which are invested in endoplasmic reticulum and closely associated with flavoprotein enzymes: NADPH-cytochrome P-450 reductase, NADH-cytochrome b_5 reductase, cytochrome b_5, and phosphatidylcholine (Coon, 1978; Hammer and Wills, 1978; Gillette *et al.*, 1972).

The presence of multiple forms of membrane heme proteins, cytochrome P-450s (Levin *et al.*, 1980; Guengerich, 1977; Imai and Sato, 1974), may be attributed at least in part to the broad range of substrate specificity of the MFO system. Multiple forms of cytochrome P-450s are differentiated by apoprotein moieties and substrate specificities and spectral properties (Lu and West, 1980). In mammals, cytochrome P-450s are found in varying concentrations in the endoplasmic reticulum of liver, kidney, small intestine, lung, adrenal glands, and other tissues (Guengerich and Manson, 1979). Cytochrome P-450 also is present in nuclear envelope, and there is evidence that distinct differences exist in the nature and reactivity between cytochrome P-450 from nuclear envelope and that from microsome (Cheng *et al.*, 1980; Mukhtar *et al.*, 1978). Cytochrome P-450 of the nuclear envelope may play an important role in carcinogen activation and metabolism.

The MFO system can be induced or inhibited by different chemicals. Two major classes of compounds are the inducers of this system. Phenobarbital is the prototype for one class of chemical which stimulates the metabolism of a wide variety of substrates and induces a number of cytochrome P-450s. Polycyclic aromatic hydrocarbons are the other class of compounds which induce subspecies of cytochrome P-450, commonly referred to as cytochrome P-448 or P_1-450. This type of inducer enhances biotransformation of a limited number of substrates. Prototypes for the latter class are 3-methylcholanthrene (3-MC) and benzo[*a*]pyrene. The induction MFO system is usually detected by a relative increase of MFO activity as determined by the *in vivo* or *in vitro* rate of drug metabolism. The induction mechanism occurs through DNA-dependent RNA synthesis, mRNAs, decreases of RNA and cytoplasmic RNase activity, and turnover of microsomal phospholipids (Smith *et al.*, 1976; Jacob *et al.*, 1974; Gelboin *et al.*, 1967). Many different compounds inhibit the MFO system either by acting as an alternative substrate or by reversible binding to a specific component of the MFO system. SKF525A (β-diethylaminoethyldiphenylpropylacetate) is the well-known inhibitor of the MFO system, and its effects on hexobarbital metabolism were recognized earlier by Cook *et al.* (1954). In the biotransformation processes some of the compounds undergo enzymatic hydrolysis, which is a vital reaction for the deactivation of certain drugs and toxicants such as degradation of potentially nucleophilic reactive epoxides (Guengrich, 1982).

The conjugation process (phase II) transforms xenobiotics to more polar compounds for excretion. It does usually follow the functionalization reaction, and it is a synthetic process which requires energy in the form of ATP, and a conjugating agent which in most cases is a nucleotide. UDP-glucuronic acid enzymatically reacts with a number of nucleophiles. Tripeptide glutathione (GSH), through the action of enzymes (GSH transferases), reacts with great varieties of electrophiles, and the products are excreted in urine in the form of mercapturic acids. Conjugation and excretion are important processes in the detoxification mechanism, and any change in the capacity of the organism to carry out these steps has a profound effect on the ultimate biological activity of toxic compounds.

Since discovery of the role of the MFO system and components in the biotransformation of chemical compounds, the effect of quality and quantity of food components on the *in vivo* and *in vitro* metabolism of xenobiotics in different species has been investigated. Macro- and micronutrients play a significant role in both phases of the metabolism of drugs and foreign compounds. Dietary nutrients may also function in a way to reduce absorption of toxic chemicals from the digestive tract. The interaction of nutrients and drugs and toxicant in the alimentary tract, or the influence of dietary nutrient on the absorption of drugs and toxic chemicals are also important aspects of foreign compound metabolism which will not be discussed in this chapter. This review will focus on the role and importance of macro- and micronutrients on detoxification processes of foreign compounds after absorption.

II. MACRONUTRIENTS IN DETOXIFICATION

A. Fat

Since dietary fat has been the major concern of public health, the effect of quantity and quality of dietary fat on the metabolism of drugs, carcinogens, and foreign compounds has drawn the attention of investigators. Dietary fat influences the fatty acid profile of cellular components in animal and human tissues (Witting *et al.*, 1961; Horwitt and Harvey, 1962). The influence of dietary fat on the susceptibility of individuals or populations to certain disorders arising from xenobiotics action has been the subject of numerous investigations.

Dietary fat might have a profound effect on the toxicity of foreign compounds and on the action of drugs through altering microsomal drug metabolism of hepatic and extrahepatic tissues or by changing bioavailability of drug or toxicants to the site of action. Phosphatidylcholine is known as an essential membranous component of the MFO system (Strobel *et al.*, 1970), and its fatty acid composition in the membrane can be altered through dietary fat treatments (Wade *et al.*, 1978; Hammer and Wills, 1978). The requirement for quality and quantity of dietary fat, for optimal activity and induction of cytochrome P-450 has been investigated both in animals and humans. Caster *et al.* (1970) have reported an increase of hexobarbital metabolism in the liver of rats fed 3% corn oil. A marked increase of cytochrome P-450 has been shown in response to phenobarbital induction in the animals fed with diets containing either herring oil or linoleic acid (Marshall and McLean, 1971), whereas feeding coconut oil in the diet was not effective on elevating cytochrome P-450. Century (1973) has reported that phenobarbital-pretreated rats which have been fed linseed or menhaden oils had the highest and animals which have been fed beef fat or low levels of corn oil had the lowest stimulation of *in vitro* drug metabolism. These results were supported by those of Marshall and McLean (1971), who reported that the addition of herring oil or linoleic acid to the diet allowed a large increase of cytochrome P-450 in response to phenobarbital pretreatment while the addition of coconut oil to the diet did not induce cytochrome P-450. Century (1973) also pointed out that without phenobarbital pretreatment, no difference was found in drug metabolism with increasing the level of corn oil. Furthermore, increased hexobarbital metabolism by feeding corn oil was not confirmed by Century's experiment. In an experiment with isolated perfused liver of rat, Lam and Wade (1980) found that clearance of hexobarbital was significantly faster in the livers from rats fed a diet with 10% corn oil than in liver from rats fed a fat-free diet, indicating that feeding 10% corn oil diet enhances hepatic hexobarbital oxidase activity. In contrast, Hopkins and West (1976a) reported that rats fed a diet containing sunflower seed oil for 4 weeks had a longer pentobarbital-induced sleeping time and a lower concentration of hepatic microsomal cytochrome P-450 than rats fed a diet containing beef tallow fat. The controversial results of animal studies might be implicated, as Hopkins and West (1976b) propounded that either the degree of saturation of dietary fat or the propensity to form lipid peroxides might be responsible for those results.

Norred and Marzuki (1984) have demonstrated that diets devoid of or low in polyunsaturated fat and high in saturated fat produced a lower level of cytosolic GSH transferase activity in rat hepatocytes. Our findings show that the relationship of dietary fat and the drug-metabolizing enzyme system appears to be species-dependent (Meydani *et al.*, 1985). We found that hexobarbital-induced sleeping time was shorter in cebus monkeys fed coconut oil diet and in squirrel monkeys fed corn oil diet for 8 years. Our findings indicate that dietary fat unsaturation in different species influences the drug-metabolizing system differently, possibly through effects on membrane phospholipids, particularly of phosphatidylcholine.

Absolute amount of fat in the diet may have a major effect on the MFO system. Presence or absence of fat in the diets of animals has been shown to have a marked effect on the activity and induction of the drug-metabolizing enzyme system. Rowe and Wills (1976) found that liver microsomal cytochrome *P*-450 content and the rate of oxidative demethylation were lowest when a fat-free diet was fed to the rats, whereas they were increased by addition of 10% lard and much more by addition of 10% corn oil. This increase was much more pronounced when phenobarbital pretreatment was used as an inducer. Relative to the 10% corn oil diet, a lower concentration of hepatic microsomal cytochrome *P*-450 is also reported from rats fed a fat-free diet for 21 days (Cheng *et al.*, 1980, 1981). Phenobarbital treatment significantly increased liver microsomal cytochrome *P*-450 concentration in rats fed both fat-free and 10% corn oil diet; the increase was significantly greater in rats fed a 10% corn oil diet than in those fed the fat-free diet. Although the microsomal cytochrome *P*-450 concentration as measured by CO-binding spectra was increased by dietary corn oil, the putative cytochrome *P*-450 protein was found to be only slightly elevated. In contrast, Sitar and Gordon (1980) found no significant difference in the total liver microsomal cytochrome *P*-450 between rats fed either 4% or 38% of total calories from fat source. Furthermore, they found that low fat intake resulted in a significant increase of a certain group of cytochrome *P*-450s which were separated by ion exchange chromatography. The level of dietary fat was found to have an insignificant effect on 3-MC induction of cytochrome *P*-450 (Cheng *et al.*, 1981). 3-MC brought about an increase of concentration of cytochrome *P*-450 (as measured by CO-binding spectra) to nearly equal levels in rats fed fat-free or 10% corn oil diet for 21 days.

The effect of dietary fat on the detoxification of foreign compounds in humans is not as extensively investigated as in animals. Anderson *et al.* (1979) studied the effect of amount and type of dietary fat on drug metabolism using antipyrine and theophylline plasma half-life ($t_{1/2}$) and clearance in human subjects. Feeding subjects with a high-fat diet (70% fat and 10% protein of total calories) for 2 weeks resulted in increase of $t_{1/2}$ for antipyrine and theophylline. That was an indication of possible depression of the MFO system. Whereas low-fat diet (30% fat and 50% protein of total calories) resulted in a lower $t_{1/2}$ for both drugs. Their results indicated that substitution of dietary protein for fat can result in acceleration of drug metabolism. In the other study, feeding human subjects with high-fat diets (60% of total calories) containing constant protein (15% of total calories) for 2 weeks had no effect on the $t_{1/2}$ of both drugs. Furthermore, changing 80%

of total fat to either form of saturated or unsaturated fat also had no significant effect on the mean plasma $t_{1/2}$ for either drug. These findings have led to the suggestion that the saturated or unsaturated fat composition of the diet does not greatly alter rates of drug oxidation by the liver in humans. Changing the proportion of saturation to unsaturation of fat in the diet of six human subjects for a short time also has been shown to have no significant effect on the metabolism of the antipyrine and debrisquine (Mucklow *et al.*, 1980).

Tumor enhancement by high-fat diet was reported as early as 50 years ago (Watson and Mellanby, 1930). The interaction of dietary fat and the MFO system on the activation or deactivation of carcinogens has been the subject of extensive investigation. Tumor-promoting action of dietary fat types through microsomal enzyme induction has been suggested for aflatoxin-induced liver tumor. Newberne *et al.* (1979) found that rats fed with beef fat had depressed p-nitroanisol demethylase activity as compared to corn oil-fed rats. Moreover, they found that when rats were treated with aflatoxin B_1 (AFB_1), p-nitroanisol demethylase activity and benzo[*a*]pyrene hydroxylase activity were increased. In the rats fed a corn oil diet the activity of both enzymes was higher than in those fed a beef fat diet, and, in addition, liver tumor incidence was lower than the groups fed the corn oil diet. Presence of the nuclear MFO system in close proximity to DNA may play an important role in the activation of carcinogens. Cheng *et al.* (1980, 1981) have found that the concentration of nuclear envelope cytochrome P-450 from 10% corn oil-fed rats was higher than rats fed the fat-free diet. They also reported that phenobarbital pretreatment induced the nuclear cytochrome P-450 level in rats fed the fat-free diet but not in rats fed the corn oil diet. However, pretreatment with 3-MC did not induce nuclear cytochrome P-450 from rats fed the fat-free diet.

Carroll and Khor (1971) reported that the type of dietary fat might have a great influence on the incidence of tumors. They have shown that rats treated with 7,12-dimethylbenz[*a*]anthracene (DMBA) and fed unsaturated fats developed more mammary tumors than those fed saturated fat at the same level in the diet. Newberne *et al.* (1978) have also shown that the addition of beef fat retarded mammary tumor induction. In contrast, Carroll and Hopkins (1979) and Hopkins and Carroll (1979) have demonstrated that animals fed diets containing saturated fat (17% coconut and 3% sunflower seed oil) and treated with DMBA had enhanced tumor incidence as much as with feeding diets containing 20% sunflower seed oil. They have also shown that a dietary essential fatty acid is required for tumor yield. These findings are supported by epidemiological data which indicate a correlation between tumor incidence and dietary fat intake (Carroll, 1980). Although animal studies indicate that dietary fat through the effect on the MFO system promotes or activates carcinogens, the few human studies do not show changes in the MFO system through dietary fat intervention.

For the proper *in vivo* or *in vitro* function of the microsomal MFO system, lipids of membrane, particularly phospholipids, are required. Phosphatidylcholine is the essential component of this system for maximum expression of activity (Strobel *et al.*, 1970). The role and mechanism by which dietary fat exerts its effect is not well established; however, it appears to function as the matrix allowing effective interaction between the NADPH-cytochrome P-450 reductase and cytochrome P-450. Since the distribution of enzymes of the MFO system is heterogeneous (Yang, 1977), possibly phospholipids provide a translational mobility to the enzymes and enhance electron transfer from reductase to a large number of cytochrome P-450 molecules (Yang, 1975, 1977).

Fatty acid composition of phospholipid in the endoplasmic reticulum might have a major effect on the activity of this enzyme system. Davison and Wills (1974) demonstrated that incorporation of linoleate into phospholipid of microsomes increases when phenobarbital or 3-MC inducers are used. Different levels of linoleate might be required for optimal activity of specific enzymes of this system. Lambert and Wills (1977) have reported a maximal *in vitro* demethylation in both induced and controlled rats fed herring oil, which was high in polyunsaturated fatty acid but contained 1.17% linoleate. Lang (1976) has shown that O-demethylation was inhibited with high levels of dietary linoleate, whereas arylhydrocarbon hydroxylase (AHH) activity was depressed with low levels of dietary fat. Increase of polyunsaturated fatty acids content in the membrane increases susceptibility of membrane to lipid peroxidation (Tien *et al.*, 1981) and exposes cytochrome P-450 to radical attack and subsequent deactivation.

Marshall and McLean (1971), on the basis of their findings on dietary fat and phenobarbital pretreatments, proposed a theoretical mechanism for the permissive effect of dietary unsaturated fatty acid on the enzyme induction by phenobarbital. They suggested that an endogenous factor which serves as a mediator between inducers and increased level of cytochrome P-450 might exist, and that it can be metabolically inactivated in the presence of an inducer. Unsaturated fatty acids might also enhance the ability of the inducer, which can in turn block inactivation of these endogenous factors and therefore enhance induction. The other proposed mechanism for the effect of lipid substances on MFO activity has been partially demonstrated by the findings that endogenous lipids such as steroids and fatty acids may occupy cytochrome P-450-binding sites, thereby displacing exogenous substances and possibly interfering with their metabolism (Campbell and Hayes, 1974). A partial stimulating effect of dietary cholesterol on the MFO system has been suggested to occur because of structural changes of the endoplasmic reticulum (Hietanen *et al.*, 1975; Laitinen, 1976; Lang *et al.*, 1976; Lambert and Wills, 1977). Cheng *et al.* (1980) speculated that dietary fat may cause perturbations in the membrane, which alters the positioning of cytochrome P-450 and renders it more active or less active as measured by the CO-binding spectrum and enzyme assay; yet concentration of cytochrome P-450 in the membrane might not be changed, as they have demonstrated by fluorescence gel scanning, and therefore qualitative alteration was the major reason for the observed quantitative changes. However, Wade and Norred (1976) presented evidence that both quality and quantity of the MFO system can be affected by dietary fat.

B. Protein

Protein intake of individuals and populations varies a great deal. The daily amount of protein synthesis and degradation in the body is considerable, and the daily requirement varies with age and with pathological and physiological states of individuals. Deficiency of protein, with or without deficiency of total calories, is one of the devastating nutritional problems among children in most of the underdeveloped countries. The pathophysiology of protein–calorie malnutrition is quite complicated and has substantial effects on the vulnerability of individuals to toxicological insults.

Amino acids of dietary protein are involved in the synthesis of numerous biological molecules, of which quite a few are involved in the absorption, binding, metabolism, and excretion of many toxic chemicals and drugs. Metabolism of toxic chemicals and drugs has been shown to be impaired by protein deprivation. Increased toxicity of chemical compounds and drugs in protein deficiency was reported as early as 1954 by Drill. Kato *et al.* (1962) for the first time demonstrated reduction of hepatic MFO activity in protein deficiency. Protein deficiency decreases the activity of the MFO system in the liver, which in turn increases the $t_{1/2}$ of numerous toxic chemicals and drugs and thereby potentiates toxicity on drug action. In protein deficiency, depending on the compound, it may either become more toxic or less toxic than the parent compound. Therefore, deficiency of protein may exacerbate or alleviate the ultimate action of chemical compounds. Quantity and quality of protein in the diet alters both phase I and phase II reactions in drug metabolism. For example, the toxicity of strychnine, zoxazolamine, and pentobarbital has been shown to be increased in protein-deprived rats (Kato *et al.*, 1968). These compounds are normally metabolized and become less toxic by the action of the MFO system. The toxicity of most pesticides such as chlorinated hydrocarbons and acetylcholinesterase inhibitors, as well as herbicides and fungicides, have been demonstrated to be increased severalfold by protein deficiency (Boyd and Krupa, 1970). Protein deficiency may also result in a decrease of toxicity of compounds such as carbon tetrachloride (McLean and McLean, 1966), octamethyl pyrophosphoramide (Kato *et al.*, 1968), and heptachlor (Weatherholtz *et al.*, 1969). These compounds are known to be metabolically activated to a more toxic compound by microsomal oxidation.

Change in the level and/or in the activity of drug-metabolizing enzymes of the liver in protein deficiency have been attributed to the altered detoxification capacity. Decreased MFO activity of enzymes with a low-protein diet has also been reported by several investigators. Clinton *et al.* (1979) have found that feeding rats a low-protein diet from weaning onward decreased hepatic cytochrome *P*-450 content. Magdalou *et al.* (1979) have shown that protein depletion decreased cytochrome *P*-450 content, total protein, and total phospholipid in the liver. In contrast, others have found that a short-term protein deficiency had no significant effect on hepatic cytochrome *P*-450 content (Hietanen, 1980). The controversial results on the effect of dietary protein on hepatic cytochrome *P*-450 might be due to the differences in the ages of animals when dietary regimen was started in the different studies.

Protein deprivation, besides decreasing the cytochrome *P*-450 content of liver, also decreases NADPH-cytochrome *P*-450 (*c*) reductase, cytochrome b_5, and numerous other enzymes (Kato *et al.*, 1968; Campbell and Hayes, 1976; Hietanen, 1980; Clinton *et al.*, 1977). Depression of MFO activity by low dietary protein has been shown to be due to decreased quantity of microsomal protein (Magdalou *et al.*, 1979) and mainly due to decreased activity of the existing enzyme system (Campbell and Hayes, 1976). Change of activity of enzymes despite a low cytochrome *P*-450 content was not found in a chronically protein-deficient monkey (Rumack *et al.*, 1973). Protein deprivation, besides its effect on phase I reactions, also increases liver UDP-glucuronyltransferase (UDPG transferase) activity, which is involved in the phase II reactions (Hietanen, 1980; Smith *et al.*, 1973; Woodcock and Wood, 1971; Wood and Woodcock, 1970).

Clearance of drugs and plasma $t_{1/2}$ of drugs are common tools which have been used for evaluation of *in vivo* status of the MFO system in humans and animals. Among the drugs, antipyrine and theophylline are widely used substrates for this purpose. Barbiturates are the inducer of antipyrine metabolism (Kahn *et al.*, 1980), whereas theophylline metabolism is not inducible by barbiturates; however, its metabolism is inducible by polycyclic hydrocarbons (Lohman and Miech, 1976; Piafsky *et al.*, 1975), which are inducers of cytochrome *P*-448 enzymes in liver. In monkeys it was found not only that $t_{1/2}$ of antipyrine increases but also that activity of aminopyrine and ethylmorphine *N*-demethylase and aniline hydroxylase were decreased in the liver by dietary protein deficiency (Sharma *et al.*, 1985; Rumack *et al.*, 1973). Isocaloric increasing of the ratio of dietary protein to carbohydrate in well-nourished volunteers has been shown to enhance clearance of antipyrine and theophylline (Kappas *et al.*, 1976). Prolonged antipyrine $t_{1/2}$ and reduced clearance of antipyrine (Wilmana *et al.*, 1979; Mucklow *et al.*, 1979) were found in Asian vegetarians, having relatively low daily dietary protein intake. Brodie *et al.* (1980) did not find any change in antipyrine, paracetamol, and phenacetin clearance in nine Caucasian vegetarians. They indicated that differences between Asian and Caucasian vegetarians on drug metabolism possibly were related to dietary protein intake.

Plasma proteins, particularly albumin, have an important role in the binding, distribution, and delivery of foreign compounds in the body. Binding and clearance of phenylbutazone from plasma has been shown to decrease as plasma protein, albumin, and microsomal cytochrome *P*-450 were decreased in protein-deficient rats (Varma, 1979). The increase of serum albumin in kwashiorkor-rehabilitated children has been found to correlate with the increased rate of metabolism and decreased $t_{1/2}$ of acetanilide (Buchanan *et al.*, 1980). Therefore, delivery and availability of a drug to the site of action and metabolism can also be affected in protein deficiency.

The effect of dietary protein on the toxicity of lead, an environmental pollutant, is controversial. Baernstein and Grand (1942) showed that lead toxicity can be increased by feeding low dietary protein. Verlangieri *et al.* (1982) have reported that chronic lead ingestion significantly increased locomotor activity of both sexes of low protein status. However, both high and low dietary protein may increase the lead content of different tissues (Levander, 1979).

High intake of dietary protein may exert a protective effect against toxicity of foreign compounds and enhance the adaptability of individuals and animals to toxic insults by increasing the activity level of the drug-metabolizing enzyme system. Kato *et al.* (1968) demonstrated that a high-protein diet containing 50% casein significantly increased the activity of several enzymes of the MFO system in young male rats but not in female rats. Kato *et al.* (1980) indicated that the activity of the MFO enzyme system increases as the protein content of the diet increases, up to 35%. Czygan *et al.* (1974) also noted that rats fed a high-protein diet had a high level of hepatic cytochrome *P*-450. Others have also demonstrated the enhancement of MFO activities by high dietary protein intake (Venkatesan *et al.*, 1970; Sachan, 1976; Clinton *et al.*, 1977). Activity of AHH, an enzyme which metabolizes carcinogenic polycyclic aromatic hydrocarbons, has been shown to increase as protein content of the diet was increased (Clinton *et al.*, 1979). Decreased antipyrine and theophylline $t_{1/2}$ as an indicator of increased activities of the MFO system with high dietary protein intake in humans (Anderson *et al.*, 1982) also supports the protective effect of dietary protein as an inducer of the drug-metabolizing system.

Rats fed an 18% gluten diet, as compared to rats fed an 18% casein diet supplemented with methionine, have shown a decreased level of cytochrome *P*-450 and depressed *in vitro* metabolism of ethylmorphine and aniline with increased hexobarbital-induced sleeping time (Miranda and Webb, 1973). These effects were not detected in guinea pigs fed 30% of the same proteins in their diet (Chadwick *et al.*, 1973). Kato *et al.* (1981a) have examined the effect of several proteins from animal and vegetable sources and found that a gelatin diet induces a very low activity of the MFO system. However, despite poor protein quality of the diet in their experiment, feeding polychlorated biphenyls (PCB) apparently caused a higher aniline hydroxylase and cytochrome *P*-450 activity. Kato *et al.* (1981a,b, 1982) also discovered that methionine-supplemented soy protein depressed aniline hydroxylase activity but slightly increased the activity of aminopyrine *N*-demethylase and NADPH-cytochrome *c* reductase and the level of cytochrome *P*-450. They concluded that in general the relative biological values of proteins were positively correlated with aniline hydroxylase, cytochrome P-450, and NADPH-cytochrome c reductase. Edes *et al.* (1979) have shown that methionine and cysteine deficiency results in the reduction of intestinal and hepatic MFO enzyme activity. Rats fed 48% less than the required sulfur amino acids, of methionine, and cysteine have shown a decreased cytochrome P-450 and increase of UDPG transferase activity (Magdalou *et al.*, 1979). Depression of hepatic MFO activity by marginal methionine, folic acid, and choline deficiency has also been demonstrated by other investigators (Suit *et al.*, 1977; Poireir *et al.*, 1977; Campbell *et al.*, 1978).

Glutathione peroxidase (GSH-Px), which metabolically reduces toxic peroxides and protects cells from free-radical injuries, is a selenoenzyme (Flohe *et al.*, 1973). Quality of dietary protein affects selenium metabolism. At the suboptimal dietary methionine intake, metabolism of selenium might be altered and consequently less selenium would be available for GSH-Px biosynthesis in the cells (Sunde *et al.*, 1981). Therefore, dietary methionine and quality of dietary protein are important for the optimal utilization of selenium from plant origin and may have consequences for the detoxification of compounds which are metabolized through GSH-Px or GSH transferase action.

Sulfur amino acids of dietary protein participate in the biosynthesis of GSH, which is the major nonprotein thiol compound found in all types of living cells. The thiol group of GSH is the most chemically active group in the molecule and has important biological functions. GSH has a potent oxidation–reduction capability and protects cells against hydroperoxide damage and prevents the formation of hydroxy radicals (Sunde and Hoekstra, 1980). GSH also serves as a coenzyme for several enzymes and can be conjugated with reactive products of cytochrome P-450. Reduction in the rat liver GSH pool in protein deficiency has been demonstrated (Edwards and Westerfeld, 1952). Mainigi and Campbell (1981) found that feeding a low-protein diet to rats reduces hepatic GSH within hours and the low level remains for at least 6 weeks. Mainigi and Campbell (1981) noted that the level of the hepatic GSH increases with addition of AFB_1 to the diet, regardless of dietary protein level and animal sex. They found that acute AFB_1 lesions in the liver were much more pronounced in the rats fed a high-protein diet. These findings, together with findings of others, indicate that the relationship between dietary protein and GSH level and protection against lesions of liver is not simple and probably other factors are involved.

Methionine deficiency has been shown to reduce GSH level in liver of mice and to increase acetaminophen hepatotoxicity (Reicks and Hathcock, 1984), whereas rats fed diets containing either 40% or 140% of requirements of sulfur amino acids for 5 weeks had no significant changes in liver GSH level (Meydani and Hathcock, 1984). Further, addition of atrazine, a herbicide which is mainly conjugated with GSH and cysteine and is excreted as mercapturic acid, was not effective in reduction of liver GSH. Although isolated hepatocytes have been shown to be capable of biosynthesis of GSH from exogenous methionine (Thor *et al.,* 1979), feeding rats or mice with excess methionine did not affect such biosynthetic pathways (Meydani and Hathcock, 1984; Reicks and Hathcock, 1984). Furthermore, Campbell *et al.* (1978) have shown that the level of GSH in the liver was not affected after 90 days of dietary methionine deficiency, while the activity of MFO enzymes was depressed. A similar observation was made by Poirer *et al.* (1977).

In the case of marginal methionine deficiency, a possible adaptive mechanism could be involved for regeneration and preservation of GSH, rather than conjugation and excretion processes. However, pathophysiological evidence from our study indicates that nontoxic levels of excess dietary methionine alleviate toxicity of methylmercury and atrazine in rats. The protective effect of dietary methionine supplementation on copper in chicks (Jensen and Maurice, 1979) and toxicity of paracetamol in rats (McLean and Day, 1975) has been demonstrated. The other protective effect of dietary sulfur amino acids is related to sulfoconjugation of toxic chemicals. In rabbits, the sulfur amino acids have been found to be better precursors of sulfate esters than organic sulfate (Bray *et al..* 1952). Magdalou *et al.* (1979) have indicated that, in methionine deficiency, decrease of sulfoconjugate might be related to the decrease of its precursor, sulfur amino acids, which also causes a compensatory increase of UDPG acid and UDPG transferase activity.

The substances whose mutagenicity and carcinogenicity are dependent on cytochrome *P*-450-mediated microsomal activation have been suggested to be most likely affected by dietary protein. Toxicity and carcinogenicity of foreign compounds is dependent on the extent of covalent bonding of their highly reactive metabolites to critical macromolecules (Gillette, 1974). Activities of drug-metabolizing enzymes can alter the quality or quantity of these metabolites. For example, although reactive metabolites of aryl hydrocarbons are formed from the action of the MFO system, the majority of them are conjugated in the phase II processes, and thus critical macromolecules such as DNA and RNA are protected. The steady state of reactive metabolites depends on the rate of formation and removal by the drug-metabolizing enzyme system (Campbell and Hayes, 1976). McLean and Magee (1970) have shown that protein deficiency decreased hepatic microsomal oxidases in rats and prevented the induction of hepatic tumors by dimethylnitrosamine (DMN) while incidence of renal tumor was enhanced. Czygan *et al.* (1974) have demonstrated a decreased DMN mutagenicity of live microsomes from rats fed decreasing levels of protein in their diet. DMN requires metabolic activation to exert mutagenicity and carcinogenicity, whereas *N*-nitrosomethylurea does not. Therefore, carcinogenicity and mutagenicity of *N*-nitrosomethylurea are enhanced by a protein-free diet (Swann and McLean, 1971). Madhaven and Gopalan (1968) have indicated that rats fed 20% protein were less sensitive to the aflatoxin hepatocarcinogenicity than those fed low dietary protein.

The influence of several dietary amino acids such as methionine, tryptophan, phenylalanine, and tyrosine on tumor induction has been investigated. Several experiments on the marginal deficiency of methionine together with choline defidiency in the diet have shown an enhancement of carcinogenicity of many compounds such as aflatoxin, nitrosamines, acetaminofluorine, and ethionine (Newberne and McConnell, 1980). Since proteins become hydrolyzed to their component amino acids in the gut before absorption, Newberne and McConnell (1980) have suggested that quality or source of dietary protein with well-balanced amino acids would have no significant influence on the carcinogenicity of a compound.

Thus, it does appear that induction and activity of the drug-metabolizing enzyme system in the liver in relation to dietary protein and amino acids plays an important role in detoxification of foreign compounds. However, the relationship or interaction is not simple. Reduced DNA replication associated with protein deficiency in male rats has been purported to lower quantity of microsomal protein and activity of enzyme per unit of tissue (Mgbodile and Campbell, 1972). An altered ratio of phosphatidylcholine to cytochrome P-450 in protein deficiency has been attributed to the decreased cytochrome P-450 content (Hayes *et al.*, 1973). Therefore, the important mechanisms by which protein exerts its effect on the detoxification process might be through change in the biosynthesis of microsomal protein and changing ratio of phosphatidylcholine to cytochrome P-450 of the endoplasmic reticulum in the hepatocyte. In this respect, the effect of dietary protein on the other factors such as cytosolic enzymes and cosubstrates of the drug metabolism system, as well as the effect on the plasma protein concentration, should be well recognized.

C. Carbohydrate

Prolonged phenobarbital hypnosis with iv administration of glucose is one of the earliest observations on the effect of carbohydrate on drug metabolism (Lamson *et al.*, 1951). Activity of several hepatic MFO enzymes has also been shown to be markedly decreased by feeding rats with sucrose instead of the standard chow diet for 1–3 days (Kato, 1966, 1967). A decrease of cytochrome P-450 and cytochrome b_5 contents in both male and female rats was also observed in Kato's studies.

Reduction of hexobarbital metabolism by a high intake of glucose has been demonstrated in mice (Strother *et al.*, 1971). Relative to a starch diet, sucrose increases the lethality to rats of benzylpenicillin due to the reduced rate of its metabolism (Boyd *et al.*, 1970). Dickerson *et al.* (1971) have reported that feeding a sugar diet to rats decreased the activity of several MFO enzymes and lowered cytochrome P-450 levels.

In most of the studies on the effect of dietary fat and protein on drug and toxicant metabolism, substitution of carbohydrate for fat or protein nutriture has been employed without regard to the possible effect of carbohydrate modification. Using antipyrine and theophylline $t_{1/2}$ in plasma, Alvares *et al.* (1976), Kappas *et al.* (1976), and Anderson *et al.* (1982) have found that a high-carbohydrate diet had no significant effect on drug metabolism as compared to a normal diet in humans. Sonawane *et al.* (1983) have indicated that the relative quantities of carbohydrate and fat in the diet are more important than the quality of carbohydrate in the modification of MFO system. A specific role for carbohydrate in the detoxification processes is not established yet. Williams (1978) has indicated involvement of glucose in the phase II process of biotransformation. Based on the inhibitory effect of carbohydrate on δ-aminolevulinate synthetase, a rate-limiting enzyme in liver heme synthesis, Anderson *et al.* (1982) suggested that reduction of cytochrome *P*-450 content possibly is interrelated with depression of heme biosynthesis by carbohydrate.

III. MICRONUTRIENTS IN DETOXIFICATION

A. Vitamins

1. Vitamin E

Large bodies of clinical and experimental evidence indicate that vitamin E has widespread biological effects in the maintaining the health of the reproductive, circulatory, muscular, skeletal, immune, and nervous systems (Nelson, 1980). Dietary vitamin E has influence on the toxicity and/or carcinogenicity of some chemical compounds.

Vitamin E is a well-known stabilizer of biological membranes (Kurokawa *et al.*, 1970; Lucy, 1972) and, through providing a suitable environment for the synthesis and activity of membrane-associated enzymes, protects organisms against toxic substances. Some of the protective effect of vitamin E emerges directly from its antioxidant property and some through its influence on the drug-metabolizing enzyme system (Zannoni and Sato, 1976). The antioxidative function of vitamin E has been proposed in CCL_4-induced liver injury (Gallagher, 1962), while others have presented evidence that lipid peroxidation is not an important mechanism in CCl_4 toxicity (McLean, 1967; Green *et al.*, 1969). The mechanism by which vitamin E partially prevents CCl_4 hepatotoxicity is yet to be explored.

Two well-identified urban air pollutants, namely, ozone and nitrogen dioxide, cause lung injuries in humans and animals. Menzel (1970) and Roehm *et al.* (1971) indicated that ozone and nitrogen dioxide promote lipid peroxidation through free-radical formation. Several studies have shown that pretreatment with vitamin E might provide partial protection against toxicity of ozone and nitrogen dioxide (Roehm *et al.*, 1971, 1972; Chow and Tappel, 1972; Fletcher and Tappel, 1973). Evidence has been presented that deficiency of dietary vitamin E markedly enhances lipid peroxidation and changes lipid composition in tissues.

The toxicity of paraquat, a herbicide which causes lung injury through peroxidation of unsaturated lipids, has been shown to be enhanced in vitamin E-deficient mice. Vitamin E supplementation had a reversal effect and protected mice against paraquat toxicity (Bus *et al.*, 1975, 1976).

A possible antioxidative effect of vitamin E on cardiotoxicity of adriamycin, a drug used in the treatment of cancer (Blum and Carter, 1974), has attracted the attention of investigators. Pretreatment with large doses of vitamin E has resulted in decreased severity of cardiomyopathy in rats (Sonneveld, 1978) and increased survival of mice, and has protected against adriamycin-induced myocardial lipid peroxidation (Myers *et al.*, 1976, 1977). However, Van Vleet *et al.* (1980) failed to demonstrate the cardioprotective effect of vitamin E in adriamycin-treated dogs.

It appears that the protective effect of vitamin E in lead toxicity is mainly attributed to its antioxidant property. Evidence has emerged from the work of Levander and co-workers (1975, 1977a,c, 1978; Levander, 1979), who observed severe anemia, splenomegaly, and increased fragility of the red blood cell in lead toxicity of E-deficient rats. A higher level of dietary vitamin E provided greater protection against the lead-induced deformation of red blood cells (Levander *et al.*, 1977a). Disturbed biosynthesis of heme, as detected by decreased activity of δ-aminolevulinic acid dehydratase (ALAD) and increased excretion of aminolevulinic acid in urine, are known mechanisms in lead toxicity (Haeger-Aronsen, 1960). Vitamin E has been suggested to function as a regulator of heme synthesis at one of the rate-limiting steps, particularly, ALAD (Zannoni and Sato, 1976). Bartlett *et al.* (1974) examined the influence of vitamin E on ALAD activity and found vitamin E-deficient weanling rabbits had enhanced lead-induced anemia compared to those who have been receiving 1 mg/day of α-tocopherol per kilogram of body weight. However, a higher vitamin E supplementation did not eliminate lead toxicity.

Mercury is another environmental pollutant whose toxicity might be reduced with dietary vitamin E. Welsh (1974) was the first to show that vitamin E has a protective effect against methylmercury toxicity in fowl. Later, Welsh and Soares (1976), Welsh (1976, 1977), Sunde (1976), and Chang *et al.* (1977) demonstrated that when vitamin E is given to quail and rats, it reduces the toxic effects of methylmercury in these animals and produces better growth rates and longer life spans. Kasuya (1975) showed that vitamin E has a direct protective effect against toxicity of methylmercury in neuronal cultures. Histological evidence also has supported the protective effect of vitamin E on nervous tissue (Chang *et al.*, 1978). The precise protective mechanism of vitamin E against the toxicity of methylmercury is not well understood. Ganther (1978) has proposed that vitamin E would modify mercury toxicity either by acting as a free-radical scavenger or through stabilizing cell membranes where mercury binds and initiates free-radical formation and lipid peroxidation (Stacey and Kappus, 1982; Yonaha *et al.*, 1980; Ribarov and Benov, 1981).

Carpenter (1968) reported that vitamin E-deficient rats had decreased hepatic activity of microsomal oxidative demethylation for codeine and aminopyrine but showed no changes in cytochrome P-450 or cytochrome b_5. Carpenter (1972) noted that enzyme activity was restored by feeding α-tocopherol, while actinomycin D, an inhibitor of protein synthesis, blocked the restoration.

Earlier studies have shown that activity of ALAD, a key enzyme in heme synthesis, as well as hepatic cytochrome P-450 and cytochrome b_5 were decreased in vitamin E deficiency (Murty *et al.*, 1970; Carpenter, 1972; Horn *et al.*, 1976). However, Chen *et al.* (1982) found no changes on cytochrome b_5 content and cytochrome c reductase activity, while concentration of cytochrome P-450 and activity of ethylmorphine N-demethylase and benzo[*a*]pyrene hydroxylase in vitamin E-deficient rats were decreased. Decreased activity of cytochrome P-450 in vitamin E deficiency has also been noted by Jensen and Clausen (1981), and they have speculated that destruction of proteins by toxic free radicals and hydroperoxide formation in vitamin E deficiency could be responsible for the low level of cytochrome P-450. Therefore, the ability of vitamin E to scavenge free radicals and inhibit lipid peroxidation probably plays an important role in the function of hepatic drug metabolism.

2. Vitamin A

Vitamin A is required for normal epithelial cell differentiation and is involved in regulating the stability of biological membrane (Lotan, 1980). Activity of several oxidative enzymes as well as cytochrome P-450 content of rat liver has been shown to be decreased by vitamin A deficiency, while NADPH-cytochrome c reductase activity remained unaffected (Becking, 1973). In agreement with Becking's findings, Colby *et al.* (1975) suggested that decline of drug metabolism in vitamin A deficiency is related to depression of specific activity of oxidative enzymes.

Depending on the animal species and type of tissue investigated, it has been found that vitamin A deficiency has differential effect on MFO activity. Feeding male guinea pigs with a vitamin A-deficient diet for 9 months has resulted in depressed AHH and 7-ethoxycoumarin deethylase activities in liver, whereas specific activity of these enzymes as well as aminopyrine demethylase was increased in the small intestine (Miranda *et al.*, 1979). In other species such as rabbit they have found that vitamin A deficiency decreased hepatic aniline hydroxylase and 7-ethoxycoumarin deethylase activities, but increased intestinal aminopyrine demethylase activity. However, the activity of enzymes in the lungs of both species was not affected by vitamin A deficiency.

With low intake of dietary vitamin A, incidence of lung cancer in men having smoking habits is relatively high (Bjelke, 1975). Possible involvement of vitamin A in the metabolism of benzo[*a*]pyrene, a chemical carcinogen which is found in cigarette smoke, has been investigated and results are inconsistent. Deficiency of retinoid has been shown to enhance binding of benzo[*a*]pyrene metabolites to the tracheal epithelial DNA in hamsters (Genta *et al.*, 1974). In contrast, lowered benzo[*a*]pyrene hydroxylase activities have been reported for lung tissue of vitamin A-deficient rabbits (Miranda and Chhabra, 1981). Furthermore, activities of microsomal epoxide hydrase, and cytosolic GSH *S*-transferase of lung, liver, and intestine in guinea pigs and rabbits have been shown not to be affected by vitamin A deficiency (Miranda *et al.*, 1979).

Regeneration of epithelial cells in the terminal bronchioles of hamsters exposed to nitrogen dioxide diminishes in vitamin A deficiency, whereas adequate and excess dietary vitamin A have been shown to exert a harmful effect which predisposes hamsters to nitrogen dioxide toxicity, as detected by hypertrophy and hyperplasia of terminal bronchiole cells (Kim, 1977, 1978).

Natural retinoids, due to their inadequate tissue distribution and excessive toxicity features (Hathcock, 1976), have only limited usefulness for cancer chemoprevention. The protective effect of natural dietary vitamin A (not synthetic analogs) against carcinogens has proved to be inconsistent, (Sporn *et al.*, 1976; Lotan, 1980), and it seems that synthetic analogs are promising alternatives.

3. Vitamin C

Vitamin C has long been regarded as a detoxifying agent. The protective effect of ascorbic acid on the phenol, phenylqumoline carboxylic acid, and barbiturate toxicity were reported almost 45 years ago (Calabrese, 1979). Ascorbic acid has a protective effect against ozone-induced pulmonary edema, oxygen toxicity, and CCl_4. Calabrese (1979) listed several toxic substances, including pesticides, heavy metals, and hydrocarbons, whose toxicity and/or carcinogenicity has been shown to be modified by ascorbic acid.

Increased excretion of ascorbic acid in urine of animals exposed to drugs or toxicants was the first finding which triggered investigations on the possible antidotal effect of vitamin C. Initially, Zilva (1935) noticed that excretion of ascorbic acid in the urine of guinea pigs increased when ether was administered as a general anesthetic drug. Conney *et al.* (1961) and Evans *et al.* (1960) suggested that enhancement in conversion of hexose into vitamin C and precursors D-glucuronate and L-gluconate by barbital and chloretone is initiated in the pathway before or at the stage of D-glucuronic acid synthesis with concomitant increase in ascorbic acid excretion.

Richards *et al.* (1941) noted that ascorbic acid-deficient guinea pigs slept longer than controls after pentabarbital administration. Conney *et al.* (1961) for the first time showed that the increased paralysis time in ascorbic acid-deficient guinea pigs treated with zoxazolamine, was due to reduced metabolism of drugs by the hepatic MFO system. Decreased hydroxylation of acetanilid, aniline, and antipyrine in rats maintained on ascorbic acid-deficient diets has also been demonstrated (Axelrod *et al.*, 1954). Large reduction in hydroxylation of coumarin has been found to be related to ascorbic acid deficiency (Degkwitz *et al.*, 1974). In addition, numerous studies have confirmed that activity of several microsomal enzymes decreases with the ascorbic acid deficiency, and is reversible and can be enhanced by vitamin C administration (Kato *et al.*, 1969; Zannoni and Lynch, 1973; Sikic *et al.*, 1977; Kuinzig *et al.*, 1977; Zannoni and Sato, 1975). However, in rats, AHH, epoxide hydrase, and NADPH-cytochrome *c* reductase were reported not affected by vitamin C deficiency (Sikic *et al.*, 1977; Kuinzig *et al.*, 1977).

Ascorbic acid prevents the nitrosamine formation from nitrite in the alimentary tract (Mirvish, 1975; Calabrase, 1979). Therefore, an inhibitory effect of ascorbic acid on nitrosation of many drugs and foreign chemicals can play an important role in protection against some form of cancer (Newberne and McConnell, 1980). A protective effect of dietary ascorbic acid against the environmental pollutants such as lead and cadmium was also reported in rats (Suzuki and Yoshida, 1978, 1979). However, it was not curative when toxicity was already established.

Increasing dietary ascorbic acid (Kato *et al.*, 1982) has been shown to reduce the growth retardant effect of PCB in rats. Furthermore, dietary ascorbic acid increases acetaminophen $t_{1/2}$ and reduces mortality (Kato *et al.*, 1982; Peterson and Knodell, 1984). Conversion of *N*-acetyl-*p*-benzyquinomine, a reactive metabolite of acetaminophen, back to acetaminophen by ascorbic acid was found responsible for prolongation of $t_{1/2}$. Blanchard and Hochman (1984) demonstrated that the pharmacokinetics of caffeine were influenced by dietary vitamin C in young but not in aged guinea pigs. In addition, ascorbic acid modifies elimination of several biologically reactive intermediates such as superoxide anions and quinones (Deamer *et al.*, 1971). This vitamin also introduces some beneficial effects by inhibiting covalent binding of reactive metabolites to critical protein molecules (Mulder *et al.*, 1978; Dybing *et al.*, 1976; Hinson, 1980).

Ascorbic acid has been assumed to be nontoxic even in grams per day quantities (Hathcock, 1976), and very high ascorbic acid intake may have a cancer-preventive effect. However, it may have a deleterious effect on the MFO activities and cytochrome *P*-450 content. Montgomery *et al.* (1982) reported a synergistic interaction between ascorbate and paraquat which causes disruption of subcellular energy metabolism. The *in vivo* potentiation of paraquat toxicity by ascorbate has been reported by Montgomery *et al.* (1982).

Degkwitz and Staudinger (1974) have suggested that reduction of cytochrome *P*-450 in ascorbic acid-deficient animals results from impaired heme biosynthesis. Sikic *et al.* (1977) have hypothesized that ascorbic acid may influence the incorporation of ferrous iron into the heme moiety of cytochrome *P*-450. However, biosynthesis of heme has been reported to be unaffected by ascorbic acid deficiency (Rikans *et al.*, 1977). Nevertheless, various levels of dietary vitamin C may facilitate metabolic degradation of xenobiotics by liver microsomal enzymes. Foreign compounds increase vitamin C excretion in urine. Thus, the human requirement for vitamin C (since humans, like monkeys and guinea pigs, do not synthesize this vitamin in the body) may be of importance, especially if there is chronic exposure to drugs, toxicants, and environmental pollutants.

4. Riboflavin

Riboflavin is a component of the coenzymes in various flavoprotein enzymes which are required for oxidation–reduction reactions. Liver microsomal flavoprotein, NADPH-cytochrome c reductase, supplies reducing equivalents to cytochrome P-450. It does contain 1 mol of FAD and 1 mol of FMN (Iyanagi and Mason, 1973). The requirement for riboflavin in the drug-metabolizing enzyme system was recognized earlier by Mueller and Miller (1950). Later Patel and Pawar (1974) and Yang (1974), in support of other studies (Rivilin *et al.*, 1968), showed that this vitamin exerts its effect on the drug-metabolizing enzyme system via NADPH-cytochrome c reductase.

The reports on the activity of the MFO system in riboflavin deficiency are contradictory. Patel and Pawar (1974) reported that prolonged riboflavin deficiency in adult rats has resulted in reduction of aminopyrine, ethylmorphine (type I substrates), aniline, and acetanilide (type II substrates) metabolism. They found that NADPH-cytochrome c reductase, cytochrome b_5, and cytochrome P-450 activities were decreased and concluded that reductions in enzyme activity might be related to the changes in the ultrastructure of the endoplasmic reticulum. Furthermore, cytochrome P-450 content and activity of AHH have been found to decrease in riboflavin deficiency (Catz *et al.*, 1970; Yang, 1974). *In vitro* addition of flavins has also been shown to stimulate the reduction of nitro and azo compounds (Fouts *et al.*, 1957; Williams *et al.*, 1970; Shargel and Mazel, 1973). Conversely, a change in riboflavin status may enhance toxicity of certain compounds.

Studies on the influence of riboflavin on the toxicity and carcinogenicity of compounds in experimental animals have shown that the toxicity of dieldrin was potentiated marginally in riboflavin-deficient rats (Tinsley, 1966). Roe *et al.* (1972) reported that the toxicity of boric acid was alleviated by riboflavin supplementation in riboflavin-deficient rats, guinea pigs, and chicks. Riboflavin may have a beneficial effect on reduction of nitrite-induced methemoglobinemia (Matsuki *et al.*, 1978; Kaplan and Chirouze, 1978).

As noted earlier, riboflavin may facilitate the destruction of azo dye in liver by the MFO system and provide protection against azo dye-induced cancer. For example, the incidence of azo dye-induced cancer has been shown to be inversely related to riboflavin content of diet and liver (Lambooy, 1970; Williams *et al.*, 1970). In addition, Kensler (1948) demonstrated the importance of flavins in the reductive pathway and showed a direct correlation between hepatic flavin content and ability of rat liver slice to reduce the carcinogenic azo dye, dimethylaminoazobenzene. Deficiency of this vitamin may provide protection against toxicity of a compound such as acetaminophen, while it predisposes the animal to the deleterious effects of carcinogenic compounds such as dimethyl benzanthracene, whose metabolic intermediates are shown to be carcinogenic in mice (Wynder *et al.*, 1985; Raheja *et al.*, 1983).

The kinetic studies suggested a separate role for the two species of flavins in the reductase (Iyanagi *et al.*, 1974). FAD serves as an electron acceptor for NADPH and FMN as an electron donor in the cytochrome *P*-450 system (Vermilion and Coon, 1978; Vermilion *et al.*, 1981). Hara and Taniguchi (1982) presented evidence that riboflavin deficiency results in an abnormal NADPH-cytochrome *c* reductase due to unbalanced content of FAD and FMN in the microsome. They observed that the amount of FMN in the livers of riboflavin-deficient rats was not enough to saturate the binding site of flavoprotein molecules in the microsome, while a relatively excess amount of FAD was available to be inserted to the FMN-binding site of the molecules,

The above evidence indicates that riboflavin nutritional status markedly influences xenobiotic metabolism in the body, and individuals having low riboflavin status such as oral contraceptive drug users might be at great risk if they are exposed to environmental pollutants in their daily life.

5. *Thiamin (Vitamin B_1)*

Thiamin is required for carbohydrate metabolism, and multiple factors such as eating habits, low thiamin intake, or alcoholism may contribute to thiamin deficiency in the human population. Deficiency of thiamin has been shown to increase heptachlor and aniline metabolism in the liver microsome, whereas thiamin supplementation significantly decreases metabolism of these substrates (Wade *et al.*, 1969). These findings later on were attributed to the decrease of cytochrome *P*-450 and b_5 content of hepatic microsomes in thiamin-supplemented rats (Grosse and Wade, 1971). In their studies they also observed reduction of NADPH-cytochrome *c* reductase activity. Wade *et al.* (1975) have indicated that the reduction of cytochrome *P*-450 in high-thiamin treatment was due to the types of carbohydrate used in the experiments and have noted that rats fed high thiamin with sucrose had a decreased cytochrome *P*-450 content, whereas rats fed high thiamin with starch had no depressed cytochrome *P*-450 content. However, enzymatic activity with both types of carbohydrate was depressed. Wade *et al.* (1983) indicated that the capacity to respond to phenobarbital induction is in part regulated by the level of thiamin intake.

Bratton *et al.* (1981) have shown that treatment of cattle with 100 mg/day per calf of thiamin hydrochloride prevented clinical signs of lead poisoning and death. They found that thiamin had no protective effect on the ability of lead to inhibit δ-aminolevulinic acid dehydratase activity in erythrocytes. Therapeutic use of thiamin might be of value in the prevention and treatment of lead toxicity. It may interact with lead in some way to prevent tissue accumulation of lead and reduce poisoning. On the other hand, dietary deficiency of thiamin can protect against toxicity of aflatoxin in chickens (Ruchirawat *et al.*, 1978; Hamilton *et al.*, 1974).

These findings indicate that deficiency or excess of dietary thiamin may have a considerable influence on the drug-metabolizing enzyme systems but also interact with toxic compounds with different mechanisms.

6.   Vitamin B_6 (Pyridoxine)

Vitamin B_6 serves as a coenzyme and has an essential role in protein metabolism. Subclinical deficiency of vitamin B_6 in humans might be found among pregnant women, uremic patients, chronic alcoholics, and patients with chronic liver disease (Snider, 1980).

Supplemental intake of this vitamin may have a harmful effect as it has been shown to reduce milk production in nursing mothers and to increase cadmium toxicity in rats (Greentree, 1979).

Beneficial effects of vitamin B_6 therapy have been demonstrated in isoniazid, ethylene glycol, and decaborane toxicities (Wason *et al.*, 1981). Deficiency of vitamin B_6 has been reported in patients undergoing isonizid therapy (Biehl and Vilter, 1954). Seizure activity due to decreased α-aminobutyric acid in isoniazid-overdosed patients has been shown to be reversed by vitamin B_6 without any adverse side effects. Wason *et al.* (1981) have stated that pyridoxine prevents the reducing effect of isoniazid on the activity of glutamic acid decarboxylase, thereby preventing reduction of GABA in the brain.

Toxic compounds, such as carbon disulfide, PCB, and penicillamine, have been shown to disrupt normal function of vitamin B_6 in intermediary metabolism (Fujiwara and Kuriyama, 1977; Rumsby and Shepherd, 1981). Chronic exposure to these compounds may result in vitamin B_6 deficiency, and individuals with a nutritional deficiency of this vitamin will be more susceptible to toxicity of these compounds. Penicillamine, which is commonly used in rheumatoid arthritis and other diseases, reacts with pyridoxal 5'-phosphate or inhibits its synthesis, and chronic intake of this drug may produce vitamin B_6 deficiency. Penicillamine induced vitamin B_6 deficiency can be readily reversed by administration of pyridoxine (Gibbs and Walshe, 1969).

7.   Vitamin B_{12}

Vitamin B_{12} serves also as a coenzyme for several important biochemical pathways. Strict vegetarians and oral contraceptive users, as well as ruminants grazed on cobalt-deficient pastures have been shown to develop deficiency of this vitamin (Chanarin, 1980; Shojania, 1982; Herbert, 1976).

Vitamin B_{12} has been recognized to be involved in detoxification of cyanide (Mushett *et al.*, 1952). Injection of large doses of vitamin B_{12} has been reported to cure dimness of vision (amblyopia) in tobacco smokers, which was recognized to be due to chronic cyanide toxicosis (Heaton *et al.*, 1958; Chisolm *et al.*, 1976). Hydroxycobalamin is a specific antidote for cyanide toxicity, and it has been used for reduction of elevated cyanide toxicity in humans during sodium nitroprusside (a vasodilator used after cardiac surgery) administration (Cottrell *et al.*, 1978).

Hydroxycobalamin has one less cyanide radical than cyanocobalamin, thereby allowing cyanide to combine and form cyanocobalamin, which is then excreted in the urine (Kaplan and Finlayson, 1981). Therefore, hydroxycobalamin may play a significant role in the overall detoxification of cyanide by complementing usual detoxification mechanisms such as the formation of thiocyanate.

This vitamin plays an important role in nervous tissue. The methylated form, methylcobalamin, has been shown to inhibit the toxic effect of mehtylmercuric chloride on nervous fiber of rat cerebellum explants (Kasuya, 1980). Methylcobalamin possibly exerts its effect on methylmercuric chloride toxicity through increasing phosphatidylcholine synthesis and increasing lipid metabolism.

A beneficial effect of vitamin B_{12} in combination with vitamin C in lead and CCl_4 toxicities has been also reported (Kao and Forbes, 1973; Kasbekar *et al.,* 1959). When combined with inositol and choline, it has a curative effect on aflatoxin-induced fatty liver (Reed *et al.,* 1968).

Nitrous oxide (laughing gas), which was once regarded as a chemically inert gas, inactivates this vitamin and influences pathways mediated by vitamin B_{12}, and can cause megaloblastic anemia (Chanarin, 1980). Therefore, evaluation of the vitamin B_{12} status of dental patients undergoing frequent anesthesia with this gas is recommended.

B. Minerals

1. Iron

Iron has a central role in the several heme-containing molecules such as hemoglobin and cytochrome P-450s. Iron deficiency usually results in anemia, and it is prevalent among children and young women.

Iron deficiency may alter the metabolism of xenobiotics in the body. Although it seems that iron deficiency would reduce cytochrome P-450's content and thereby decrease detoxification capacity, experimental studies have shown differently. Catz *et al.* (1970) have found that iron depletion in adult mice had no effect on AHH or nitroreductase activities, while metabolism of type I substrates such as aminopyrine and hexobarbital was increased. It has been shown that aniline metabolism is the most sensitive metabolic pathway to iron deficiency of rats in drug metabolism. In iron depletion studies of rats, Becking (1972, 1976) found no effect on cytochrome P-450 and cytochrome b_5 levels. However, increased hydroxylase activity was noted as early as 18 days, and NADPH-cytochrome c reductase activity increased after 25–35 days. Becking (1976) also indicated that all enzymatic activities in formerly deficient rats were returned to control levels by feeding iron-containing diet for 7 days.

Chetty *et al.* (1979) have shown that the reduced liver microsomal NADPH-cytochrome c reductase, NADPH-dehydrogenase, cytochrome P-450, and aniline metabolism in cobalt-induced toxicity of iron-deficient rats were completely reversed when animals were transferred to iron-sufficient diets. They also noted that rats which had received iron-sufficient diet and high concentration of cobalt (200 ppm) did not show any alteration in the microsomal electron transfer system.

Fouts and Pohl (1971) have shown that ferric iron had an inhibitory effect while ferrous iron had a stimulatory effect on the *in vitro* activity of NADPH-- cytochrome *c* reductase. Change of intracellular ferric/ferrous ratio has been suggested for the increased rate of drug metabolism in iron-depleted rats (Becking, 1976).

Supplementation with iron in mice has been shown to decrease aminopyrine metabolism and decrease cytochrome *P*-450 content in rats (Wills, 1972; Maines and Kappas, 1977a,b). Increase of lipid peroxidation due to excess iron was proposed to be responsible for reduced MFO activity (Wills, 1972). Others suggested increase of heme oxygenase activity, which degrades heme of cytochrome *P*-450 might be responsible to a decreased MFO activity in iron-overloading state (Maines and Kappas, 1977a,b; Paine and Legg, 1978; Maines, 1979). Chronic iron treatment may increase sensitivity of organisms to subsequent exposure to the other metals and potentiates the acute effects of secondary metal on heme metabolism. In this respect, interaction of lead and iron is well documented. Iron deficiency increases susceptibility of rats to lead toxicity (Mahaffey and Goyer, 1972). Mahaffey and Rader (1980) also indicated that iron clinically prevents accumulation of the body burden of lead rather than stimulating lead metabolism.

2. *Magnesium*

Magnesium as a prosthetic ion is essential in many enzymatic reactions. Its interrelationships with calcium and parathyroid hormone have been well documented (Shils, 1976). Dietary magnesium alters *in vivo* and *in vitro* MFO systems in rats. Becking (1976) have found that content of cytochrome *P*-450 and NADPH-cytochrome *c* reductase, hydroxylation of aniline, and N-demethylation of aminopyrine were reduced after 12 days of feeding rats with a magnesium-deficient diet. *In vitro* addition of magnesium to the rat hepatic microsomal preparation have been shown to increase activity of NADPH oxidase and NADPH-cytochrome *c* reductase (Peters and Fouts, 1970a,b). The same workers found that the effect of magnesium deficiency on the drug-metabolizing enzyme system was reversed by feeding a magnesium-supplemented diet. Further increases of magnesium concentration enhanced the activity of NADPH-cytochrome *c* reductase while NADPH oxidation was inhibited. They speculated that magnesium may enhance the flow of electrons to substrate in the MFO system. Alternatively, it may protect tissue from oxidative damage by maintaining the GSH concentration as it is demonstrated in the erythrocytes (Hsu *et al.*, 1982).

3. *Selenium*

Selenium is the required component of GSH-Px enzyme, whose antioxidant activity serves to maintain the integrity of cellular and subcellular membranes (Hoekstra, 1975). Selenium deficiency does not alter the activity of cytochrome P-450, cytochrome b_5, and NADPH-cytochrome c reductase without induction of the system (Burk *et al.*, 1974; Burk and Masters, 1975). Mackinnon and Simon (1976) have indicated that selenium deficiency decreases heme synthesis. In agreement with this, Maines and Kapas (1976a,b) demonstrated that injection of 5 μmol selenium per 100 gm body weight did not change cytochrome P-450 content, whereas synthesis of aminolevulinic acid and heme oxygenase activity were rapidly increased. Burk and Correia (1977) have indicated that selenium deficiency can accelerate heme degradation.

Selenium is known to interact with toxic metals such as lead, mercury, and cadmium. Selenium supplementation of rats has been shown to reduce retention of lead in tissue slightly (Levander *et al.*, 1977b; Sifri and Hoekstra, 1978). In lead toxicity, selenium supplementation provides protection through antioxidative effects of GSH-Px or via effects on heme synthesis. Nevertheless, Levander *et al.* (1977b) emphasized that although selenium in vitamin E-deficient rats has some protective effect against lead toxicity, the excess selenium required to demonstrate such an effect can be toxic and harmful. Parizek and Ostadalova (1967) have shown that selenium counteracts mercuric chloride toxicity. Selenium in some way alters the transfer of mercury from protein to GSH and increases its biliary excretion (Ganther *et al.*, 1972; Stillings *et al.*, 1974; Sell and Horani, 1976; Alexander and Norseth, 1979). Selenium also increases the biliary excretion of cadmium in cadmium toxicity (Stowe, 1976). The exact mechanism or mechanisms involved in biliary excretion of mercury and cadmium is yet to be elucidated.

Selenium administration has been shown to prevent cadmium-induced reduction of microsomal cytochrome P-450 content and microsomal binding of both ethylmorphine and aniline *in vivo* but not *in vitro* (Early and Schnell, 1981). This effect of selenium is speculated to occur throughout the protecting endoplasmic reticulum from cadmium-induced lipid peroxidation. By the same effect of cytochrome P-450 systems, selenium may enhance DMN toxicity via increasing biotransformation of this compound to a more toxic metabolite. Such enhancement has been reported by Skaare and Nafstad (1978).

Increased susceptibility to several toxic compounds in selenium deficiency can be interpreted via changes in the activity of GSH-Px and peroxidation of membrane lipids. For example, in selenium deficiency in which activity of GSH-Px decreases, paraquat toxicity manifests by increasing lipid peroxidation (Bus *et al.*, 1976). Conversely, dietary selenium protects chicks against acute paraquat and nitrofurantoin (urinary tract antimicrobial drug) toxicity (Peterson *et al.*, 1982; Combs and Peterson, 1983). Selenium deficiency also increases susceptibility of animals to ozone-induced oxidative stress (Chow, 1977). Synthesis of GSH in isolated rat hepatocytes has been shown to be accelerated by selenium deficiency. Therefore, selenium deficiency may facilitate detoxification of those compounds whose metabolism requires GSH conjugation (Hill and Burk, 1982). Selenium may render the toxic effect of numerous substances by possibly affecting heme synthesis or stabilizing biological membrane and providing the proper environment for the enzymes' activities which are involved in detoxification processes.

4. Zinc

Deficiency or excess of dietary zinc may influence metabolism and detoxification of various compounds. Zinc does stabilize biological membrane and provides protection against peroxidative damages. In the drug-metabolizing system, deficiency of zinc depresses the activity of several enzymes (Becking and Morrison, 1970), whereas supplementation decreases cytochrome P-450 content (Maines and Kappas, 1976b). Zinc protects animals from the hepatotoxic effects of CCL_4, as indicated by a decreased level of lipid peroxidation and enhanced stability of lysosomes (Chvapil et al., 1973). Since the GSH level in blood (Mills et al., 1981) and probably other tissues decreases in zinc deficiency, the protective effect of zinc against lipid peroxidative agents might be attributed to the maintenance of a level of the reduced form of GSH. The protective effect of zinc in ethanol toxicity was claimed to be due to the effect on NADPH oxidations and an increased level of alcohol dehydrogenase activity in liver (Chvapil et al., 1976).

5. Copper

Williams (1978) listed copper as a necessary nutrient in components of the oxidizing system in the functionalization process of drug metabolism. However, copper deficiency has been found to have no effect on rat hepatic microsomal cytochrome P-450 content, with or without phenobarbital induction, while increased microsomal heme oxygenase has been observed (Williams et al., 1981; Moffitt and Murphy, 1973). In addition, Moffitt and Murphy (1973) have reported that activities of aniline hydroxylase and hexobarbital oxidase were depressed, while benzo[a]pyrene hydroxylase activity was unaffected in copper deficiency.

IV. CONCLUSION

The relationship of nutrients and metabolism of xenobiotics is complex. Biotransformation of xenobiotics as well as endogenous substances are markedly affected by the component of dietary regimen, and in this review some of the relevant observations are described. Human and animal studies have revealed the importance of some nutrients in the detoxification process, and some may have promising effects on chemical carcinogenesis.

As cofactors or prosthetic groups for some enzymes, micronutrients play an important role in detoxification process. Interaction of nutrients with each other at absorptive or metabolic levels complicates interpretation of *in vivo* studies. Manipulation of nutrients in *in vitro* studies has provided some valuable information in the metabolism of toxicants. The complexity of studies arises also when change of a nutrient requires substitution with others to maintain total caloric intake. However, valuable information has been accumulated mostly using animal models for the *in vivo* and *in vitro* studies. Further studies in this area should be encouraged.

REFERENCES

Alexander, J., and Norseth, T. (1979). The effect of selenium on the biliary excretion and organ distribution of mercury in the rat after exposure to methylmercury chloride. *Acta Pharmacol. Toxicol.* **44,** 168–176.

Alvares, A. P., Anderson, K. E., Conney, A. H., and Kappas, A. (1976). Interactions between nutritional factors and drug biotransformations in man. *Proc. Natl. Acad. Sci. U.S.A.* **73,** 2501–2504.

Anderson, K. E., Conney, A. H., and Kappas, A. (1979). Nutrition and oxidative drug metabolism in man: Relative influence of dietary lipids, carbohydrate and protein. *Clin. Pharmacol. Ther.* **26,** 493–501.

Anderson, K. E., Conney, A. H., and Kappas, A. (1982). Nutritional influences on chemical biotransformations in humans. *Nutr. Rev.* **40,** 161–171.

Axelrod, J., Undernfriend, S., and Brodie, B. B. (1954). Ascorbic acid in aromatic hydroxylation. III. Effect of ascorbic acid on hydroxylation of acetanilide, aniline and antipyrine in vivo. *J. Pharmacol. Exp. Ther.* **111,** 176–181.

Baernstein, H. D., and Grand, J. A. (1942). The relation of protein intake to lead poisoning in rats. *J. Pharmacol Exp. Ther.* **74,** 18–24.

Bartlett, R. S., Rousseau, J. R., Jr., Frier, H. I., and Hall, R. C., Jr. (1974). Effect of vitamin E on delta-aminolevulinic acid dehydratase activity in weanling rabbits with chronic plumbism. *J. Nutr.* **104,** 1637–1645.

Becking, G. C. (1972). Influence of dietary iron levels on hepatic drug metabolism in vivo and in vitro in the rat. *Biochem. Pharmacol.* **21,** 1585–1593.

Becking, G. C. (1973). Vitamin A status and hepatic drug metabolism in the rat. *Can. J. Physiol. Pharmacol.* **51,** 6–11.

Becking, G. C. (1976). Hepatic drug metabolism in iron-, magnesium- and potassium-deficient rats. *Fed. Proc., Fed. Am. Soc. Exp. Biol.* **35,** 2480–2485.

Becking, G. C., and Morrison, A. B. (1970). Role of dietary magnesium in the metabolism of drug by NADPH-dependent rat liver microsomal enzymes. *Biochem. Pharmacol.* **19,** 2639–2644.

Biehl, J. P., and Vilter, R. W. (1954). Effect of isoniazid on vitamin B_6 metabolism; its possible significance in producing isoniazid neuritis. *Proc. Soc. Exp. Biol. Med.* **85,** 389–394.

Bjelke, E. (1975). Dietary vitamin A and human lung cancer. *Int. J. Cancer* **15,** 561–565.

Blanchard, J., and Hochman, D. (1984). Effects of vitamin C on caffeine pharmacokinetics in young and aged guinea pigs. *Drug-Nutr. Interact.* **2**, 243–255.

Blum, R. H., and Carter, S. K. (1974). Adriamycin—A new anti-cancer drug with significant clinical activity. *Ann. Intern. Med.* **80**, 249.

Boyd, E. M., and Krupa, V. (1970). Protein-deficient diet and diuron toxicity. *Agric. Food Chem.* **18**, 1104–1107.

Boyd, E. M., Dobos, I., and Taylor, F. (1970). Benzylpenicillin toxicity in albino rats fed synthetic high starch versus high sugar diets. *Chemotherapy (Basel)* **15**, 1–11.

Bratton, G. R., Zmudzki, J., Bell, M. C., and Warnock, L. G. (1981). Thiamin (vitamin B_1) effects on lead intoxication and deposition of lead in tissues: Therapeutic potential. *Toxicol. Appl. Pharmacol.* **59**, 164–172.

Bray, M. G., Humphris, B. G., Thorpe, W. V., White, K., and Wood, P. B. (1952). Kinetic studies of the metabolism of foreign organic compounds. 4. The conjugation of phenols with sulphuric acid. *Biochem. J.* **52**, 419–423.

Brodie, M. J., Boobis, A. R., Toverud, E.-L., Ellis, W., Murray, S., Dollery, C. T., Webster, S., and Harrison, R. (1980). Drug metabolism in white vegetarians. *Br. J. Clin. Pharmacol.* **9**, 523–524.

Buchanan, N., Davis, M. D., Henderson, D. B., Mucklow, J. C., and Rawlins, M. D. (1980). Acetanilide pharmacokinetics in kwashiorkor. *Br. J. Clin. Pharmacol.* **9**, 525–526.

Burk, R. F., and Correia, M. A. (1977). Accelerated hepatic haem catabolism in the selenium-deficient rat. *Biochem. J.* **168**, 105–111.

Burk, R. F., and Master, B. S. S. (1975). Some effects of selenium deficiency on the hepatic microsomal cytochrome *P*-450 system in the rat. *Arch. Biochem. Biophys.* **170**, 124–131.

Burk, R. F., MacKinnon, A. M., and Simon, F. R. (1974). Selenium and hepatic microsomal hemoproteins. *Biochem. Biophys. Res. Commun.* **56**, 431–436.

Bus, J. S., Aust, S. D., and Gibson, J. E. (1975). Lipid peroxidation: A possible mechanism for paraquat toxicity. *Res. Commun. Chem. Pharmacol.* **11**, 31–38.

Bus, J. S., Aust, S. D., and Gibson, J. E. (1976). Paraquat toxicity: Proposed mechanism of action involving lipid peroxidation. *Environ. Health Perspect.* **16**, 139–146.

Calabrese, E. J. (1979). Should the concept of the recommended dietary allowance be altered to incorporate interactive effects of ubiquitous pollutants? *Med. Hypotheses* **5**, 1273–1285.

Campbell, T. C., and Hayes, J. R. (1974). Role of nutrition in the drug metabolizing enzyme system. *Pharmacol. Rev.* **26**, 171–197.

Campbell, T. C., and Hayes, J. R. (1976). The effect of quantity and quality of dietary protein on drug metabolism. *Fed. Proc., Fed. Am. Soc. Exp. Biol.* **35**, 2470–2474.

Campbell, T. C., Hayes, J. R., and Newberne, P. M. (1978). Dietary lipotropes, hepatic microsomal mixed-function oxidase activities, and in vivo covalent binding of aflatoxin B_1 in rats. *Cancer Res.* **38**, 4569–4573.

Carpenter, M. P. (1968). Role of α-tocopherol in microsomal hydroxylation. *Fed. Proc., Fed. Am. Soc. Exp. Biol.* **27**, 677.

Carpenter, M. P. (1972). Vitamin E and microsomal drug hydroxylations. *Ann. N.Y. Acad. Sci.* **203**, 81–92.

Carroll, K. K. (1980). Lipids and carcinogenesis. *J. Environ. Pathol. Toxicol.* **3**, 253–271.

Carroll, K. K., and Hopkins, G. J. (1979). Dietary polyunsaturated fat versus saturated fat in relation to mammary carcinogenesis. *Lipids* **14**, 155–158.

Carroll, K. K., and Khor, H. T. (1971). Effect of level and type of dietary fat on incidence of mammary tumors induced in female Sprague-Dawley rats by 7,12-dimethylbenz[*a*]anthracene. *Lipids* **6**, 415–420.

Caster, W. O., Wade, A. E., Greene, F. E., and Meadows, J. S. (1970). Effect of different levels of corn oil in the diet upon the rate of hexobarbital, heptachlor and aniline metabolism in the liver of the male white rat. *Life Sci.* **9**, 181–190.

Catz, C. S., Juchau, M. R., and Yaffe, S. J. (1970). Effects of iron, riboflavin and iodide deficiencies on hepatic drug-metabolizing enzyme systems. *J. Pharmacol. Exp. Ther.* **174,** 197–205.

Century, B. (1973). A role of the dietary lipid in the ability of phenobarbital to stimulate drug detoxification. *J. Pharmacol. Exp. Ther.* **185,** 185–194.

Chadwich, R., Peoples, A., and Cranmer, M. (1973). The effect of protein quality and ascorbic acid deficiency on stimulation of hepatic microsomal enzymes in guinea pigs. *Toxicol. Appl. Pharmacol.* **24,** 603–611.

Chanarin, I. (1980). Cobalamins and nitrous oxide: A review. *J. Clin. Pathol.* **33,** 909–916.

Chang, L. W., Gilbert, M. M., and Sprecher, J. (1977). Morphological evidence on the protective effects of vitamin E against methylmercury toxicity in nervous sytem. *Fed. Proc., Fed. Am. Soc. Exp. Biol.* **36,** 404.

Chang, L. W., Gilbert, M. M., and Sprecher, J. (1978). Modification of methylmercury neurotoxicity by vitamin E. *Environ. Res.* **17,** 356–366.

Chen, J., Goetchius, M. P., Combs, G. F., Jr., and Campbell, T. C. (1982). Effects of dietary selenium and vitamin E on covalent binding of aflatoxin to chick liver cell macromolecules. *J. Nutr.* **112,** 350–355.

Cheng, K. C., Ragland, W. L., and Wade, A. E. (1980). Effect of lipid ingestion on the induction of drug metabolizing enzymes of nuclear envelope and microsomes by phenobarbital. *J. Environ. Pathol. Toxicol.* **4,** 219–235.

Cheng, K. C., Ragland, W. L., and Wade, A. E. (1981). Dietary fat and 3-MC induction of hepatic nuclear and microsomal cytochrome *P*-450. *Drug-Nutr. Interact.* **1,** 163–174.

Chetty, K. N., Drummond, L., SubbaRao, D. S. V., and Desaiah, D. (1979). Inhibition of rat hepatic microsomal cytochrome *P*-450 system by cobaltous chloride and reversal of inhibition by iron in vivo. *Drug Chem. Toxicol.* **2,** 375–381.

Chisholm, I. A., Bronte-Stewart, J., and Foulds, W. S. (1967). Hydroxycobalamin versus cyanocobalamin in the treatment of tobacco amblyopia. *Lancet* **2,** 450–451.

Chow, C. K. (1977). Effect of dietary selenium and vitamin E on the biochemical responses in the lungs of ozone-exposed rats. *Fed. Proc., Fed. Am. Soc. Exp. Biol.* **36,** 1094.

Chow, C. K., and Tappel, A. L. (1972). An enzymatic protective mechanism against lipid peroxidation damage to lung of ozone exposed rats. *Lipids* **7,** 518–524.

Chvapil, M., Ryan, J. N., Elias, S. L., and Peng, Y. H. (1973). Protective effect of zinc on CCl_4-induced liver injury in rats. *Exp. Mol. Pathol.* **19,** 186–196.

Chvapil, M., Ludwig, J. C., Sipes, I. G., and Misiorowski, R. L. (1976). Inhibition of NADPH oxidation and related drug oxidations in liver microsomes by zinc. *Biochem. Pharmacol.* **25,** 1787–1791.

Clinton, S. K., Truex, C. R., and Visek, W. J. (1977). Effects of protein deficiency and excess on hepatic mixed function oxidase activity in growing and adult female rats. *Nutr. Rep. Int.* **16,** 463–477.

Clinton, S. K., Truex, C. R., and Visek, W. J. (1979). Dietary protein, aryl hydrocarbon hydroxylase and chemical carcinogenesis in rats. *J. Nutr.* **109,** 55–62.

Colby, H. D., Kramer, R. E., Greiner, J. W., Robinson, D. A., Krause, R. F., and Canady, W. J. (1975). Hepatic drug metabolism in retinol-deficient rats. *Biochem. Pharmacol.* **24,** 1644–1646.

Combs, G. F., Jr., and Peterson, F. J. (1983). Protection against acute paraquat toxicity by dietary selenium in chick. *J. Nutr.* **113,** 538–545.

Conney, A. H., Bray, G. A., Evans, C., and Burns, J. J. (1961). Metabolic interactions between L-ascorbic acid and drugs. *Ann. N.Y. Acad. Sci.* **92,** 115–127.

Cook, L., Toner, J. J., and Fellows, E. J. (1954). The effect of β-diethylaminoethyl-diphenylpropylacetate hydrochloride (SKF No. 525-A) on hexobarbital. *J. Pharmacol. Exp. Ther.* **111,** 131–141.

Coon, M. J. (1978). Oxygen activation in the metabolism of lipids. drugs and carcinogens. *Nutr. Rev.* **36,** 319–328.

Cottrell, J. E., Casthely, P., Brodie, J. D., Patel, K., Klein, A., and Turndorf, H. (1978). Prevention of nitroprusside-induced cyanide toxicity with hydroxycobalamin. *N. Engl. J. Med.* **298,** 809–811.

Czygan, P., Greim, H., Carro, A., Schaffner, F., and Popper, H. (1974). The effect of dietary protein deficiency on the ability of isolated microsomes to alter the mutagenicity of a primary and a secondary carcinogen. *Cancer Res.* **34,** 119–123.

Davison, S. C., and Wills, E. D. (1974). Studies on the lipid composition of the rat liver endoplasmic reticulum after induction with phenobarbitone and 20-methylantheren. *Biochem. J.* **140,** 461–468.

Deamer, D. W., Heikkila, R. E., Panganamala, R. V., Cohen, G., and Cornwall, D. G. (1971). Alloxan–dialuric acid cycle and the generation of hydrogen peroxide. *Physiol. Chem. Phys.* **3,** 426–430.

Degkwitz, E., and Staudinger, H. J. (1974). Role of vitamin C on microsomal cytochromes. *In* "Vitamin C: Recent Aspects of its Physiological and Technological Importance" (G. S. Birch and K. J. Parker, eds.), pp. 161–177. Wiley, New York.

Dickerson, J. W. T., Basu, T. K., and Parke, D. V. (1971). Activity of drug-metabolizing enzymes in the liver of growing rats fed on diets high in sucrose, glucose, fructose or an equimolar mixture of glucose and fructose. *Proc. Nutr. Soc.* **30,** 27A–28A.

Drill, V. A. (1954). Lipotropic effects of vitamin B_{12} and other factors. *Ann. N. York. Acad Sci.* **57,** 654–663.

Dybing, E., Nelson, S. D., Mitchell, J. R., Sasame, H. A., and Gillette, J. R. (1976). Oxidation of α-methyldopa and other catechols by cytochrome *P*-450 generated superoxide anion: Possible mechanism of methyldopa hepatitis. *Mol. Pharmacol.* **12,** 911–920.

Early, J. L., Jr., and Schnell, R. C. (1981). Selenium antagonism of cadmium-induced inhibition of hepatic drug metabolism in the male rat. *Toxicol. Appl. Pharmacol.* **58,** 57–66.

Edes, T. E., Clinton, S. K., Truex, C. R., and Visek, W. J. (1979). Intestinal and hepatic mixed function oxidase activity in rats fed methionine and cysteine-free diets (40620). *Proc. Soc. Exp. Biol. Med.* **162,** 71–74.

Edwards, S., and Westerfeld, W. W. (1952). Blood and liver glutathione during protein deprivation. *Proc. Soc. Exp. Biol. Med.* **79,** 57–59.

Evans, C., Conney, A. H., Trousof, N., and Burns, J. J. (1960). Metabolism of D-galactose to D-glucuronic acid, L-gulonic acid and L-ascorbic acid. *Biochim. Biophys. Acta* **41,** 9–14.

Fletcher, B. L., and Tappel, A. L. (1973). Protective effects of dietary α-tocopherol in rats exposed to toxic levels of ozone and nitrogen dioxide. *Environ. Res.* **6,** 165–175.

Flohe, L., Gunzler, W. A., and Schock, H. M. (1973). Glutathione peroxidase: a selenoenzyme. *FEBS Letters* **32,** 132–134.

Fouts, J. R., and Pohl, R. J. (1971). Further studies on the effects of metal ions on rat liver microsomal reduced nicotinamide adenine dinucleotide phosphate-cytochrome *P*-450 reductase. *J. Pharmacol. Exp. Ther.* **179,** 91–100.

Fouts, J. R., Kamm, J. J., and Brodie, B. B. (1957). Enzymatic reduction of prontasil and other azo dyes. *J. Pharmacol. Exp. Ther.* **120,** 291–300.

Fujiwara, M., and Kuriyama, K. (1977). Effect of PCB (polychlorobiphenyls) on L-ascorbic acid, pyridoxal phosphate and riboflavin contents in various organs and on hepatic metabolism of L-ascorbic acid in the rat. *Jpn. J. Pharmacol.* **27,** 621–627.

Gallagher, C. H. (1962). The effect of antioxidants on poisoning by carbon tetrachloride. *Aust. J. Exp. Biol.* **40,** 241–254.

Ganther, H. E. (1978). Modification of methylmercury toxicity and metabolism by selenium and vitamin E: Possible mechanisms. *Environ. Health Perspect.* **25,** 71–76.

Ganther, H. E., Goudi, C., Sunde, M. L., Kopecky, M. J., Wagner, P., Oh, S. H., and Hoekstra, W. G. (1972). Selenium: Relation to decreased toxicity of methylmercury added to diets containing tuna. *Science* **175**, 1124–1125.

Gelboin, H. V., Wartham, J. S., and Wilson, R. G. (1967). 3-methylcholantherene and phenobarbital stimulation of rat liver RNA polymerase. *Nature (London)* **214**, 281–283.

Genta, V. M., Kaufman, D. G., Harris, C. C., Smith, J. M., Sporn, M. B., and Saffiotti, U. (1974). Vitamin A deficiency enhances the binding of benzo[*a*]pyrene to tracheal epithelial DNA. *Nature (London)* **247**, 48–49.

Gibbs, K., and Walshe, J. M. (1969). Interruption of the tryptophan–nicotinic acid pathway by penicillamine-induced pyridoxine deficiency in patients with Wilson's disease and in experimental animals. *Ann. N.Y. Acad. Sci.* **166**, 158–169.

Gillette, J. R. (1974). A perspective on the role of chemically reactive metabolite of foreign compounds in toxicity. I. correlation of changes in covalent binding of reactive metabolites with changes in the incidence and severity of toxicity. *Biochem. Pharmacol.* **23**, 2785–2794.

Gillette, J. R., Davis, D. C., and Sasame, H. A. (1972). Cytochrome P-450 and its role in drug metabolism. *Annu. Rev. Pharmacol.* **12**, 57–82.

Green, J., Bunyan, J., Cawthorne, M. A., and Diplock, A. T. (1969). Vitamin E and hepatotoxic agents. 1. Carbon tetrachloride and lipid peroxidation in the rat. *Br. J. Nutr.* **23**, 297–307.

Greentree, L. B. (1979). Dangers of vitamin B_6 in nursing mothers. *N. Engl. J. Med.* **300**, 141–142.

Grosse, W., III, and Wade, A. E. (1971). The effect of thiamin consumption on liver microsomal drug-metabolizing pathways. *J. Pharmacol. Exp. Ther.* **176**, 758–765.

Guengerich, F. P. (1977). Separation and purification of multiple forms of microsomal cytochrome P-450. Activities of different forms of cytochrome P-450 towards several compounds of environmental interest. *J. Biol. Chem.* **25**, 3970–3979.

Guengerich, F. P. (1982). Epoxide hydrolase: Properties and metabolic role. *Rev. Biochem. Toxicol.* **4**, 5–30.

Guengerich, F. P., and Manson, P. S. (1979). Immunologic comparison of hepatic and extrahepatic cytochrome P-450. *Mol. Pharmacol.* **15**, 154–164.

Haeger-Aronsen, B. (1960). Studies on urinary excretion of delta-aminolaevulinic acid and other haem precursors in lead workers and lead intoxicated rabbits. *Scand. J. Clin. Lab. Invest.* **12**, 1–28.

Hamilton, P. B., Tung, H. T., Wyatt, R. D., and Donaldson, W. E. (1974). Interaction of dietary aflatoxin with some vitamin deficiencies. *Poult. Sci.* **53**, 871–877.

Hammer, C. T., and Wills, E. D. (1978). The role of lipid components of the diet in the regulation of the fatty acid composition of rat liver endoplasmic reticulum and lipid peroxidation. *Biochem. J.* **174**, 585–593.

Hara, T., and Taniguchi, M. (1982). Abnormal NADPH-cytochrome P-450 reductase in the liver microsomes of riboflavin-deficient rats. *Biochem. Biophys. Res. Commun.* **104**, 394–401.

Hathcock, J. N. (1976). Nutrition: Toxicology and pharmacology. *Nutr. Rev.* **34**, 65–70.

Hayes, J. R., Mgbodile, M. U. K., and Campbell, T. C. (1973). Effect of protein deficiency on the inducibility of the hepatic microsomal drug-metabolizing enzyme system. I. *Biochem. Pharmacol.* **22**, 1005–1014.

Heaton, J. M., McCormick, A. J. A., and Freeman, A. G. (1958). Tobacco amblyopia: A clinical manifestation of vitamin B_{12} deficiency. *Lancet* **2**, 286–290.

Herbert, V. (1976). Vitamin B_{12}. *In* "Nutrition Reviews. Present Knowledge in Nutrition" (D. M. Hegsted, C. A. Chester, W. J. Darby, K. W. McNutt, R. M. Stalvy, and E. H. Stotz, eds.), 4th ed., pp. 191–302. Nutr. Found., Inc., New York.

Hietanen, E. (1980). Modification of hepatic drug metabolizing enzyme activities and their induction by dietary protein. *Gen. Pharmacol.* **11**, 443–450.

Hietanen, E., Laitinen, M., Vainio, H., and Hanninen, O. (1975). Dietary fats and properties of endoplasmic reticulum. II. Dietary lipid induced changes in activities of drug metabolizing enzymes in liver and duodenum of rat. *Lipids* **10,** 467–472.

Hill, K. E., and Burk, F. (1982). Effect of selenium deficiency and vitamin E deficiency on glutathione metabolism in isolated rat hepatocytes. *J. Biol. Chem.* **257,** 10668–10672.

Hinson, J. (1980). Biochemical toxicology of acetaminophen. *Rev. Biochem. Toxicol.* **2,** 103–129.

Hoekstra, W. G. (1975). Biochemical function of selenium and its relation to vitamin E. *Fed. Proc., Fed. Am. Soc. Exp. Biol.* **34,** 2083–2089.

Hopkins, G. J., and Carroll, K. K. (1979). Relationship between the amount and type of dietary fat in the promotion of mammary carcinogenesis induced by 7,12-dimethylbenz[a]anthracene. *JNCI, J. Natl. Cancer Inst.* **62,** 1009–1012.

Hopkins, G. J., and West, C. E. (1976a). Effect of dietary fats on pentobarbital-induced sleeping times and hepatic microsomal cytochrome *P*-450 in rats. *Lipids* **11,** 736–740.

Hopkins, G. J., and West, C. E. (1976b). Possible role of dietary fats in carcinogenesis. *Life Sci.* **19,** 1103–1116.

Horn, L. R., Machlin, L. J., Barker, M. O., and Brin, M. (1976). Drug metabolism and hepatic heme proteins in the vitamin E deficient rat. *Arch. Biochem. Biophys.* **172,** 270–277.

Horwitt, M. K., and Harvey, C. C. (1962). Rate of fatty acid change in plasma, erythrocyte and depot fat in humans ingesting different fats. *Am. J. Clin. Nutr.* **10,** 351–352.

Hsu, J. M., Rubenstein, B., and Puleker, A. G. (1982). Role of magnesium in glutathione metabolism of rat erythrocytes. *J. Nutr.* **112,** 488–496.

Imai, Y., and Sato, R. (1974). A gel-electrophoretically homogeneous preparation of cytochrome *P*-450 from liver microsomes of phenobarbital pretreated rabbits. *Biochem. Biophys. Res. Commun.* **60,** 8–14.

Iyanagi, T., and Mason, H. S. (1973). Some properties of hepatic reduced nicotinamide adenine dinucleotide phosphate-cytochrome *c* reductase. *Biochemistry* **12,** 2297–2308.

Iyanagi, T., Makino, N., and Mason, H. S. (1974). Redox properties of the reduced nicotinamide adenine dinucleotide phosphate-cytochrome *P*-450 and reduced nicotinamide adenine dinucleotide-cytochrome b_5 reductases. *Biochemistry* **13,** 1701–1710.

Jacob, S. T., Scharf, M. B., and Vesell, E. S. (1974). Role of RNA in induction of hepatic microsomal mixed function oxidases. *Proc. Natl. Acad. Sci. U.S.A.* **71,** 704–707.

Jensen, G. E., and Clausen, J. (1981). Subcellular distribution of the cytochrome *P*-450 complex and glutathione peroxidase activity in vitamin E and essential fatty acid deficiency. *Lipids* **16,** 137–141.

Jensen, L. S., and Maurice, D. V. (1979). Influence of sulfur amino acids on copper toxicity in chicks. *J. Nutr.* **109,** 91–97.

Kahn, G. C., Boobis, A. R., Blair, I., Brodie, M. J., and Davies, D. S. (1980). Antipyrine as an in vitro probe of mixed function oxidase activity. *Br. J. Clin. Pharmacol.* **9,** 284P.

Kao, R. L. C., and Forbes, R. M. (1973). Lead and vitamin effects on heme synthesis. *Arch. Environ. Health* **27,** 31–35.

Kaplan, J. A., and Finlayson, D. L. (1981). Cyanide antagonist. *Can. Anaesth. Soc. J.* **28,** 290.

Kaplan, J. C., and Chirouze, M. (1978). Therapy of recessive congenital methemoglobinemia by oral riboflavin. *Lancet* **2,** 1043–1044.

Kappas, A., Anderson, K. E., Conney, A. H., and Alvares, A. P. (1976). Influence of dietary protein and carbohydrate on antipyrine and theophylline metabolism in man. *Clin. Pharmacol. Ther.* **20,** 643–653.

Kasbekar, K. K., Lavate, W. V., Rege, D. V., and Sreenivasen, A. (1959). A study of vitamin B_{12} protection in experimental liver injury to the rat by carbon tetrachloride. *Biochem. J.* **72,** 384–389.

Kasuya, M. (1980). The effect of methylcobalamin on the toxicity of methylmercury and mercuric chloride on nervous tissue in culture. *Toxicol. Lett.* **7,** 87–93.

Kato, N., Tani, T., and Yoshida, A. (1980). Effect of dietary level of protein on liver microsomal drug-metabolizing enzymes, urinary ascorbic acid and lipid metabolism in rats fed PCB-containing diets. *J. Nutr.* **110,** 1686–1694.

Kato, N., Tani, T., and Yoshida, A. (1981a). Effect of dietary quality of protein on liver microsomal mixed function oxidase system, plasma cholesterol and urinary ascorbic acid in rats fed PCB. *J. Nutr.* **111,** 123–133.

Kato, N., Kawai, K., and Yoshida, A. (1981b). Effect of dietary level of ascorbic acid on the growth, hepatic lipid peroxidation, and serum lipids in guinea pigs fed polychlorinated biphenyls. *J. Nutr.* **111,** 1727–1733.

Kato, N., Mochizuki, S., Kawai, K., and Yoshida, A. (1982). Effect of dietary level of sulfur-containing amino acids on liver drug-metabolizing enzymes, serum cholesterol and urinary ascorbic acid in rats fed PCB. *J. Nutr.* **112,** 848–854.

Kato, R. (1966). Possible role of *P*-450 in the oxidation of drugs in liver microsomes. *J. Biochem. (Tokyo)* **59,** 574–583.

Kato, R. (1967). Effects of starvation and refeeding on the oxidation of drugs by liver microsomes. *Biochem. Pharmacol.* **16,** 871–887.

Kato, R., Chiesara, E., and Vassanelli, P. (1962). Factors influencing induction of hepatic microsomal drug-metabolizing enzymes. *Biochem. Pharmacol.* **11,** 211–220.

Kato, R., Oshima, T., and Tomizawa, S. (1968). Toxicity and metabolism of drugs in relation to dietary protein. *Jpn. J. Pharmacol.* **18,** 356–466.

Kato, R., Takanaka, A., and Oshima, T. (1969). The effect of vitamim C deficiency on the metabolism of drugs and NADPH-linked electron transport system in liver microsomes. *Jpn. J. Pharmacol.* **19,** 25–33.

Kensler, C. J. (1948). The influence of diet on the ability of rat liver slices to destroy the carcinogen *N,N*-dimethyl-*p*-aminobenzene. *Cancer (Philadelphia)* **1,** 483–488.

Kim, J. C. S. (1977). Virus activation by vitamin A and NO_2 gas in hmasters. *Environ. Health Perspect.* **19,** 317–330.

Kim, J. C. S. (1978). The effect of dietary vitamin A on NO_2 exposure on the hamster lung. *Environ. Res.* **17,** 116–130.

Kuinzig, W., Tkaczeuski, V., Kamm, J. J., Conney, A. M., and Burn, J. J. (1977). The effect of ascorbic acid deficiency on extrahepatic microsomal metabolism of drugs and carcinogens in the guinea pig. *J. Pharmacol. Exp. Ther.* **201,** 527–533.

Kurokawa, I., Kimura, T., Veno, Y., Suzuki, J., Kishi, Y., Nagai, T., and Kamimura, M. (1970). The effect of vitamin E on the preservation of blood. *J. Vitaminol.* **16,** 180–189.

Laitinen, M. (1976). Enhancement of hepatic drug metabolism with dietary cholesterol in the rat. *Acta Pharmacol. Toxicol.* **39,** 241–249.

Lam, T. C. L., and Wade, A. E. (1980). Influence of dietary lipid on the metabolism of hexobarbital by the isolated, perfused rat liver. *Pharmacology* **21,** 64–67.

Lambert, L., and Wills, E. D. (1977). The effect of dietary lipids on 3,4-benzo[*a*]pyrene metabolism in the hepatic endoplasmic reticulum. *Biochem. Pharmacol.* **26,** 1423–1427.

Lambooy, J. P. (1970). Riboflavin protection against azo dye hepatoma induction in the rat. *Proc. Soc. Exp. Biol. Med.* **134,** 192–194.

Lamson, P. D., Greig, M. E., and Hobdy, C. J. (1951). Modification of barbiturate anesthesia by glucose, intermediary metabolites and certain other substances. *J. Pharmacol. Exp. Ther.* **103,** 460–470.

Lang, M. (1976). Depression of drug metabalism in liver microsomes after treating rats with unsaturated fatty acids. *Gen. Pharmacol.* **7,** 415–419.

Lang, M., Laitinen, M., Hietanen, E., and Vainio, H. (1976). Modification of microsomal membrane components and induction of hepatic drugs biotransformation in rats on a high cholesterol diet. *Acta Pharmacol. Toxicol.* **39,** 273–288.

Levander, O. A. (1979). Lead toxicity and nutritional deficiencies. *Environ. Health Perspect.* **29,** 115–125.

Levander, O. A., Morris, V. C., Higgs, D. J., and Ferretti, R. J. (1975). Lead poisoning in vitamin E-deficient rats. *J. Nutr.* **105,** 1481–1485.

Levander, O. A., Morris, V. C., and Ferretti, R. J. (1977a). Filterability of erythrocyte from vitamin E-deficient lead-poisoned rats. *J. Nutr.* **107,** 363–372.

Levander, O. A., Ferretti, R. J., and Morris, V. C. (1977b). Osmotic and peroxidative fragilities of erythrocytes from vitamin E-deficient lead poisoned rats. *J. Nutr.* **107,** 373–377.

Levander, O. A., Morris, V. C., and Ferretti, R. J. (1977c). Comparative effects of selenium and vitamin E in lead-poisoned rats. *J. Nutr.* **107,** 378–382.

Levander, O. A., Morris, V. C., and Ferretti, R. J. (1978). Effects of cell age on the filterability of erythrocytes from vitamin E-deficient lead poisoned rats. *J. Nutr.* **108,** 145–151.

Levin, M., Botelho, L. H., Thomas, P. E., and Ryam, D. E. (1980). *In* "Microsomes, Drug Oxidation and Chemical Carcinogenesis" (M. J. Coon, A. H. Conney, R. W. Estabrook, H. V. Gelboin, J. R. Gillette and P. J. O'Brien, eds.), pp. 47–57. Academic Press, New York.

Lohman, S. M., and Miech, R. P. (1976). Theophylline metabolism by the rat liver microsomal system. *J. Pharmacol. Exp. Ther.* **196,** 213–225.

Lotan, R. (1980). Effects of vitamin A and its analogs (Retinoids) on normal and neoplastic cells. *Biochim. Biophys. Acta* **605,** 33–91.

Lu, A. Y. H., and West, S. B. (1980). Multiplicity of mammalian microsomal cytochromes *P*-450. *Pharmacol. Rev.* **31,** 227–295.

Lucy, J. A. (1972). Functional and structural aspects of biological membranes: A suggested structural role for vitamin E in the control of membrane permeability and stability. *Ann. N.Y. Acad. Sci.* **203,** 4–11.

MacKinnon, A. M., and Simon, F. R. (1976). Impaired hepatic heme synthesis in the phenobarbital-stimulated selenium deficient rat. *Proc. Soc. Exp. Biol. Med.* **152,** 568–572.

McLean, A. E. M. (1967). The effect of diet and vitamin E on liver injury due to carbon tetrachloride. *Br. J. Exp. Pathol.* **48,** 632–636.

McLean, A. E. M., and Day, P. A. (1975). The effect of diet on the toxicity of paracetamol and the safety of paracetamol–methionine mixtures. *Biochem. Pharmacol.* **24,** 37–42.

McLean, A. E. M., and McLean, E. K. (1966). The effect of diet and 1,1,1-trichloro 2,2-bis-(*p*-chlorophenyl) ethane (DDT) on microsomal hydroxylating enzymes and on the sensitivity of rats to carbon tetrachloride poisoning. *Biochem. J.* **100,** 564–571.

McLean, A. E. M., and Magee, P. N. (1970). Increased renal carcinogenesis by dimethylnitrosamine in protein-deficient rats. *Br. J. Exp. Pathol.* **51,** 587–590.

Madhaven, T. V., and Gopalan, C. (1968). The effect of dietary protein on carcinogenesis of aflatoxin. *Arch. Pathol.* **85,** 133–138.

Magdalou, J., Steimetz, D., Balt, A.-M., Poullain, B., Siest, G., and Debry, G. (1979). The effect of dietary sulfur-containing amino acids on the activity of drug-metabolizing enzymes in rat liver microsomes. *J. Nutr.* **109,** 864–871.

Mahaffey, K. R., and Rader, J. I. (1980). Metabolic interactions: Lead, calcium and iron. *Ann. N.Y. Acad. Sci.* **355,** 130–139.

Mahaffey-Six, K., and Goyer, R. A. (1972). The influence of iron deficiency on tissue content of toxicity of ingested lead in the rat. *J. Lab. Clin. Med.* **79,** 128–136.

Maines, M. D. (1979). Role of trace metals in regulation of cellular heme and hemoprotein metabolism: Sensitizing effects of chronic iron treatment on acute gold toxicity. *Drug Metab. Rev.* **9,** 237–255.

Maines, M. D., and Kappas, A. (1976a). Selenium regulation of hepatic heme metabolism: Induction of delta-aminoleuvulinate synthetase and heme oxygenase. *Proc. Natl. Acad. Sci. U.S.A.* **73,** 4428–4431.

Maines, M. D., and Kappas, A. (1976b). Studies on the mechanism of induction of heme oxygenase by cobalt and other metal ions. *Biochem. J.* **154**, 125–131.

Maines, M. D., and Kappas, A. (1977a). Regulation of cytochrome *P*-450-dependent microsomal drug-metabolizing enzymes by nickel, cobalt and iron. *Clin. Pharmacol. Ther.* **22**, 780–790.

Maines, M. D., and Kappas, A. (1977b). Metals as regulators of heme metabolism. *Science* **198**, 1215–1221.

Mainigi, K. D., and Campbell, T. C. (1981). Effects of low dietary protein and dietary aflatoxin on hepatic glutathione levels in F-344 rats. *Toxicol. Appl. Pharmacol.* **59**, 196–203.

Marshall, W. J., and McLean, A. E. M. (1971). A requirement for dietary lipids for induction of cytochrome *P*-450 by phenobarbitone in rat liver microsomal fraction. *Biochem. J.* **122**, 569–573.

Matsuki, T., Yubisui, T., Tomoda, A., Yoneyama, Y., Takeshita, M., Hirano, M., Kobayashi, K., and Tani, Y. (1978). Acceleration of methemoglobin reduction by riboflavin in human erythrocytes. *Br. Haematol.* **39**, 523–528.

Menzel, D. B. (1970). Toxicity of ozone, oxygen, and radiation. *Annu. Rev. Pharmacol.* **10**, 379–391.

Meydani, M., and Hathcock, J. N. (1984). Effect of dietary methionine on methylmercury and atrazine toxicity. *Drug-Nutr. Interact.* **2**, 217–233.

Meydani, M., Blumberg, J. B., and Hayes, K. C. (1985). Dietary fat unsaturation enhances drug metabolism in cebus but not in squirrel monkeys. *J. Nutr.* **115**, 573–578.

Mgbodile, M. U. K., and Campbell, J. C. (1972). Effect of protein deprivation of male weanling rats on the kinetics of hepatic microsomal enzyme activity. *J. Nutr.* **102**, 53–60.

Mills, B. J., Lindeman, R. D., and Lang, C. A. (1981). Effect of zinc deficiency on blood glutathione levels. *J. Nutr.* **111**, 1098–1102.

Miranda, C. L., and Chhabra, R. S. (1981). Effects of high dietary vitamin A on drug-metabolizing enzyme activities in guinea pig and rabbit. *Drug-Nutr. Interact.* **1**, 55–61.

Miranda, C. L., and Webb, R. E. (1973). Effects of dietary protein quality on drug metabolism in the rat. *J. Nutr.* **103**, 1426–1430.

Miranda, C. L., Mukhtar, H., Bend, J. R., and Chhabra, R. S. (1979). Effects of vitamin A deficiency on hepatic and extrahepatic mixed-function oxidase and epoxide-metabolizing enzymes in guinea pigs and rabbits. *Biochem. Pharmacol.* **28**, 2713–2716.

Mirvish, S. S. (1975). Blocking the formation of *N*-nitroso compounds with ascorbic acid in-vitro and in-vivo. *Ann. N.Y. Acad. Sci.* **258**, 175–180.

Moffitt, A. E., Jr., and Murphy, S. K. (1973). Effect of excess and deficient copper intake on rat liver microsomal enzyme activity. *Biochem. Pharmacol.* **22**, 1463–1476.

Montgomery, M. R., Furry, J., Gee, S. J., and Krieger, R. I. (1982). Ascorbic acid and paraquat: Oxygen depletion with concurrent oxygen activation. *Toxicol. Appl. Pharmacol.* **63**, 321–329.

Mucklow, J. C., Caraher, M. T., Henderson, D. B., and Rawlins, M. B. (1979). The effect of individual dietary constituents on antipyrine clearance in Asian immigrants. *Br. J. Clin. Pharmacol.* **7**, 416–417.

Mucklow, J. C., Caraher, M. T., Idle, J. R., Rawlins, M. D., Sloan, T., Smith, R. L., and Wood, P. (1980). The influence of changes in dietary fat on the clearance of antipyrine and 4-hydroxylation of debrisquine. *Br. J. Clin. Pharmacol.* **9**, 283P.

Mueller, G. C., and Miller, J. A. (1950). The reductive cleavage of 4-dimethyl-aminoazobenzene by rat liver: Reactivation of carbon dioxide treated homogenates by riboflavin-adenine din-ulceotide. *J. Biol. Chem.* **185**, 145–154.

Mukhatar, H., Elmamlouk, T. H., Philpot, R. M., and Bend, J. R. (1978). Rat hepatic nuclear cytochrome *P*-450 and epoxide hydrase in membranes prepared by two methods: Similarities with the microsomal wnzymes. *Mol. Pharmacol.* **15**, 192–196.

Mulder, G. J., Hinson, J. A., and Gillette, J. R. (1978). Conversion of the *N-O*-glucuronide and

N-O-sulfate conjugates of *N*-hydroxyphenacetin to reactive intermediates. *Biochem. Pharmacol.* **27**, 1641–1649.

Murty, H. S., Caasi, P. I., Brooks, S. D., and Nair, P. P. (1970). Biosynthesis of heme in the vitamin E-deficient rat. *J. Biol. Chem.* **245**, 5498–5504.

Mushett, C. W., Kelley, K. L., Boxer, G. E., and Rickards, J. C. (1952). Antidotal efficacy of vitamin B_{12} (hydroxycobalamin) in experimental cyanide poisoning. *Proc. Soc. Exp. Biol. Med.* **8**, 539–543.

Myers, C. E., McGuire, W., and Young, R. (1976). Adriamycin: Amelioration of toxicity by alpha-tocopherol. *Cancer Treat. Rep.* **60**, 961–962.

Myers, C. E., McGuire, W. P., Liss, R. H., Ifrim, I., Grotzinger, K., and Young, R. C. (1977). The role of lipid peroxidation in cardiac toxicity and tumor response. *Science* **197**, 165–167.

Nelson, J. S. (1980). Pathology of vitamin E deficiency. *In* "Vitamin E: A Comprehensive Treatise." (L. J. Machline, ed.), pp. 397–428. Dekker, New York.

Newberne, P. M., and McConnell, R. G. (1980). Nutrient deficiencies in cancer causation. *J. Environ. Pathol. Toxicol.* **3**, 323–356.

Newberne, P. M., Gross, R. L., and Roe, D. A. (1978). Drug, toxin and nutrient interactions. *World Rev. Nutr. Diet* **29**, 130–169.

Newberne, P. M., Weigert, J., and Kula, N. (1979). Effect of dietary fat on hepatic-mixed function oxidases and hepatocellular carcinoma induced by aflatoxin B_1 in rats. *Cancer Res.* **39**, 3986–3991.

Norred, W. P., and Marzuki, A. (1984). Effects of dietary saturated or polyunsaturated fat on hepatic glutathione *S*-transferase activity. *Drug-Nutr. Interact.* **3**, 11–20.

Paine, A. J., and Legg, R. F. (1978). Apparent lack of correlation between the loss of cytochrome *P*-450 in hepatic parenchymal cell culture and the stimulation of haem oxygenase activity. *Biochem. Biophys. Res. Commun.* **81**, 672–679.

Parizek, J., and Ostadalova, I. (1967). The protective effect of small amount of selenite in sublimate intoxication. *Experimentia* **23**, 142–143.

Patel, J. M., and Pawar, S. S. (1974). Riboflavin and drug metabolism in adult male and female rats. *Biochem. Pharmacol.* **23**, 1467–1477.

Peters, M. A., and Fouts, J. R. (1970a). The influence of magnesium and some other divalent cations on hepatic microsomal drugs metabolism *in vitro*. *Biochem. Pharmacol.* **19**, 533–544.

Peters, M. A., and Fouts, J. R. (1970b). A study of some possible mechanisms by which magnesium activates hepatic microsomal drug metabolism *in vitro*. *J. Pharmacol. Exp. Ther.* **173**, 233–241.

Peterson, F. J., and Knodell, R. G. (1984). Ascorbic acid protects against acetaminophen and cocaine-induced hepatic damage in mice. *Drug-Nutr. Interact.* **3**, 33–42.

Peterson, F. J., Combs, G. F., Jr., Holtman, J., and Mason, R. P. (1982). Effect of selenium and vitamin E deficiency on nitrofurantoin toxicity in the chick. *J. Nutr.* **112**, 1741–1746.

Piafsky, K. M., Sitar, D. S., and Ogilvie, R. I. (1975). Effect of phenobarbital administration on theophylline kinetics. *Clin. Res.* **23**, 610A.

Poirier, L. A., Grantham, P. H., and Rogers, A. E. (1977). The effect of marginally lipotrope-deficient diet on the hepatic levels of delta-adenosylmethionine and on the urinary metabolites of 2-acetylaminofluorine in rats. *Cancer Res.* **37**, 744–748.

Raheja, K. L., Turkki, P. R., Linscheer, W. G., and Cho, C. (1983). Effects of riboflavin status on acetaminophen toxicity in the rat. *Drug-Nutr. Interact.* **2**, 183–191.

Reed, J. R., Deacon, L. E., Farr, F., and Couch, J. R. (1968). Inositol and the fatty liver syndrome. *Proc. Annu. Tex. Nutr. Conf.* **23**, 204–209.

Reicks, M. M., and Hathcock, J. N. (1984). Effects of dietary methionine and ethanol on acetaminophen hepatatoxicity in mice. *Drug-Nutr. Interact.* **3**, 43–52.

Ribarov, S. R., and Benov, L. C. (1981). Relationship between the hemolytic action of heavy metals and lipid peroxidation. *Biochim. Biophys. Acta* **640**, 721–726.

Richards, R. K., Kueter, K., and Klatt, T. J. (1941). Effect of vitamin C deficiency on action of different types of barbiturates. *Proc. Soc. Exp. Biol. Med.* **48,** 403–409.

Rikans, L. E., Smith, C. R., and Zannoni, V. G. (1977). Ascorbic acid and the heme synthesis in deficient guinea pig liver. *Biochem. Pharmacol.* **26,** 797–799.

Rivilin, R. S., Menendex, C., and Langdon, R. G. (1968). Biochemical similarities between hypothyroidism and riboflavin deficiency. *Endocrinology (Baltimore)* **83,** 461–469.

Roe, D. A., McCormick, D. B., and Lin, R. T. (1972). Effects of riboflavin on boric acid toxicity. *J. Pharm. Sci.* **61,** 1081–1085.

Roehm, J. N., Hadley, J. G., and Menzel, D. B. (1971). Antioxidants vs. lung disease. *Arch. Intern. Med.* **128,** 88–93.

Roehm, J. N., Hadley, J. G., and Menzel, D. (1972). The influence of vitamin E on the lung fatty acids of rats exposed to ozone. *Arch. Environ. Health* **24,** 237–242.

Rowe, L., and Wills, E. D. (1976). The effect of dietary lipids and vitamin E on lipid peroxide formation, cytochrome *P*-450 and oxidative demethylation in the endoplasmic reticulum. *Biochem. Pharmacol.* **25,** 175–179.

Ruchirawat, M., Mahathanatrakul, W., Sinrashatanant, Y., and Kittikool, D. (1978). Effects of thiamine deficiency on the metabolism and acute toxicity of dimethylnitrosamine in the rat. *Biochem. Pharmacol.* **27,** 1783–1786.

Rumack, B. H., Holtzman, J., and Chase, H. P. (1973). Hepatic drug metabolism and protein malnutrition. *J. Pharmacol. Exp. Ther.* **186,** 441–446.

Rumsby, P. C., and Shepherd, D. M. (1981). The effect of penicillamine on vitamin B_6 function in man. *Biochem. Pharmacol.* **30,** 3051–3053.

Sachan, D. S. (1976). Induction of microsomal drug-metabolizing enzymes by oral contraceptives in protein-malnourished rats. *J. Nutr.* **106,** 1569–1576.

Sell, J. L., and Horani, F. G. (1976). Influence of selenium on toxicity and metabolism of methylmercury in chicks and quail. *Nutr. Rep. Int.* **14,** 439–447.

Shargel, L., and Mazel, P. (1973). Effect of riboflavin deficiency on phenobarbital and 3-methylcholanthrene induction of microsomal drug metabolizing enzymes of the rat. *Biochem. Pharmacol.* **22,** 2365–2373.

Sharma, B., Mehta, S., Nain, C. K., and Mathur, V. S. (1985). Pharmacokinetic profile of antipyrine in young rhesus monkeys (*Macaca mulatta*) with protein energy malnutrition. *Drug-Nutr. Interact.* **3,** 93–98.

Shils, M. E. (1976). Magnesium. *In* "Nutrition Reviews. Present Knowledge in Nutrition," (D. M. Hegsted, C. A. Chester, W. J. Darby, K. W. McNutt, R. M. Stalvy, and E. H. Stotz, eds.), 4th ed., pp. 247–258. Nutr. Found., Inc., New York.

Shojania, A. M. (1982). Oral contraceptives: Effect on folate and vitamin B_{12} metabolism. *Can. Med. Assoc. J.* **126,** 244–247.

Sifri, M., and Hoekstra, W. G. (1978). Effect of lead on lipid peroxidation in rats deficient or adequate in selenium and vitamin E. *Fed. Proc., Fed. Am. Soc. Exp. Biol.* **37,** 757.

Sikic, B. J., Mimnaugh, E. G., Litterst, G. L., and Gram, T. E. (1977). The effects of ascorbic acid deficiency and repletion on pulmonary, renal, and hepatic drug metabolism in the guinea pig. *Arch. Biochem. Biophys.* **179,** 663–671.

Sitar, D. S., and Gordon, E. R. (1980). Effect of diet and drug on the qualitative and quantitative distribution of cytochrome *P*-450 in rat liver. *Can. J. Physiol. Pharmacol.* **58,** 331–335.

Skaare, J. U., and Nafstad, I. (1978). Interaction of vitamin E and selenium with the hepatotoxic agent dimethylnitrosamine. *Acta Pharmacol. Toxicol.* **43,** 119–128.

Smith, J. A., Butler, T. C., and Poole, D. T. (1973). Effect of protein deprivation in guinea pigs on glucuronate conjugation of chloramphenicol by liver microsomes. *Biochem. Pharmacol.* **22,** 981–983.

Smith, S. J., Liu, D. K., Leonard, T. B., Duceman, B. W., and Vesell, E. S. (1976). Phenobarbital-induced increase in methylation of ribosomal precursor ribonucleic acid. *Mol. Pharmacol.* **12,** 820–831.

Snider, D. E. (1980). Pyridoxine supplementation during isoniazid therapy. *Tubercle* **61,** 191–196.

Sonawane, B. R., Coates, P. M., Yaffe, S. J., and Koldovsky, O. (1983). Influence of dietary carbohydrates (α-saccharides) on hepatic drug metabolism in male rats. *Drug-Nutr. Interact.* **2,** 7–16.

Sonneveld, P. (1978). Effect of α-tocopherol on the cardiotoxicity of adriamycin in the rat. *Cancer Treat. Rep.* **62,** 1033–1036.

Sporn, M. B., Dunlop, N. M., Newton, D. L., and Smith, J. M. (1976). Prevention of chemical carcinogenesis by vitamin A and its synthetic analogs (retinoids). *Fed. Proc., Fed. Am. Soc. Exp. Biol.* **35,** 1332–1338.

Stacey, N. H., and Kappus, H. (1982). Cellular toxicity and lipid peroxidation in response to mercury. *Toxicol. Appl. Pharmacol.* **63,** 29–35.

Stillings, B. R., Lagally, H., Baversfeld, P., and Soares, J. (1974). Effects of cysteine, selenium and fish protein on the toxicity and metabolism of methylmercury in rats. *Toxicol. Appl. Pharmacol.* **30,** 243–254.

Stowe, H. D. (1976). Biliary excretion of cadmium by rats: Effects of zinc, cadmium, and selenium pretreatments. *J. Toxicol. Environ. Health* **2,** 45–54.

Strobel, L., Lu, A. H. Y., Heidema, J., and Coon, M. J. (1970). Phosphatidylcholine requirement in the enzymatic reduction of heam protein *P*-450 and in fatty acid, hydrocarbon, and drug hydroxylation. *J. Biol. Chem.* **245,** 4851–4854.

Strother, A., Throckmorton, J. K., and Herzer, C. (1971). The influence of high sugar consumption by mice on the duration of action of barbiturates and in vitro metabolism of barbiturates, aniline, and *p*-nitroanisole. *J. Pharmacol. Exp. Med.* **179,** 490–498.

Suit, J., Rogers, A. E., Jettern. M. E. R., and Luria, S. E. (1977). Effects of diet on conversion of aflatoxin B_1 to bacterial mutagens by rats in vivo and by rat hepatic microsomes in vitro. *Mutat. Res.* **46,** 313–323.

Sunde, M. L. (1976). "Effect of Vitamin E on Mercury Toxicity," Annu. Rep., p. 384. Food Res. Inst., University of Wisconsin, Madison.

Sunde, R. A., and Hoekstra, W. G. (1980). Structure, synthesis and function of glutathione peroxidase. *Nutr. Rev.* **38,** 265–273.

Sunde, R. A., Gutzke, G. E., and Hoekstra, W. G. (1981). Effect of dietary methionine on the biopotency of selenite and selenomethionine in the rat. *J. Nutr.* **111,** 76–86.

Suzuki, T., and Yoshida, A. (1978). Long-term effectiveness of dietary iron and ascorbic acid in the rat preventions and cure of cadmium toxicity in rats. *Am. J. Clin. Nutr.* **31,** 1491–1498.

Suzuki, T., and Yoshida, A. (1979). Effectiveness of dietary iron and ascorbic acid in the prevention and cure of moderately long-term lead toxicity in rats. *J. Nutr.* **109,** 1974–1978.

Swann, P. F., and McLean, A. E. M. (1971). Cellular injury and carcinogenesis. The effect of protein-free high carbohydrate diet on the metabolism of dimethylnitrosamine in the rat. *Biochem. J.* **124,** 283–288.

Thor, H., Moldius, P., and Orrenius, S. (1979). Metabolic activation and hepatotoxicity: Effect of cysteine, *N*-acetylcysteine, and methionine on glutathione biosynthesis and bromobenzene toxicity in isolated hepatocytes. *Arch. Biochem. Biophys.* **192,** 405–413.

Tien, M., Suingen, B. A., and Aust, S. D. (1981). Superoxide dependent lipid peroxidation. *Fed. Proc., Fed. Am. Soc. Exp. Biol.* **40,** 179–82.

Tinsley, I. J. (1966). Nutritional interactions in dieldrin toxicity. *J. Agric. Food Chem.* **14,** 563–566.

Van Vleet, J. F., Ferrans, V. J., and Weirich, W. E. (1980). Cardiac disease induced by chronic adriamycin administration in dogs and an evaluation of vitamin E and selenium as cardioprotectants. *Am. J. Pathol.* **99,** 13–42.

Varma, D. R. (1979). Influence of dietary protein on the anti-inflammatory and ulcerogenic effects and on the pharmacokinetics of phenylbutazone in rats. *J. Pharmacol. Exp. Ther.* **211**, 388–344.

Venkatesan, N., Arcos, J. C., and Argus, M. F. (1970). Amino acid induction and carbohydrate repression of dimethylnitrosamine demethylase in rat liver. *Cancer Res.* **30**, 2563–2567.

Verlangieri, A. J., Meyer, J. J., Barnes, T. B., and Kapeghian, J. C. (1982). Effects of dietary protein content on locomotor activity during chronic lead exposure in male and female rats. *Toxicologist* **2**, 54.

Vermilion, J. L., and Coon, M. J. (1978). Identification of the high and low potential flavins of liver microsomal NADPH-cytochrome *P*-450 reductase. *J. Biol. Chem.* **253**, 8812–8819.

Vermilion, J. L., Ballou, D. P., Massey, V., and Coon, M. J. (1981). Separate role for FMN and FAD in catalysis by liver microsomal NADPH-cytochrome *P*-450 reductase. *J. Biol. Chem.* **256**, 266–277.

Wade, A. E., and Norred, W. P. (1976). Effect of dietary lipid on drug-metabolizing enzymes. *Fed. Proc., Fed. Am. Soc. Exp. Biol.* **35**, 2475–2479.

Wade, A. E., Greene, F. E., Ciordia, R. M., Meadows, J. S., and Caster, W. O. (1969). Effects of dietary thiamine intake on hepatic drug metabolism in the male rat. *Biochem. Pharmacol.* **18**, 2288–2291.

Wade, A. E., Wu, B., and Lee, J. (1975). Nutritional factors affecting drug metabolizing enzymes of the rat. *Biochem Pharmacol.* **24**, 785–789.

Wade, A. E., Norred, W. P., and Evans, J. S. (1978). Lipids in drug detoxication. *In* "Nutrition and Drug Interrelations" (J. N. Hathcock and J. Coon, eds.), pp. 475–503. Academic Press, New York.

Wade, A. E., Evans, J. S., Holmes, D., and Baker, M. T. (1983). Influence of dietary thiamin on phenobarbital induction of rat hepatic enzymes responsible for metabolizing drugs and carcinogens. *Drug-Nutr. Interact.* **2**, 117–130.

Wason, S., Lacouture, P. G., and Lovejoy, F. H. (1981). Single high-dose pyridoxine treatment for isoniazid overdose. *JAMA, J. Am. Med. Assoc.* **246**, 1102–1104.

Watson, A. F., and Mellanby, E. (1930). Tar cancer in mice. II. The condition of skin when modified by external treatment or diet, as a factor in influencing the cancerous reaction. *Br. J. Exp. Pathol.* **11**, 311–322.

Weatherholz, W. M., Campbell, T. C., and Webb, R. E. (1969). Effect of dietary protein levels on the toxicity and metabolism of heptachlor. *J. Nutr.* **98**, 90–94.

Welsh, S. O. (1974). Physiological effects of methylmercury toxicity: Interaction of methylmercury with selenium, tellurium and vitamin E. Ph.D. Thesis, University of Maryland, College Park.

Welsh, S. O. (1976). Influence of vitamin E on mercury poisoning in rats. *Fed. Proc., Fed. Am. Soc. Exp. Biol.* **35**, 761.

Welsh, S. O. (1977). Contrasting effects of vitamin A and E on mercury poisoning. *Fed. Proc., Fed. Am. Soc. Exp. Biol.* **36**, 1146.

Welsh, S. O., and Soares, J. H. (1976). The protection effect of vitamin E and selenium against methylmercury toxicity in Japanese quail. *Nutr. Rep. Int.* **13**, 43–51.

Williams, D. M., Burk, R. F., Jenkinson, S. G., and Lawrence, R. A. (1981). Hepatic cytochrome *P*-450 and microsomal heme oxygenase in copper-deficient rats. *J. Nutr.* **111**, 979–983.

Williams, J. R., Jr., Grantham, P. H., Yamamoto, R. S., and Weisburger, J. H. (1970). Effect of dietary riboflavin on azo dye reductase in liver and in bacteria of cecal contents of rats. *Biochem. Pharmacol.* **19**, 2523–2525.

Williams, R. T. (1978). Nutrient in drug detoxification reactions. *In* "Nutrition and Drug Interrelations" (J. N. Hathcock, and J. Coon, eds.), pp. 303–318. Academic Press, New York.

Wills, E. D. (1972). Effects of iron overload on lipid peroxidation and oxidative demethylation by the liver endoplasmic reticulum. *Biochem. Pharmacol.* **21**, 239–247.

Wilmana, P. F., Brodie, M. J., Mucklow, J. C., Farser, H. S., Toverud, E. L., Davies, D. S.,

Dallery, C. T., Hillyard, C. J., McIntyre, I., and Park, B. K., (1979). Reduction of circulating 25-hydroxyvitamin D by antipyrine. *Br. J. Clin. Pharmacol.* **8,** 523–528.

Witting, L. A., Harvey, C. C., Century, B., and Horwitt, M. K. (1961). Dietary alterations of fatty acids of erythrocytes and mitochondria of brain and liver. *J. Lipid Res.* **2,** 412–417.

Wood, G. C., and Woodcock, B. G. (1970). Effect of dietary protein deficiency on the conjugation of foreign compounds in rat liver. *J. Pharm. Pharmacol.* **22,** Suppl., 605–635.

Woodcock, B. K., and Wood, G. C. (1971). Effect of protein-free diet on UDP glucuronyltransferase and sulfontransferase activities in rat liver. *Biochem. Pharmacol.* **20,** 2703–2731.

Wynder, E. L., Hoffman, D., Chan, P., and Reddy, B. (1975). Interdisciplinary and experimental approaches: Metabolic epidemiology. *In* "Persons at High Risk of Cancer: An Approach to Cancer Etiology and Control" (J. F. Fraumeni, Jr., ed.), pp. 485–500. Academic Press, New York.

Yang, C. S. (1974). Alterations of the aryl hydrocarbon hydroxylase system during riboflavin depletion and repletion. *Arch. Biochem. Biophys.* **160,** 623–630.

Yang, C. S. (1975). The association between cytochrome *P*-450 and NADPH-cytochrome *P*-450 reductase in microsomal membrane. *FEBS Lett.* **54,** 61–64.

Yang, C. S. (1977). The organization and interaction of monooxygenase enzymes in the microsomal membrane. *Life Sci.* **21,** 1047–1058.

Yonaha, M., Itoh, E., Ohbayashi, Y., and Uchiyama, M. (1980). Induction of lipid peroxidation in rats by mercuric chloride. *Res. Commun. Chem. Pathol. Pharmacol.* **28,** 105–112.

Zannoni, V. G., and Lynch, M. M. (1973). The role of ascorbic acid in drug metabolism. *Drug Metab. Rev.* **2,** 57–69.

Zannoni, V. G., and Sato, P. H. (1975). Effects of ascorbic acid on microsomal drug metabolism. *Ann. N.Y. Acad. Sci.* **258,** 119–130.

Zannoni, V. G., and Sato, P. H. (1976). The effect of certain vitamin deficiencies on hepatic drug metabolism. *Fed. Proc., Fed. Am. Soc. Exp. Biol.* **35,** 2464–2469.

Zilva, S. S. (1935). The behavior of L-ascorbic acid and chemically related compounds in the animal body. The influence of generalized ether anaesthesia on the urinary excretion. *Biochem. J.* **29,** 2366–2368.

2

Effect of Nutrition on Monooxygenation and Conjugation in the Liver

Steven A. Belinsky, Frederick C. Kauffman, and
Ronald G. Thurman

I. INTRODUCTION

Epidemiological studies suggest that diet may influence 30–40% of all cancers in men and 60% in women (for a comprehensive review, see Committee on Diet Nutrition and Cancer, 1982). The strong correlation between diet and cancer may stem from the nearly 3000 substances added to foods during processing and another 12,000 chemicals used in food packing materials. Only a small proportion of the substances added to foods have been tested for carcinogenicity. In

NUTRITIONAL TOXICOLOGY, VOL. II

Copyright © 1987 by Academic Press, Inc.
All rights of reproduction in any form reserved.

addition, food contains many naturally occurring contaminants, some of which are carcinogenic in animals (e.g., aflatoxin, *N*-nitroso compounds), that may pose a potential risk of cancer to humans. Moreover, many edible plants contain natural pesticides, some which are activated by the mixed-function oxidase (MFO) pathway to highly reactive intermediates that usually react with DNA and other cellular constituents. Many of these highly reactive intermediates are detoxified by conjugating pathways present in the cells. Dietary modifications may stimulate or inhibit the activation and/or detoxification of environmental agents by affecting these metabolic pathways. Before dietary manipulations can be used effectively to reduce the incidence of neoplasia, factors which regulate mixed-function oxidation and conjugation in intact cells must be identified.

The MFO system is a particularly complex biological system consisting of multienzymatic components that are dependent on a continuous supply of NADPH. This cofactor is generated by other multienzyme systems. Diet has profound effects on this important metabolic system. The abnormal chronic intake of most nutrients can modify the activity of drug-metabolizing systems measured *in vitro*. These effects are often due to alteration in the structure and composition of microsomal membranes. More importantly, however, has been the realization in the past decade that monooxygenases and phase II enzymes in intact cells are regulated via their respective cofactor supplies (Thurman and Kauffman, 1980). Nutrition can have profound effects on cofactor supply and can thereby influence toxicity acutely by modification of monooxygenation and conjugation reactions. In addition, it is now clear that complex interactions between nutrition and toxicity can only be studied meaningfully in whole-cell preparations such as perfused livers or isolated hepatocytes where cofactor generation systems are intact. Isolated membrane fractions where cofactors are supplied in excess have lost this important form of metabolic regulation.

II. REGULATION OF MIXED-FUNCTION OXIDATION IN THE INTACT LIVER

Considerable progress has been made in identifying the sequence of events involved in operation of the MFO system. The three major components consist of NADPH-cytochrome *P*-450 reductase, a family of cytochrome *P*-450 proteins, and phospholipid, which are components of the membranes of the endoplasmic reticulum. Many cytochromes are present for each flavoprotein, and this may account for the wide substrate specificity of the system. Oxidation of compounds via this system involves the following sequence of events: An oxidized cytochrome binds the drug substrate, which is reduced by the flavoprotein in an NADPH-dependent reaction. This P-450 $^{2+}$–drug complex then reacts with oxygen to form a $P\text{-}450^{2+}$–O_2–drug complex which is reduced by the second electron from NADPH. The breakdown of this second complex releases hydroxylated drug and water and regenerates oxidized cytochrome *P*-450. Work that has led to elucidation of the above sequence of events *in vitro* has been dealt with extensively in a number of papers and reviews (Bjorkhem, 1977; Cooper *et al.*, 1965; Estabrook *et al.*, 1977; Lu and Levin, 1974; Omura and Sato, 1964a,b).

In intact cells, mixed-function oxidation is intimately related to other cellular events involved in the generation of the reduced cofactor and the provision of activated biosynthetic intermediates needed for conjugation of oxidized products. A scheme illustrating some of the interactions that may occur is presented in Fig. 1. NADPH is generated by highly regulated multienzyme systems that exist in several intracellular compartments. For example, the major dehydrogenases of the pentose phosphate cycle are cytosolic, whereas fatty acid oxidation and the citric acid cycle are primarily intramitochondrial. The pentose shunt

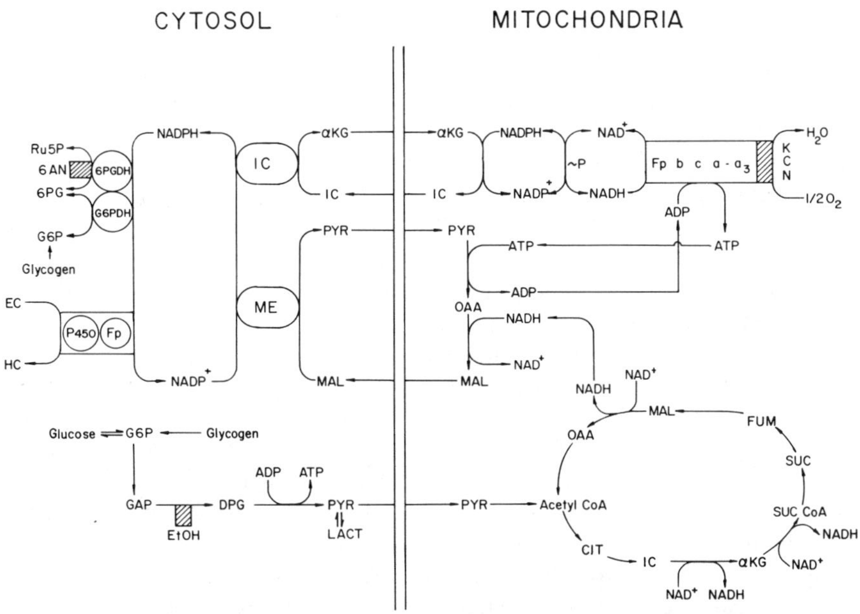

Fig. 1. Interactions between drug and intermediary metabolism in intact cells. Cytosolic reduced nicotinamide adenine dinucleotide phosphate (NADPH) may be generated by the pentose phosphate pathway in a series of reactions starting with glucose 6-phosphate (G6P) and involving the enzymes glucose-6-phosphate dehydrogenase (G6PDH) and 6-phosphogluconate dehydrogenase (6PGDH). In addition, cytosolic NADPH may be generated by a malate (MAL) shuttle, involving the egress of malate into the cytosol, and NADPH production via malic enzyme (ME). Alternatively, mitochondrial NADPH is generated by an energy (~P)-requiring transhydrogenase that carries out the reduction of NADP⁺ from NADPH. A shuttle mechanism involving isocitrate dehydrogenase (ICDH) transfers hydrogen from NADPH to α-ketoglutarate (KG) in the mitochondria and regenerates NADPH in the cytosol. Other abbreviations used: GAP (glyceraldehyde 3-phosphate); IC (isocitrate); Pyr (pyruvate); OAA (oxaloacetate); CIT (citrate); SUC-CoA, (succinyl-CoA); SUC (succinate); FUM (fumarate); FA (fatty acid); and EtOH (ethanol).

provides reducing equivalents in the cytosol directly, whereas the latter systems furnish substrates for malic enzyme and isocitrate dehydrogenase which can then form NADPH in the cytosol. Movement of reducing equivalents from the mitochondrial to the cytosolic space via specific substrates involves complex substrate shuttle mechanisms. Until recently, scant attention has been given to interactions that occur between these systems and rates of mixed-function oxidation in whole cells.

There are at least four types of regulation that can be imposed upon mixed-function oxidation in intact cells: induction, substrate and cofactor supply, activation and inhibition by effectors, and competing reactions. Metabolic events that compete for substrates and cofactors (e.g., fatty acid synthesis) undoubtedly play an important role in determining the availability of NADPH for mixed-function oxidation in intact cells.

Induction of enzyme components is generally a slow form of regulation; however, under some conditions it can occur in a few hours. In most cases, induction is not absolutely specific for unique components of the MFO system. For example, phenobarbital induces several forms of cytochrome *P*-450 (Coon *et al.*, 1977), glucuronyl transferase (Orrenius *et al.*, 1978), and several NADPH-generating enzymes (Kauffman *et al.*, 1977, 1979).

Regulation of mixed-function oxidation by the supply of substrate and cofactor may involve a number of events. For example, diffusion of oxygen, transport of drug to binding sites on cytochrome *P*-450, and delivery of NADPH to the flavoprotein may be rate-controlling. Of these three possibilities, regulation via the NADPH supply is probably the most important because delivery of oxygen and diffusion of drug is not limiting under physiological conditions. Maintenance of the oxidation–reduction state of the $NADP^+$–NADPH couple is a highly regulated process in intact cells. NADPH is formed in the cytosol via oxidation of glucose 6-phosphate, 6-phosphogluconate, malate, and isocitrate. Reducing equivalents are also formed in the mitochondria via transhydrogenation and transferred into the cytosol via specific substrate shuttle mechanisms. Once NADPH is generated in or transferred to the cytosol, a number of reactions will compete for this cofactor. In addition to fatty acid synthesis, reduction of oxidized glutathione is another reaction which competes for NADPH. At the cytochrome *P*-450 level, substrates that compete for binding sites include a wide array of xenobiotics as well as endogenous substrates such as steroid hormones, vitamin D, bilirubin, fatty acids, and prostaglandins.

Alteration of the formation of specific intermediates such as NADPH and activated substrates used in conjugation reactions provides mechanisms whereby nutritional and endocrine factors may regulate mixed-function oxidation in whole cells on both an acute and chronic basis. Nutritional factors are known to influence the levels of MFO components (Campbell and Hayes, 1983). This paper reviews methods and results of experiments on the regulation of mixed-function oxidation and conjugation in periportal and pericentral regions of the liver lobule with particular emphasis on acute interactions with nutrition.

There is considerable information concerning the catalytic properties of the MFO system *in vitro* which suggests that the rate-limiting step in drug oxidation in microsomes is at the introduction of the second electron (Bjorkhem, 1977; Imai *et al.*, 1977). Experiments supporting this conclusion were carried out in the presence of excess NADPH and are therefore not directly comparable to the intact cell where NADPH is largely bound to various dehydrogenases and may be rate-limiting for mixed-function oxidation. When concentrations of NADPH were adjusted *in vitro* to approximate those in the intact organ, rates of mixed-function oxidation were limited by the turnover of their cofactor (Holtzclaw *et al.*, 1984).

The first study to suggest that NADPH was limiting for mixed-function oxidation in the intact liver was carried out in 1969 by Thurman and Scholz. They showed that oxygen uptake of the perfused liver from a fed rat was increased markedly upon infusion of aminopyrine, a classical substrate for the MFO system. However, no increase was observed if the experiment was performed in the liver of a fasted rat in the presence of an inhibitor of the mitochondrial respiratory chain, antimycin A. In contrast, microsomes prepared from livers in these two metabolic states oxidized aminopyrine at similar rates when supplied with an active NADPH-generating system. Thus, they concluded that NADPH supply was a major rate determinant for mixed-function oxidation in the intact cell.

Further support for the hypothesis that NADPH is rate-limiting for mixed-function oxidation in the intact cell under certain conditions has been described in other experiments. For example, Thurman *et al.* (1977a) showed that linear rates of *p*-nitrophenol production occurred when *p*-nitroanisole was infused into livers from fed, normal rats or added to microsomes incubated in the presence of NADPH. In contrast, high rates of *p*-nitrophenol production by perfused livers from phenobarbital-treated rats were linear for less than 2 min and then declined to around 25% of the control value. Since oxygen and substrate were supplied in excess, it was concluded that the decrease in rates of mixed-function oxidation was due to a decline in NADPH supply.

In the cytosol, NADPH can be generated by the enzymes of the pentose cycle, glucose-6-phosphate dehydrogenase and 6-phosphogluconate dehydrogenase (Fig. 1); however, in intact cells approximately 80% of the intracellular NADPH is located in mitochondria (Bücher and Sies, 1976). One of the major sources for NADPH generation in mitochondria is an energy-dependent transhydrogenase which utilizes NADH to reduce $NADP^+$ (Hoek and Ernster, 1974). Because biological membranes are impermeable to pyridine nucleotides (Lehninger, 1975), substrate shuttle pathways are required to move reducing equivalents from the mitochondria into the cytosol. Substrate shuttle pathways transfer hydrogen to small molecules such as malate which penetrate mitochondrial membranes. NADPH is then generated in the cytosol by dehydrogenation of the carrier molecule. The two shuttle pathways involved in the transfer of hydrogen from the mitochondria to the cytosol are the "isocitrate shuttle" and the "malic enzyme shuttle."

Junge and Brand (1975) hypothesized that the supply of NADPH for mixed-function oxidation is sustained by the flux of carbon over the pentose cycle in glycogen-rich livers from fed rats because rates of NADPH generation via the pentose cycle exceed rates of mixed-function oxidation in isolated hepatocytes. This hypothesis must now be questioned in view of more recent studies. Treatment of rats with 6-aminonicotinamide, an antimetabolite which is converted into the 6-amino analog of $NADP^+$, is a potent inhibitor of the pentose cycle enzyme 6-phosphogluconate dehydrogenase (Kohler *et al.*, 1970). Inhibition of 6-phosphogluconate dehydrogenase by 6-aminonicotinamide treatment increased 6-phosphogluconate levels 700-fold (Thurman *et al.*, 1977a) and inhibited generation of NADPH by the pentose cycle by over 90% (Belinsky *et al.*, 1985). However, rates of *p*-nitroanisole O-demethylation in livers from fed rats treated with 6-aminonicotinamide were not altered (Belinsky *et al.*, 1985). There are two possible interpretations of these results. First, 6-aminonicotinamide treatment could activate NADPH generation by pathways other than the pentose cycle; second, alternative sources of NADPH may normally provide reducing equivalents for monoxygenation in the fed state. Although one cannot choose between these alternatives, these data indicate that maximal rates of mixed-function oxidation can be maintained by reducing equivalents generated from other sources, presumably of mitochondrial origin, in the absence of a functional pentose cycle. There is some support for the hypothesis that reducing equivalents generated in the mitochondria are important for the maintenance of maximal rates of mixed-function oxidation in the fed state. The infusion of potassium cyanide, an inhibitor of cytochrome oxidase, diminished rates of *p*-nitroanisole O-demethylation by 50–75% in perfused livers from fed, normal, and phenobarbital-treated rats (Reinke *et al.*, 1983). The infusion of cyanide, however, did not affect rates of NADPH generation by the pentose cycle but decreased concentrations of ATP and isocitrate, suggesting that cyanide inhibited mixed-function oxidation by diminishing the generation of NADPH from mitochondrial sources (Belinsky *et al.*, 1985).

In contrast to the fed state, where debate over the source(s) of NADPH for mixed-function oxidation exists, it is generally accepted that rates of mixed-function oxidation are sustained primarily by reducing equivalents derived from mitochondria in the fasted state. The fasted state is characterized by a lack of carbohydrate substrate for the pentose cycle (Greenbaum *et al.*, 1971), and NADPH generation by the pentose cycle is reduced by more than 90% (Belinsky *et al.*, 1985). The addition of dinitrophenol, an uncoupler of oxidative phosphorylation, inhibited *p*-nitroanisole metabolism by 70% in perfused livers from fasted, phenobarbital-treated rats, most likely by interrupting the synthesis and/or transfer of reducing equivalents from the mitochondria into the cytosol by interfering with energy-dependent NADPH synthesis and substrate shuttle pathways (Belinsky *et al.*, 1985). Ethanol, at concentrations which have minimal effects on microsomal enzymes, also inhibited rates of *p*-nitroanisole metabolism by 80% in livers from fasted rats (Reinke *et al.*, 1980). This action of ethanol has been attributed to the generation of NADH via the metabolism of ethanol and acetaldehyde, leading to redox inhibition of the citric acid cycle. Inhibition of the citric acid cycle depletes intermediates necessary for the generation of cytosolic NADPH via shuttle mechanisms. In addition, the infusion of 2-bromooctanoate, an inhibitor of the β oxidation of acyl-CoA compounds, caused a marked decrease in rates of *p*-nitroanisole metabolism and intracellular concentrations of ATP and NADH in livers from fasted rats (Danis *et al.*, 1981). 2-Bromooctanoate most likely inhibits mixed-function oxidation by diminishing the β oxidation of fatty acids. The inhibition of β oxidation results in a decreased production of NADH, depletion of acetyl-CoA for the citric acid cycle, and a subsequent decline in ATP generation. The depletion of NADH and ATP could decrease NADPH generation by the energy-dependent transhydrogenase. Thus, in the fasted state, fatty acid oxidation is important for the generation of mitochondrial NADPH. These studies with inhibitors indicate clearly that mitochondrial oxidations are the primary source of reducing equivalents for mixed-function oxidation in the fasted state and highlight the possible interactions between nutrition and monooxygenation reactions.

III. REGULATION OF GLUCURONIDATION AND SULFATION IN THE INTACT LIVER

Two major routes of conjugation in the liver are the glucuronidation and sulfation pathways. Rates of conjugation of *p*-nitrophenol were studied in livers from normal or phenobarbital-treated rats. At low concentrations ($<10 \ \mu M$) of *p*-nitrophenol, sulfation predominated over glucuronidation, whereas at concentrations over $10 \ \mu M$, glucuronidation was the major pathway of conjugation of *p*-nitrophenol (Reinke *et al.*, 1981). Since *p*-nitrophenyl sulfate formation was not influenced by either phenobarbital treatment, excess sulfate, or nutritional state, rates of sulfation may be limited by the activity of the sulfotransferases (Reinke *et al.*, 1981). In contrast to the sulfation pathway, *p*-nitrophenyl glucuronide formation was influenced by phenobarbital treatment and nutritional state. For example, glucuronidation was lowest in livers from fasted rats and highest in livers from fasted–refed rats. Differences in rates of glucuronidation correlated with the glycogen, UDP-glucose, and UDP-glucuronic acid content in livers of phenobarbital-treated rats, but not with ATP/ADP ratios or glucuronosyltransferase activity measured *in vitro* (Reinke *et al.*, 1981). These data indicate that the supply of UDP-glucuronic acid from carbohydrate reserves is an important rate determinant for glucuronidation in the intact cell.

IV. COMPARTMENTATION OF MONOOXYGENATION AND CONJUGATION IN PERIPORTAL AND PERICENTRAL REGIONS OF THE LIVER LOBULE

To study regulation of monooxygenation and conjugation in specific zones of the liver lobule, we have developed methods which allow metabolic events in periportal and pericentral regions of the lobule to be monitored. Much information already exists on the distribution of enzymes across the liver lobule (Jungerman and Katz, 1982; Rappaport, 1978). For example, key enzymes involved in glycolysis, such as glucokinase (Guder and Schmidt, 1982; Katz *et al.*, 1978), and pyruvate kinase, are concentrated in pericentral areas, while some gluconeogenic enzymes, such as phosphoenolpyruvate carboxykinase (Guder and Schmidt, 1982), fructose-1,6-diphosphatase, and glucose-6-phosphatase (Teutsch, 1981), predominate within periportal areas. Most enzymes of the MFO system are distributed unevenly across the liver lobule. Some cytochrome *P*-450 isoenzymes (Gooding *et al.*, 1978; Baron *et al.*, 1978), as well as the NADPH-generating enzymes glucose-6-phosphate dehydrogenase (Teutsch, 1981), malic enzyme (Teutsch and Reider, 1979), and isocitrate dehydrogenase (Teutsch, 1981), are more concentrated in pericentral areas. In contrast, glutathione (Smith *et al.*, 1979) and glutathione peroxidase (Yoshimura *et al.*, 1977) are slightly higher in periportal regions of the liver lobule.

Jungermann and colleagues hypothesized the existence of metabolic zonation within the liver lobule for carbohydrate metabolism (Katz and Jungerman, 1976; Sasse *et al.*, 1975). Based on the distribution and activity of enzymes across the liver lobule, they proposed that metabolic pathways such as glycolysis predominate within pericentral areas, while gluconeogenesis occurs mainly in periportal regions (Sasse *et al.*, 1975; Jungerman and Sasse, 1978). Since most metabolic processes operate far below maximal velocity and are highly regulated enzyme sequences dependent on substrate and cofactor supply as well as enzyme activity, differences in enzyme content across the liver lobule may not necessarily reflect activity of a given metabolic process in periportal or pericentral regions of the liver. Therefore, we have developed new methods employing micro-light guides and miniature oxygen electrodes to determine rates of flux in metabolic pathways noninvasively in distinct zones of the liver lobule. This approach is referred to as *s*ublobular *c*ompartmentation *of p*harmacological *e*vents (SCOPE) and is reviewed in detail elsewhere (Thurman and Kauffman, 1985). Studies of SCOPE allow quantitative information to be obtained on flux rates of metabolic processes in distinct regions of the liver lobule noninvasively using microprobes. Further work in this area should facilitate the identification of critical metabolic events resulting from alterations in nutrition which lead to cellular damage in distinct regions of the liver lobule.

A. Development of Techniques to Study Functional Aspects of Zonation

1. Micro-Light Guide

Fluorometry of tissues has been used extensively by Chance and colleagues (Chance and Thorell, 1959) to determine the localization and kinetics of reduced pyridine nucleotides in living cells. Subsequently, light guides (tip diameter of ~5 mm) containing optical fibers were used to measure NADH fluorescence and UV reflectance from the heart (Chance *et al.*, 1974) and from the rat cerebral cortex *in situ* (Mayevsky and Chance, 1974). These methods were further refined resulting in the development of micro-light guides which contain single strands of 25–80 μm diameter fibers for the measurement of NADH fluorescence and UV reflectance from mitochondrial suspensions and perfused, hemoglobin-free rat livers (Ji *et al.*, 1979).

Recently, we developed a modified micro-light guide to determine local rates of mixed-function oxidation in periportal and pericentral regions of the liver lobule in the perfused liver noninvasively (Ji *et al.*, 1981). This method involves placement of a two-stranded, 80-μm micro-light guide on specific regions of the liver lobule. One strand is connected to a light source and the other strand to a photomultiplier. The tissue is then illuminated with light from a mercury arc lamp using wavelengths selected with optical filters. Fluorescence from the tissue is transmitted by the adjacent strand through selected filters before it is detected by a photomultiplier. The signal from the photomultiplier is then filtered, amplified, and recorded. Perfusions of liver with India ink identified lightly pigmented regions as periportal areas and darkly pigmented spots as pericentral regions (Ji *et al.*, 1980; Lemasters *et al.*, 1986). Therefore, the light guide can be placed on periportal or pericentral regions of the liver lobule which permits continuous fluorometric determination of the mixed-function oxidation of model compounds. For example, fluorescence due to 7-hydroxycoumarin formation from 7-ethoxycoumarin can be measured by illuminating tissue with light at 366 nm and measuring fluorescence at 450 nm. Micro-light guides can also be used to measure the conjugation of 7-hydroxycoumarin and the intracellular NADH redox state noninvasively in periportal and pericentral regions of the liver lobule (see Section IV,B).

2. Miniature Oxygen Electrode

Measurement of oxygen tension and rates of oxygen uptake in distinct regions of the liver lobule with miniature oxygen electrodes developed in our laboratory

(Matsumura and Thurman, 1983) has also opened up new possibilities for the study of zonal hepatotoxicity. Ji *et al.* (1982) employed miniature oxygen electrodes to measure tissue oxygen tensions directly in periportal and pericentral regions of the liver lobule and measured oxygen gradients across the lobule of perfused livers. The miniature oxygen electrode can also be used to measure rates of oxygen uptake in distinct regions of the liver lobule in perfused livers by measuring rates of decrease in oxygen concentration when the outflow and inflow are stopped simultaneously ("stopped-flow O_2 uptake technique," Matsumura and Thurman, 1983). With the miniature oxygen electrode, Matsumura and Thurman (1983) showed that rates of oxygen uptake were two- to threefold greater in periportal than in pericentral regions of the liver lobule. Recently, the miniature oxygen electrode has also been used to measure rates of glycolysis in periportal and pericentral regions based on the stoichiometric changes in rates of oxygen uptake which occur during infusion of glucose. Thus, local flux rates in metabolic pathways can now be measured based on changes in regional oxygen uptake (Matsumura and Thurman, 1984).

B.   Characterization of Mixed-Function Oxidation in Periportal and Pericentral Regions

1.   *First Demonstration of SCOPE*

The first study of metabolic processes in distinct regions of the liver lobule involved measurement of cytochrome *P*-450-dependent mixed-function oxidation of 7-ethoxycoumarin to 7-hydroxycoumarin (Ji *et al.*, 1981). Rates of 7-ethoxycoumarin O-deethylation were calculated from 7-hydroxycoumarin detected in the effluent perfusate and were compared with increases in 7-hydroxycoumarin fluorescence (366 → 450 nm) measured from the liver surface with a large-tipped (2 mm diameter) light guide. This light guide excites and collects fluorescence from many periportal and pericentral regions in several lobules. As the concentration of 7-ethoxycoumarin infused into livers from fed, phenobarbital-treated rats was increased, both 7-hydroxycoumarin production and fluorescence due to 7-hydroxycoumarin from the tissue increased in a stepwise fashion (Fig. 2). A good correlation ($r = 0.98$) was observed between fluorescence of 7-hydroxycoumarin and the O-deethylation of 7-ethoxycoumarin (Ji *et al.*, 1981). We have used this correlation to convert fluorescence measured with micro-light guides into local rates of mixed-function oxidation. When 7-ethoxycoumarin was infused in perfusions in the anterograde direction, fluorescence began to increase first in periportal regions and then in pericentral areas (Ji *et al.*, 1981). The maximal fluorescence increase, expressed as a percentage of basal fluorescence, was twice as great in pericentral as in periportal areas. These fluorescence changes corresponded to local rates of mixed-function oxidation of 3.6 and 7.0 μmol/gm/hr in periportal and pericentral regions, respectively (Ji *et*

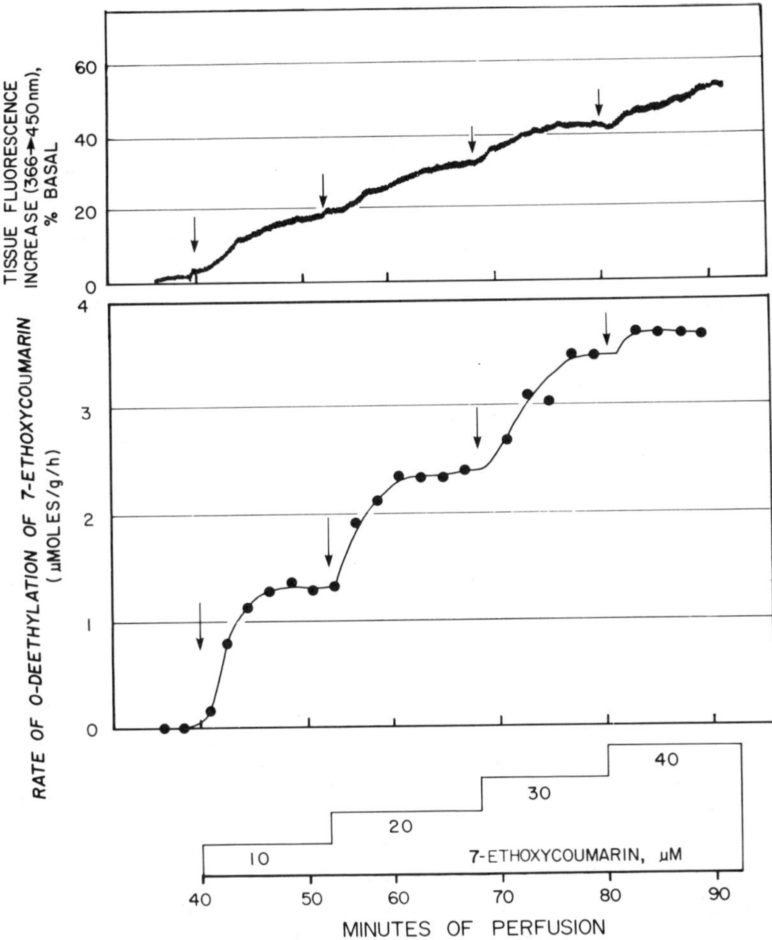

Fig. 2. Effect of 7-ethoxycoumarin concentration on the rate of O-deethylation of 7-ethoxycoumarin and on 7-hydroxycoumarin fluorescence (366 → 450 nm). The liver from a Sprague–Dawley female rat treated with sodium phenobarbital (1 mg/ml of drinking water) for 5 weeks was perfused with Krebs–Henseleit bicarbonate buffer as described elsewhere (Ji *et al.*, 1981). Infusion of 7-ethoxycoumarin is indicated by horizontal bars and vertical arrows. Glucuronide and sulfate conjugates of 7-hydroxycoumarin were measured in the perfusate by incubating samples with β-glucuronidase containing sulfatase activity. 7-Hydroxycoumarin liberated under these conditions was measured fluorometrically at wavelengths above 400 nm following excitation at 366 nm employing an Eppendorf photometer equipped with a fluorescence attachment. The rate of O-deethylation of 7-ethoxycoumarin in micromoles per gram per hour was calculated by taking the flow rate and liver wet weight into consideration. The fluorescence from the tissue was measured with a Schott light guide with a tip diameter of 2 mm placed on the surface of the left lateral lobe of the liver. The excitation light (366 nm) was from a 100-W mercury arc lamp (Illuminations Industries, Inc., Sunnyvale, California) filtered with a Corning glass filter No. 5840. The emitted light (450 nm) was detected with a photomultiplier (EMI, type 9824B) guarded with Kodak Wratten gelatin filters, nos. 2C and 47. In this particular experiment, the output voltage of the photomultiplier was adjusted to give an anode current of 66 namp when the light guide was placed on the liver surface prior to infusion of 7-ethoxycoumarin. Reproduced from Molecular Pharmacology (Ji *et al.*, 1981) with permission from Williams and Wilkins Co.

al., 1981). This technique provided the first direct evidence that rates of mixed-function oxidation are about twice as great in pericentral as in periportal regions in intact livers from phenobarbital-treated rats (Ji *et al.*, 1981). These differences in flux are due at least in part to higher concentrations of cytochrome *P*-450 in pericentral areas (Gooding *et al.*, 1978). Since the supply of NADPH is also an important determinant of rates of mixed-function oxidation in the whole liver (Thurman *et al.*, 1977b; Moldeus *et al.*, 1974; Belinsky *et al.*, 1980), it is clear that the capacity to generate NADPH in periportal and pericentral regions of the liver influences local rates of monooxygenation.

2. *Regulation of Mixed-Function Oxidation in Periportal and Pericentral Regions by NADPH Supply*

Xylitol is converted rapidly into glucose 6-phosphate and generates NADPH for mixed-function oxidation via the pentose cycle. Experiments designed to evaluate the effect of NADPH supply on mixed-function oxidation in periportal and pericentral regions of the liver lobule indicated that xylitol increased 7-hydroxycoumarin production in both regions of the lobule 80–100% (Table I). These data indicate that NADPH supply is a major determinant of rates of mixed-function oxidation in both periportal and pericentral regions of the liver lobule in the fasted state (Belinsky *et al.*, 1983).

3. *Sources of Reducing Equivalents for Mixed-Function Oxidation in Periportal and Pericentral Regions of the Liver Lobule*

The role of the pentose cycle and mitochondria in supplying NADPH for mixed-function oxidation in periportal and pericentral regions was evaluated by using 6-aminonicotinamide treatment, fasting, and potassium cyanide. Fasting depletes glycogen and glucose 6-phosphate, substrates for the pentose cycle

TABLE I

Effect of Xylitol on Rates of 7-Hydroxycoumarin Production in Periportal and Pericentral Regions of the Liver Lobule in Livers from Fasted Phenobarbital-Treated Rats

	Hydroxycoumarin production (7 mol/gm/hr)	
Addition	Periportal	Pericentral
None	2.2 ± 0.7	5.2 ± 0.7
2 mM Xylitol	3.9 ± 0.3[a]	10.8 ± 1.3

[a] $p < .05$ with respect to no addition (for details, see Belinsky *et al.*, 1983).

(Belinsky *et al.*, 1984), whereas 6-aminonicotinamide is metabolized to an analog of $NADP^+$ which inhibits 6-phosphogluconate dehydrogenase (Kohler *et al.*, 1970). Both of these treatments decreased rates of NADPH generation via the pentose cycle by greater than 90% (Belinsky *et al.*, 1985). Cyanide, an inhibitor of oxidative phosphorylation, was also used to estimate the fraction of NADPH generated by mitochondria for mixed-function oxidation. Rates of mixed-function oxidation were diminished when NADPH generation was inhibited by 6-aminonicotinamide and potassium cyanide. From the inhibitor studies summarized in Fig. 3, we conclude that the pentose cycle supplies NADPH for monooxygenation at rates two- to threefold higher in pericentral than in periportal regions in livers from phenobarbital-treated rats. These experiments also suggest that mitochondrial NADPH supply is increased by treatment with phenobarbital and β-naphthoflavone (Fig. 3).

In general, inhibitors of mitochondrial NADPH generation had a much greater effect on rates of monooxygenation than inhibitors of the pentose cycle (Fig. 3). This finding was not expected, since absolute rates of NADPH generation via the pentose cycle exceeded rates of mixed-function oxidation by at least fourfold (Junge and Brand, 1975; Belinsky *et al.*, 1985). It is important to note that a large proportion of NADPH is utilized for pathways other than mixed-function oxidation (e.g., fatty acid synthesis; Lowenstein, 1971), the reduction of oxidized glutathione (Flohe and Gunzler, 1976), and flavoprotein-dependent monooxygenation (Ziegler *et al.*, 1969). Therefore, it is reasonable to suggest that several NADPH-utilizing systems compete for NADPH and are therefore diminished when NADPH synthesis by either the pentose cycle or mitochondrial oxidations is inhibited. Although maximal rates of NADPH synthesis via the mitochondria and pentose cycle greatly exceeded rates of monooxygenation, 7-ethoxycoumarin metabolism still declined in the presence of cyanide because other reactions compete for NADPH in the cell. Thus, the MFO pathway can serve as a qualitative indicator of rates of NADPH generation in periportal and pericentral regions of the liver lobule.

C. Conjugation in Periportal and Pericentral Regions

1. *Sulfation*

The isolated perfused liver has also been used as a model to study conjugation reactions which are regulated by a number of metabolic factors, including substrate concentrations, activities of enzymes, and the supply of cofactors. Sulfation of phenolic substrates (Reinke *et al.*, 1981) has been shown to be a low-capacity, high-affinity system dependent on added sulfate, whereas glucuronidation occurs with lower affinity but has a much higher capacity (Thurman *et al.*, 1981). Studies employing hepatotoxins to destroy regions of the liver lobule selectively suggested that glucuronosyltransferases are localized predominantly

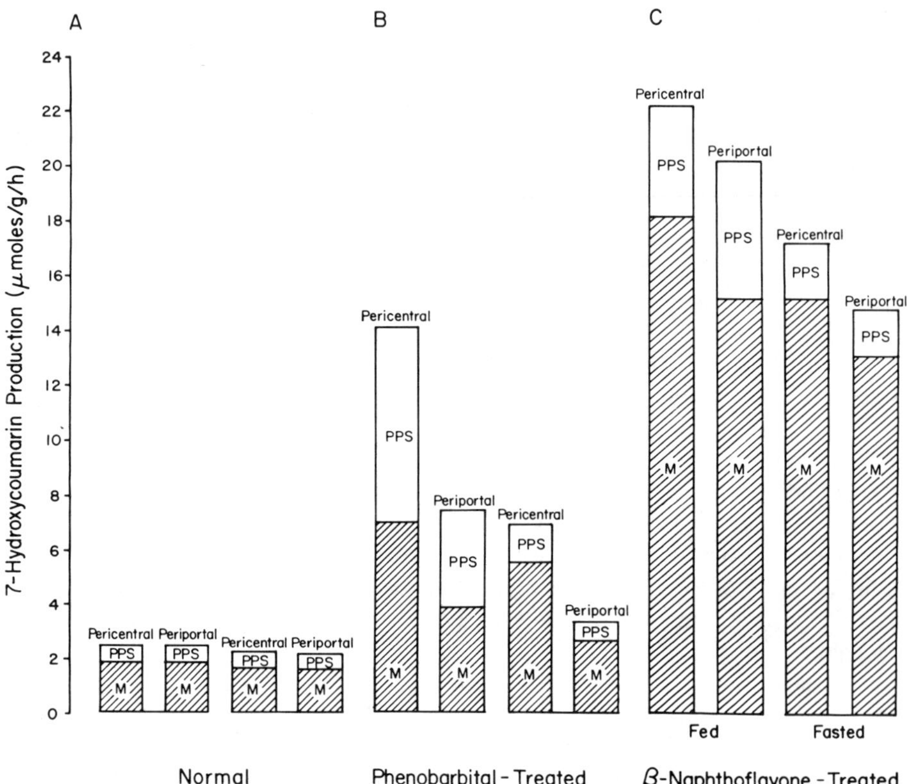

Fig. 3. Sources of reducing equivalents for mixed-function oxidation in periportal and pericentral regions of the liver from normal (A), phenobarbital-treated (B), and β-naphthoflavone-treated (C) rats. The contribution of the pentose cycle (PPS) and mitochondrial oxidations (M) to NADPH supply for the mixed-function oxidation of 7-ethoxycoumarin in periportal and pericentral regions of the liver lobule was estimated. Rates of NADPH generation by the pentose cycle and mitochondria were determined from the decrease in local rates of 7-hydroxycoumarin production produced by 6-aminonicotinamide and cyanide, respectively.

in periportal regions (James *et al.*, 1981). Pharmacokinetic modeling also suggested that sulfation of acetaminophen generated from phenacetin by the perfused rat liver was greater in periportal than in pericentral regions (Pang and Terrell, 1981). Although such studies provide useful information, they do not provide quantitative data on rates of conjugation in specific sublobular zones of the liver. Quantitative information on these processes can, however, be obtained using micro-light guides and miniature oxygen electrode technology (Conway *et al.*, 1982; Lemasters *et al.*, 1986).

Micro-light guides were used to quantitate rates of conjugation in periportal and pericentral areas of the perfused liver (Conway *et al.*, 1982). During infusion of up to 30 μM 7-hydroxycoumarin, fluorescence of free 7-hydroxycoumarin was detected only in periportal regions during perfusion in the anterograde direction and in pericentral areas during perfusion in the retrograde direction. Thus, conjugates are formed in only one region of the liver lobule with relatively low concentrations of substrate. By measuring conjugates of 7-hydroxycoumarin in the effluent perfusate when perfusion was in the anterograde or retrograde direction, rates of sulfation and glucuronidation can be estimated in periportal and pericentral regions of the lobule. Sulfation predominated over glucuronidation when 2–10 μM 7-hydroxycoumarin was infused in the anterograde direction; however, with 20–30 μM 7-hydroxycoumarin, glucuronidation predominated. In contrast, rates of glucuronidation and sulfation were similar when low concentrations of 7-hydroxycoumarin were infused in the retrograde direction; however, glucuronidation predominated at higher substrate concentrations. Thus, at low concentrations of 7-hydroxycoumarin, sulfation predominated over glucuronidation in periportal regions but not in pericentral areas of the liver lobule. When livers were perfused with sulfate-free media, the glucuronide was the predominant conjugate formed in both regions of the liver lobule. Taken together, these data indicate that sulfation competes successfully with glucuronidation for 7-hydroxycoumarin at low substrate concentrations. Furthermore, maximal rates of sulfation were twofold greater in periportal than in pericentral regions of the liver lobule (Conway *et al.*, 1982). Differences in sulfation across the liver lobule could reflect differences in either the activities of the sulfotransferases and sulfatases or 3'-phosphoadenosine 5'-phosphosulfate supply.

2. *Glucuronidation*

Previous work discussed above demonstrated that rates of glucuronidation of 7-hydroxycoumarin could be measured in specific zones of the liver lobule with low substrate (<20 μM) concentrations (Conway *et al.*, 1982). However, glucuronosyltransferases have a relatively high K_m for substrate (<50 μM); therefore, experiments were designed to study glucuronidation at high substrate concentrations. A new method employing micro-light guides was developed to determine rates of glucuronidation of 7-hydroxycoumarin in specific zones of the liver lobule when 7-hydroxycoumarin ranging from 20 to 120 μM was infused. These studies were performed using livers perfused with sulfate-free buffer under normoxic conditions where fluorescence of free 7-hydroxycoumarin was monitored from the tissue (Conway *et al.*, 1984). The formation of nonfluroescent 7-hydroxycoumarin glucuronide was then inhibited completely by perfusion with N_2-saturated perfusate containing 20 mM ethanol. Under these conditions, fluorescence recorded from the surface was directly proportional to the concentration of substrate infused. Thus, the difference in 7-hydroxycoumarin fluorescence between N_2 plus ethanol and normoxic perfusions was due to glucuronidation. Maximal rates of glucuronidation in periportal and pericentral regions of the liver lobule calculated with this new method were 10 and 35 μmol/gm/hr,

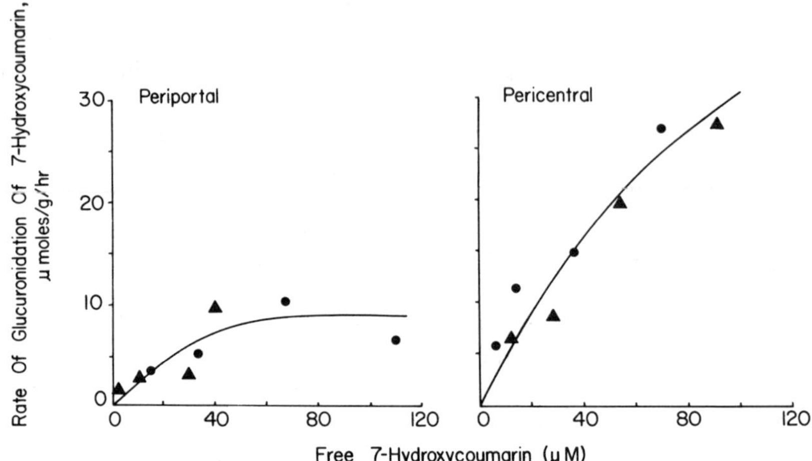

Fig. 4. Sublobular rates of glucuronidation of 7-hydroxycoumarin. The concentration of glucuronide conjugates formed in each region during anterograde and retrograde perfusions was derived from fluorescence measurements of free 7-hydroxycoumarin in the tissue (Conway *et al.*, 1984). Rates were calculated using flow rate and the wet weight of each sublobular region (wet weight/2). Reproduced from *Molecular Pharmacology* with permission from Williams and Wilkins Co.

respectively (Fig. 4), and were half-maximal with 25–50 μM 7-hydroxycoumarin in both regions of the liver lobule. The maximal capacity of the glucuronidation system is about threefold greater in pericentral than in periportal regions of the liver lobule. This difference correlates well with activity of the transferase measured in the two zones of the lobule in the perfused liver (Table II).

3. Regulation of Glucuronidation in Periportal and Pericentral Regions by UDP-Glucuronic Acid

Rates of glucuronidation in periportal and pericentral regions were 8–19 μmol/gm/hr, respectively, during infusion of 80 μM 7-hydroxycoumarin in livers of fasted rats (Conway *et al.*, 1985). Fasting for 24 hr prior to perfusion decreases rates to 3 and 9 μmol/gm/hr in periportal and pericentral regions. Infusion of glucose (20 mM) had no effect on rates of glucuronidation in livers from fed rats; however, glucose increased rates of glucuronidation rapidly in periportal and pericentral regions to 7 and 17 μmol/gm/hr, respectively, in livers from starved rats. These results indicate that the rapid synthesis of the cofactor UDP-glucuronic acid derived from glucose is an important rate determinant for glucuronidation of 7-hydroxycoumarin in both periportal and pericentral regions of livers from starved rats.

TABLE II

**Glucuronsyltransferase Activity in Microdissected Periportal
and Pericentral Regions of the Liver Lobule in Perfused Livers
from Phenobarbital-Treated, Fed Rats[a]**

Liver[b]	Glucuronosyltransferase activity (μmol/gm wet wt/hr)		Pericentral and periportal
	Periportal	Pericentral	
1	14.9 ± 0.7	50.4 ± 2.4[c]	3.4
2	29.4 ± 2.4	73.3 ± 2.0[c]	2.5
3	17.4 ± 0.9	61.8 ± 2.4[c]	3.6
K_m for	Periportal	Pericentral	
7-Hydroxycoumarin	54 μM	55 μM	
UDPGA	230 μM	200 μM	

[a]Reproduced from *Molecular Pharmacology* with permission from Williams and Wilkins Co.

[b]For livers 1, 2, and 3, values are averages ± SEM of 6–8 periportal and pericentral regions assayed from each liver with 100 μM 7-hydroxycoumarin and 9 mM UDPGA. To determine K_m values, about 50 periportal and pericentral regions were pooled from one liver. Assays were performed with a range of UDPGA concentrations (50–800 μM) in the presence of 100 μM 7-hydroxycoumarin and a range of 7-hydroxycoumarin (10–110 μM) concentrations in the presence of 9 mM UDPGA.

[c]$p < .001$, for comparison between periportal and pericentral regions in the same liver.

V.   FUTURE DIRECTIONS

Work reviewed above indicates that nutrients supplied to the liver can influence the metabolism and toxicity of several model compounds both on an acute and chronic basis. Information has been presented indicating that the regulation of xenobiotic metabolism and toxicity differ in sublobular zones of the liver. New technology has become available in the form of micro-light guides and miniature oxygen electrodes that permit the effects of nutrients on metabolic events in sublobular zones of the liver to be studied noninvasively. Thus, new opportunities exist to determine the effects of chronic and acute dietary manipulations on metabolic events in specific hepatic regions under near-physiological conditions. Important questions concerning effects of specific diets, such as high fat or vitamin deficiency or excess, on metabolism and toxicity of environmental agents need to be studied using the approaches described above. Experiments aimed at describing the actions of nutrients on events in sublobular zones of the liver will lead to new understanding of mechanisms of hepatotoxicity. This information may be applied ultimately to modification of hepatic injury and disease.

ACKNOWLEDGMENTS

Supported, in part, by grants CA-23080, CA-20807 from NCI, ES-02759 from NIEHS, and AA-03629 from NIAAA.

The authors gratefully acknowledge support from NCI, NIEHS, and NIAAA, and the assistance of numerous students, fellows, and colleagues in the work reviewed here. A list of these individuals and the current addresses follows: Dr. James G. Conway, Chemical Industry Institute of Toxicology, Research Triangle Park, NC 27709; Dr. John J. Lemasters, Department of Anatomy, University of North Carolina, Chapel Hill, NC 27514; Dr. Sungchul Ji, Department of Pharmacology, Rutgers University, Piscataway, NJ 08854; Dr. Takakatsu Matsumura, First Department of Medicine, Osaka University Medical School, 1-1-50, Fukushima, Fukushima-Ku, Osaka, 553, Japan; Dr. Toru Kashiwagi, Osaka Koseinenkin Hospital, 4-2-78, Fukushima, Fukushima-Ku, Osaka, 553, Japan.

REFERENCES

Baron, J., Redick, J. A., and Guengerich, F. P. (1978). Immunohistochemical localization of cytochrome *P*-450 in rat liver. *Life Sci.* **23**, 2627–2632.

Belinsky, S. A., Reinke, L. A., Kauffman, F. C., and Thurman, R. G. (1980). Inhibition of mixed-function oxidation of *p*-nitroanisole in perfused rat liver by 2,4-dinitrophenol. *Arch. Biochem. Biophys.* **204**, 207–213.

Belinsky, S. A., Kauffman, F. C., Ji, S., Lemasters, J. J., and Thurman, R. G. (1983). Stimulation of mixed-function oxidation of 7-ethoxycoumarin in periportal and pericentral regions of the perfused rat liver by xylitol. *Eur. J. Biochem.* **137**, 1–6.

Belinsky, S. A., Kauffman, F. C., and Thurman, R. G. (1984). Reducing equivalents for mixed-function oxidation in periportal and pericentral regions of the liver lobule in perfused livers from normal and phenobarbital-treated rats. *Mol. Pharmacol.* **26**, 574–581.

Belinsky, S. A., Reinke, L. A., Scholz, R., Kauffman, F. C., and Thurman, R. G. (1985). Rates of pentose cycle flux in perfused rat liver. Evaluation of the role of reducing equivalents from the pentose cycle for mixed-function oxidation. *Mol. Pharmacol.* 371–376.

Bjorkhem, I. (1977). Rate-limiting step in microsomal cytochrome *P*-450-catalyzed hydroxylations. *Pharmacol. Ther., Part A* **1**, 327–348.

Bücher, T., and Sies, H. (1976). Nicotinamide/nucleotide systems and drug oxidation in the liver cell. *In* "Liver Cells and Kidney Tubules in Metabolic Studies," pp. 41–48. North-Holland Publ., Amsterdam.

Campbell, T. C., and Hayes, J. R. (1983). The effect of quantity and quality of dietary protein on drug metabolism. *Fed. Proc., Fed. Am. Soc. Exp. Biol.* **35**, 2470–2474.

Chance, B., and Thorell, B. (1959). Localization and kinetics of reduced pyridine nucleotides in living cells by microfluorometry. *J. Biol. Chem.* **234**, 3044–3050.

Chance, B., Oshino, N., Sugano, T., and Mela, L. (1974). Factors in oxygen delivery to tissue. *Microvasc. Res.* **8**, 276–282.

Committee on Diet Nutrition and Cancer (1982). "Diet, Nutrition and Cancer." Assembly of Life Sciences, National Research Council, National Academy Press, Washington, D.C.

Conway, J. G., Kauffman, F. C., Ji, S., and Thurman, R. G. (1982). Rates of sulfation and glucuronidation of 7-hydroxycoumarin in periportal and pericentral regions of the liver lobule. *Mol. Pharmacol.* **25,** 487–493.

Conway, J. G., Kauffman, F. C., Tsukada, T., and Thurman, R. G. (1984). Glucuronidation of 7-hydroxycoumarin in periportal and pericentral regions of the liver lobule. *Molec. Pharmacol.* **25,** 487–493.

Conway, J. G., Kauffman, F. C., and Thurman, R. G. (1985). Effect of glucose on 7-hydroxycoumarin glucuronide production in periportal and pericentral regions of the liver lobule. *Biochem. J.* **226,** 749–756.

Coon, M. J., Ballou, D. P., Haugen, D. A., Kzezoski, S. O., Nordblom, G. D., and White, R. E. (1977). Purification of membrane bound oxygenases: Isolation of two electrophoretically homogeneous forms of liver microsomal cytochrome *P*-450. *In* "Microsomes and Drug Oxidations" (V. Ullrich, A. Hildebrandt, I. Roots, R. W. Estabrook, and A. H. Conney, eds.), pp. 82–94. Pergamon, Oxford.

Cooper, D. Y., Levin, S., Narasimihulu, S., Rosenthal, O., and Estabrook, R. W. (1965). Photochemical action spectrum of the terminal oxidase of mixed-function oxidase systems. *Science* **147,** 400–402.

Danis, M., Kauffman, F. C., Evans, R. K., and Thurman, R. G. (1981). Role of reducing equivalents from fatty acid oxidation in mixed-function oxidation: Studies with 2-bromooctanoate in the perfused rat liver. *J. Pharmacol. Exp. Ther.* **219,** 383–388.

Estabrook, R. W., and Werringloer, J. (1977). Cytochrome *P*-450—its role in oxygen activation for drug metabolism. *In* "Drug Metabolism Concepts" (D. M. Jerina, ed.), pp. 16–26. Am. Chem. Soc., Washington, D.C.

Flohe, L., and Gunzler, W. A. (1976). Glutathione-dependent enzymatic oxidoreduction reactions. *In* "Glutathione Metabolism and Function" (I. Arias and W. Jacoby, eds.), pp. 17–34. Raven Press, New York.

Gooding, P. E., Chayen, J., and Sawyer, B. (1978). Cytochrome *P*-450 distribution in rat liver and effect of sodium phenobarbitone administration. *Chem.-Biol. Interact.* **20,** 229–310.

Greenbaum, A. L., Gumaa, K. A., and McClean, P. (1971). The distribution of hepatic metabolites and the control of the pathways of carbohydrate metabolism in animals of different dietary and hormonal status. *Arch. Biochem. Biophys.* **143,** 617–663.

Guder, W. G., and Schmidt, U. (1982). Liver cell heterogeneity. *Hoppe-Seyler's Z. Physiol. Chem.*

Hoek, J. B., and Ernster, L. (1974). Mitochondrial transhydrogenase and the regulation of cytosolic reducing power. *In* "Alcohol and Aldehyde Metabolizing Systems" (R. G. Thurman, T. Yonetani, J. R. Williamson, and B. Chance, Vol. 1, pp. 351–364. Academic Press, New York.

Holtzclaw, W. D., Thurman, R. G., and Kauffman, F. C. (1984). Mitochondrial–microsomal interactions *in vitro*: Use of microsomal 7-ethoxycoumarin *O*-deethylase to study succinate-stimulated malate efflux from mitochondria. *Arch. Biochem. Biophys.* **233,** 345–353.

Imai, Y., Sato, R., and Iyanagi, T. (1977). Rate limiting step in the reconstituted microsomal drug hydroxylase system. *J. Biochem. (Tokyo)* **82,** 1237–1246.

James, R., Desmond, P., Kupfer, A., Schenker, S., and Branch, R. A. (1981). The differential localization of various drug metabolizing systems within rat liver lobule as determined by the hepatotoxins allyl alcohol, carbon tetrachloride and bromobenzene. *J. Pharmacol. Exp. Ther.* **217,** 127–132.

Ji, S., Chance, B., Nishiki, K., Smith, T., and Rich, T. (1979). Micro-light guides: A new method for measuring tissue fluorescence and reflectance. *Am. J. Physiol.* **236,** C144–C156.

Ji, S., Lemasters, J. J. and Thurman, R. G. (1980). A non-invasive method to study metabolic events within sublobular regions of hemoglobin-free perfused liver. *FEBS* Lett. **113,** 37–41.

Ji, S., Lemasters, J. J., and Thurman, R. G. (1981). A Fluorometric method to measure sublobular rates of mixed-function oxidation in the hemoglobin-free perfused rat liver. *Mol. Pharmacol.* **19,** 513–516.

Ji, S., Lemasters, J. J., Christenson, V., and Thurman, R. G. (1982). Periportal and pericentral pyridine nucleotide fluorescence from the surface of the perfused liver: Evaluation of the hypothesis that chronic treatment with ethanol produces pericentral hypoxia. *Proc. Natl. Acad. Sci. U.S.A.* **79,** 5415–5419.

Junge, O., and Brand, K. (1975). Mixed-function oxidation of hexobarbital and generation of NADPH by hexose-monophosphate shunt in isolated rat liver cells. *Arch. Biochem. Biophys.* **171,** 398–406.

Jungerman, K., and Katz, N. (1982). Functional hepatocellular heterogeneity. *Hepatology* **2,** 385–395.

Jungerman, K., and Sasse, D. (1978). Heterogeneity of liver parenchymal cells. *Trends Biochem. Sci.* **3,** 198–202.

Katz, N., and Jungerman, K. (1976). Autoregulatory shift from fructolysis to lactate gluconeogenesis in rat hepatocyte suspensions. *Hoppe-Seyler's Z. Physiol. Chem.* **357,** 359–375.

Katz, N., Teutsch, H. F., and Jungerman, K. (1978). Heterogeneous reciprocal localization of fructose-1,6-bisphosphatase and glucokinase in the liver lobule. *Eur. J. Biochem.* **129,** 611–617.

Kauffman, F. C., Evans, R. K., and Thurman, R. G. (1977). Alterations in nicotinamide and adenine nucleotide systems during mixed-function oxidation of *p*-nitroanisole in perfused liver from normal and phenobarbital-treated rats. *Biochem. J.* **167,** 583–592.

Kauffman, F. C., Evans, R. K., Reinke, L. A., and Thurman, R. G. (1979). Regulation of *p*-nitroanisole O-demethylation in perfused rat liver: Adenine nucleotide inhibition of NADP$^+$-dependent dehydrogenases and NADPH-cytochrome *c* reductase. *Biochem. J.* **184,** 675–681.

Kohler, E., Barrach, H. J., and Neubert, D. (1970). Inhibition of NADP$^+$-dependent oxidoreductase by the 6-aminonicotinamide analog of NADP. *FEBS Lett.* **6,** 225–230.

Lehninger, A. L. (1975). Phosphorylation coupled to oxidation of dihydrophosphopyridine nucleotide. *J. Biol. Chem.* **190,** 345–359.

Lemasters, J., Ji, S., and Thurman, R. G. (1986). Approaches to studying sublobular structure and function in the isolated, perfused rat liver. *In* "Regulation of Hepatic Metabolism: Intra- and Intercellular Compartmentation" (R. G. Thurman, F. C. Kauffman, and K. Jungermann, eds.), pp. 159–184. Plenum Press, New York.

Lowenstein, J. M. (1971). Effect of (−)-hydroxycitrate on fatty acid synthesis by rat liver *in vivo*. *J. Biol. Chem.* **246,** 629–632.

Lu, A. Y. H., and Levin, W. (1974). The isolation and reconstruction of the liver microsomal hydroxylation system. *Biochim. Biophys. Acta* **344,** 205–250.

Matsumura, T., and Thurman, R. G. (1983). Measuring rates of oxygen uptake in periportal and pericentral regions of the liver lobule: Stop-flow experiments with perfused liver. *Am. J. Physiol.* **244,** G656–G659.

Matsumura, T., and Thurman, R. G. (1984). Predominance of glycolysis in pericentral regions of the liver lobule. *Eur. J. Biochem.* **140,** 229–234.

Mayevsky, A., and Chance, B. (1974). A new long-term method for the measurement of NADH fluorescence in intact rat brain with chronically implanted cannula. *In* "Oxygen Transport to Tissue" (H. I. Bicher and D. F. Bruly, eds.), pp. 239–244. Plenum, New York.

Moldeus, P., Grundin, R., Vadi, H., and Orrenius, S. (1974). A study of drug metabolism linked to cytochrome *P*-450 in isolated rat liver cells. *Eur. J. Biochem.* **46,** 351–360.

Omura, T., and Sato, R. (1964a). The carbon monoxide-binding pigment of liver microsomes. I. Evidence for its hemoprotein nature. *J. Biol. Chem.* **239,** 2370–2378.

Omura, T., and Sato, R. (1964b). The carbon monoxide-binding pigment of liver microsomes. II. Solubilization, purification and properties. *J. Biol. Chem.* **239,** 2379–2385.

Orrenius, S., Anderson, B., Jernström, B., and Moldeus, P. (1978). Isolated hepatocytes as an experimental tool in the study of drug conjugation reactions. *In* "Conjugation Reactions in

Drug Biotransformation" (A. Aitio, ed.), pp. 273–282. Elsevier/North-Holland Biomedical Press, Amsterdam.

Pang, K. S., and Terrell, J. A. (1981). Retrograde perfusion to probe the heterogeneous distribution of hepatic drug metabolizing enzymes in the rat. *J. Pharmacol. Exp. Ther.* **216,** 339–346.

Rappaport, A. M. (1978). Physioanatomical basis of toxic liver injury. *In* "Toxic Injury of the Liver" (E. Farber and M. Fisher, eds.), pp. 1–58. Dekker, New York.

Reinke, L. A., Kauffman, F. C., Belinsky, S. A., and Thurman, R. G. (1980). Interactions between ethanol metabolism and mixed-function oxidation in perfused rat liver: Inhibition of *p*-nitroanisole O-demethylation. *J. Pharmacol. Exp. Ther.* **213,** 70–78.

Reinke, L. A., Belinksy, S. A., Evans, R. K., Kauffman, F. C., and Thurman, R. G. (1981). Conjugation of *p*-nitrophenol in the perfused rat liver: The effect of substrate concentration and carbohydrate reserves. *J. Pharmacol. Exp. Ther.* **217,** 863–870.

Reinke, L. A., Kauffman, F. C., Belinsky, S. A., and Thurman, R. G. (1983). Inhibition of *p*-nitroanisole O-demethylation in perfused rat liver by potassium cyanide. *Arch. Biochem. Biophys.* **225,** 313–319.

Sasse, D., Katz, N., and Jungerman, K. (1975). Functional heterogeneity of rat liver parenchyma and of isolated hepatocytes. *FEBS Lett.* **57,** 83–88.

Smith, M. T., Loveridge, N., and Wills, E. (1979). The distribution of glutathione in the rat liver lobule. *Biochem. J.* **182,** 103–108.

Teutsch, H. F. (1981). Chemomorphology of liver parenchyma. *Prog. Histochem. Cytochem.* **14,** 1–92.

Teutsch, H. F., and Reider, R. (1979). NADP-dependent dehydrogenases in rat liver parenchyma. *Histochemistry* **60,** 43–52.

Thurman, R. G., and Kauffman, F. C. (1980). Factors regulating drug metabolism in intact hepatocytes. *Pharmacol. Rev.* **31,** 229–251.

Thurman, R. G., and Kauffman, F. C. (1985). Sublobular Compartmentation of Pharmacological Events (SCOPE): Measurement of metabolic fluxes in periportal and pericentral regions of the liver lobule with microflurometric and micropolargraphic techniques. *Hepatology* **5,** 144–151.

Thurman, R. G., and Scholz, R. (1969). Mixed-function oxidation in perfused rat liver. Oxygen uptake following aminopyrine addition. *Eur. J. Biochem.* **10,** 459–467.

Thurman, R. G., Larguin, M., Evans, R., and Kauffman, F. C. (1977a). The role of reducing equivalents generated in mitochondria in hepatic mixed function oxidation. *In* "Microsomes and Drug Oxidations" (V. Ullrich, A. Hildebrandt, I. Roots, R. W. Estabrook, and A. H. Conney, eds.), pp. 315–322. Pergamon, Oxford.

Thurman, R. G., Mazazzo, D. P., Jones, L. S., and Kauffman, F. C. (1977b). The continuous kinetic determination of *p*-nitroanisole in hemoglobin-free perfused rat liver. *J. Pharmacol. Exp. Ther.* **201,** 498–506.

Thurman, R. G., Reinke, L. A., Belinsky, S. A., Evans, R. K., and Kauffman, F. C. (1981). Co-regulation of mixed-function oxidation and glucuronidation of *p*-nitrophenol in the perfused rat liver by carbohydrate reserves. *Arch. Biochem. Biophys.* **209,** 137–142.

Yoshimura, S., Komatsu, N., and Watanabe, K. (1977). Purification and immunohistochemical localization of rat liver glutathione peroxidase in micro-dissected periportal and perivenous rat liver tissue. *FEBS Lett.* **83,** 272–276.

Ziegler, D. M., Mitchell, C. H., and Jollow, D. (1969). The properties of a purified hepatic microsomal mixed-function amino oxidase. *In* "Microsomes and Drug Oxidations" (J. R. Gillette, A. H. Conney, G. J. Cosmides, R. W. Estabrook, J. R. Fouts, and G. J. Mannering, eds.), pp. 172–188. Academic Press, New York.

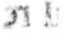

3

Metabolic and Nutritional Effects of Ethanol

Helmut K. Seitz and Ulrich A. Simanowski

I. INTRODUCTION

Ethanol has to be considered one of the most important toxins consumed regularly and in high quantities by humans. Throughout history, alcoholic beverages have been widely used for their pleasing taste and their mood-altering effects. However, during the last few decades alcohol consumption has steadily increased worldwide, and alcoholism has become one of the major health problems. In large urban areas, one of the complications of alcohol abuse—cirrhosis of the liver—is now the second most common cause of all deaths in the 25–44 age group and the third in the 45–64 age group (City of New York, Department of Health, 1981). Cirrhosis of the liver due to alcohol abuse accounts for at least

NUTRITIONAL TOXICOLOGY, VOL. II

POLYTECHNIC OF NORTH LONDON
LIBRARY & INFORMATION SERVICE

Copyright © 1987 by Academic Press, Inc.
All rights of reproduction in any form reserved.

50% of the 35,000 cirrhosis-related deaths that occur in the United States yearly (Burnett and Sorrell, 1981). Autopsy studies place the incidence of cirrhosis among alcoholics, an imprecisely defined group, between 2 and 30%, with 10% a commonly quoted figure (Burnett and Sorrell, 1981). However, the reason why not every alcoholic develops hepatic cirrhosis is still obscure. According to recent epidemiological studies, a daily ethanol consumption of more than 40 gm in males and more than 20 gm in females is already associated with an increased risk for developing alcoholic cirrhosis of the liver (Pequignot and Tuyns, 1980).

Heavy alcohol consumption exerts a deleterious effect on almost every organ and tissue of the human body. The most important ethanol-related diseases besides hepatic cirrhosis are pancreatitis, cardiomyopathy, hematological and neurological disorders, tuberculosis, and tumor development. Pathophysiological mechanisms associated with chronic alcohol consumption include physicochemical (Taraschi and Rubin, 1985), immunological (Paronetto, 1985), and metabolic (Lieber, 1985) alterations of the hepatocyte and many other cells which have been elucidated during the last decades. This chapter will focus on metabolic effects of ethanol closely related to alcohol metabolism and to the pathogenesis of alcoholic liver disease. Hepatic metabolic alterations due to ethanol may be the cause for disturbances in lipid, carbohydrate, hormone, and porphyrin metabolism. The main emphasis, however, will be on microsomal ethanol metabolism and its consequences.

Unquestionably, the progess in understanding such ethanol-mediated metabolic effects was only made possible by using adequate animal models. The technique of feeding ethanol as part of a totally liquid diet was devised and introduced into the field of alcohol research by Lieber and DeCarli (1970c). Since a great deal of information on the effect of ethanol on the metabolism of the hepatocyte has been collected by using this technique, a brief characterization of this animal model seems necessary and may help to relate ethanol intake and potential consequences in rats and baboons to that in humans (Lieber and De-Carli, 1982). In the rat, ethanol is administered as 36% of total calories incorporated into a liquid diet containing 11% carbohydrates, 18% proteins, and 35% lipids. These diets are supplemented by a variety of vitamins and trace elements. When rats are given nothing to drink or to eat but this ethanol-containing liquid diet formula, their intake of ethanol is sufficient to sustain a high daily ethanol ingestion of 10 gm/kg body weight and more (Lieber and DeCarli, 1982). This is two to three times more than achieved through the drinking water technique, provided ethanol is introduced in progressively increasing concentrations up to approximately 5%, which is comparable to concentrations in strong beer. For humans of 70 kg body weight, this would be equivalent to an ethanol intake of 700 gm or more per day (approximately six bottles of wine, 12%). However, since the rat metabolizes ethanol approximately three times faster than humans (Seitz et al., 1984b), such an alcoholic intake results in ethanol blood levels of 100–150 mg/dl, comparable to or even lower than in heavy drinkers (Lieber and DeCarli, 1982). As a consequence of this feeding technique, various complications, also observed in the alcoholic, are reproducible in the rat model, including fatty liver, hyperlipemia, various metabolic and endocrine disorders, tolerance to ethanol and other drugs, physical dependence, and the fetal alcohol syndrome. However, in the rat, ethanol-associated liver injury does not progress beyond the fatty liver stage and fibrosis or cirrhosis never have been described. These pathological features can be produced by chronic ethanol administration of 50% of total calories in the baboon (Lieber and DeCarli, 1974). Under these conditions, despite nutritionally adequate diets, an incidence, sequence, and histopathological changes of alcoholic liver disease similar to those in humans can be found in this animal species (Popper and Lieber, 1980).

II. METABOLIC EFFECTS OF ETHANOL

Small quantities of ethanol can be synthesized endogeneously in the liver and by gastrointestinal bacteria (McManus *et al.*, 1966; Krebs and Perkins, 1970; Levitt *et al.*, 1982; Bode *et al.*, 1984). However, in humans oral intake of alcoholic beverages is the main source of ethanol. Only 2–10% of the absorbed ethanol is excreted unchanged via lungs and kidney, while more than 90% is oxidized mainly in the liver. No storage mechanism and no feedback control of ethanol oxidation exists.

Pathogenesis of metabolic disorders and alcoholic liver disease is closely related to the metabolism of ethanol. As shown in Fig. 1, the hepatocyte contains three major pathways for ethanol metabolism, each located in a different subcellular compartment: the alcohol dehydrogenase (ADH) pathway of the cytosol, the microsomal ethanol-oxidizing system (MEOS) located in the smooth endoplasmic reticulum (SER), and catalase, located in the peroxisomes. Hepatic and extrahepatic metabolism of ethanol results in the production of acetaldehyde and reduced nicotinamide adenine dinucleotide (NADH). Both products contribute to an alteration of the intermediary metabolism of the liver and of other tissues observed after alcohol ingestion (Lieber, 1984a,1985). In addition, alcoholism leads to an induction of microsomal enzymes involved in the activation and degradation of many drugs, xenobiotics, toxins, and procarcinogens (Lieber, 1984a, 1985; Sato *et al.*, 1985; Seitz, 1985).

A. Ethanol Metabolism by Alcohol Dehydrogenase (ADH) and Its Consequences on Hepatic Intermediary Metabolism

1. *Alcohol Dehydrogenase (ADH)*

Because of its low K_m (0.2–2.0 mM), ADH is the major enzyme involved in ethanol metabolism. Highest ADH activity is present in the liver, although the enzyme has been found in lungs, kidney, prostate, and gastrointestinal tract (Spencer *et al.*, 1964; Smith *et al.*, 1972; Jörnvall and Pietruszko, 1972;

A. $C_2H_5OH + NAD^+ \xrightarrow{\text{ADH}} CH_3CHO + NADH + H^+$

B. $C_2H_5OH + NADPH + H^+ + O_2 \xrightarrow{\text{MEOS}} CH_3CHO + NADP^+ + 2H_2O$

C. $C_2H_5OH + H_2O_2 \xrightarrow{\text{CATALASE}} CH_3CHO + 2H_2O$

$$NADP^+ + H_2O_2 \xleftarrow{\text{NADPH OXIDASE}} NADPH + H^+ + O_2$$

D. $C_2H_5OH + H_2O_2 \xrightarrow{\text{CATALASE}} CH_3CHO + 2H_2O$

$$XANTHINE + H_2O_2 \xleftarrow{\text{XANTHINE OXIDASE}} HYPOXANTHINE + H_2O + O_2$$

Fig. 1. The three metabolic pathways of ethanol oxidation: (A) alcohol dehydrogenase (ADH); (B) microsomal ethanol-oxidizing system (MEOS); (C,D) catalase.

Pestalozzi *et al.*, 1983; Seitz *et al.*, 1984b). The enzyme has a broad spectrum of substrate specificity which includes the dehydrogenation of steroids (Okuda and Takigawa, 1970) and ω oxidation of fatty acids (Björkhem, 1972). These compounds are probably the physiological substrate for ADH, although small amounts of endogenous ethanol could play such a role. ADH is a zinc-dependent enzyme which is a dimer consisting of three subunits (α, β, γ) (Agarwal and Goedde, 1984).

ADH is located in the cytosol of the hepatocyte, and a variety of isoenzymes do exist. These isoenzymes have different biochemical properties and therefore may affect the rate of ethanol metabolism (Tipton *et al.*, 1983). For example, an atypical form of ADH has been described by von Wartburg *et al.* (1965) which exhibits five times higher activity at pH 8.8 than normal ADH. The incidence of this atypical ADH is 5–15% in Europe, while in Asia up to 90% of the populations possess this enzyme (Agarwal and Goedde, 1984).

The ADH reaction generates an excess of reducing equivalents in the cytosol primarily as NADH. Therefore acute ethanol administration results in a marked shift of the cytosolic redox potential as measured by the changes in the lactate and pyruvate ratio (Veech *et al.*, 1972; Domschke *et al.*, 1974). This altered redox state of the hepatocyte is responsible for a variety of metabolic abnormalities observed after alcohol ingestion. Some of these metabolic disturbances may predominantly occur in the perivenular (pericentral) area of the hepatic lobule because of the uneven ADH distribution, which is located chiefly in the pericentral zone (Buehler *et al.*, 1982).

2. *Effect of Ethanol-Induced Redox Shift on Lactate and Uric Acid Metabolism*

The altered redox state of the hepatocyte favors the conversion of pyruvate to lactate (Fig. 2), which results in increased concentrations of lactate in liver and serum (Jorfeldt and Juhlin-Dannfelt, 1978). A reduced utilization of extra-hepatically produced lactate, depending on the metabolic state of the liver, may additionally contribute to lactate serum elevation (Kreisberg *et al.*, 1971; Krebs, 1968). This is of special importance in patients with essential chronic lactic acidosis (Sussman *et al.*, 1970) and in diabetic patients treated with biguanides (Daughaday *et al.*, 1962).

Hyperlactacidemia also has clinical consequences with respect to uric acid metabolism. Increased concentrations of serum lactate result in a decreased renal excretion of uric acid (Lieber *et al.*, 1962). The decreased intratubular pH due to acidosis is associated with reduced dissociation of the uric acid molecule and therefore leads to an increased tubular reabsorption of uric acid. Fasting and ethanol consumption (a situation typical for the alcoholic) are both additive in the production of hyperuricemia. However, ketosis may result not only from fasting. In the alcoholic ketosis may also be present because of an increased production of β-hydroxybutyrate, a precursor of acetone (Lefevre *et al.*, 1970).

Alcoholics also exhibit an increased generation of uric acid deriving from an enhanced catabolism of nucleotides, which may further contribute to hyper-uricemia. Chronic ethanol ingestion in the rat increases adenosine triphosphate (ATP) breakdown by an enhanced ATPase activity, leading to the accumulation of uric acid (Bernstein *et al.*, 1973). This enhanced mitochondrial catabolism of ATP will be discussed later in detail.

Furthermore, hepatocellular necrosis frequently observed in alcoholic hepatitis is associated with an increased breakdown of hepatic nucleotides and with an enhanced release of uric acid into the circulation.

Although serum uric acid concentrations increase during and after seizures, the exact mechanism of delirium tremens on uric acid metabolism is still obscure (Lieber, 1985). The complex effect of alcohol on uric acid metabolism may explain why ethanol was found to exacerbate gout in patients with apparent hyperproduction of uric acid (Faller and Fox, 1982).

3. *Effect of Ethanol-Induced Redox Shift on Lipid Metabolism*

Metabolic effects of ethanol with respect to lipid metabolism include the appearance of fatty liver and hyperlipemia.

a.   Alcoholic Fatty Liver. The accumulation of lipids in the hepatocyte is one of the earliest and most striking manifestations of alcoholic liver injury. The lipids that accumulate are mainly triacylglycerols. However, increases in phos-pholipids (Lieber *et al.*, 1965: French, 1967), free cholesterol (Vasdev *et al.*, 1974), and cholesteryl esters (DeCarli and Lieber, 1967) have been found after chronic ethanol consumption. Excessive accumulation of hepatic fat might result from an increased supply of lipids to the liver from the diet (Lieber and Spritz, 1966), from the intestine (Baraona, 1985), or from adipose tissue (Lieber and Spritz, 1966; Baraona, 1985). Increased hepatic synthesis and decreased hepatic oxidation as well as impaired hepatic secretion by release into plasma lipoproteins (Baraona *et al.*, 1977, 1980) or by biliary excretion of cholesterol and phospholipids (Marin *et al.*, 1973, 1975; Maddrey and Boyer, 1973) may also contribute to fatty liver. However, it is beyond the scope of this review to discuss all these mechanisms in detail, which have been reviewed by Baraona (1985). Emphasis will be placed on alterations of lipid metabolism due to the increased hepatic NADH/NAD ratio following ethanol ingestion (Fig. 2).

Hepatic synthesis of fatty acids and of glycerolipids are found to be increased due to the altered redox state of the liver (Fig. 2). The increased incorporation of acetate into fatty acids is most likely due to stimulation of the mitochondrial system for elongation of fatty acids in response to the high reduced NADH/NAD ratio generated not only by ethanol but also by acetaldehyde oxidation (Baraona, 1985). This may provide a mechanism for attenuation of the redox shift. In addition, the redox state during ethanol oxidation favors the reduction of dihydroxyacetone phosphate to glycerol 3-phosphate, one of the precursors for the synthesis of glycerolipids (Nikkilä and Ojala, 1963). Ethanol-fed rats incorporated significantly more labeled glycerol in hepatic triacylglycerols and phospholipids than did the pair-fed controls (Mendenhall *et al.*, 1969), although ethanol decreases the hepatic uptake of glycerol (Lundquist *et al.*, 1965). The induction of microsomal lipid-synthesizing enzymes by ethanol ingestion may additionally contribute to the increased production of triglycerides and cholesterol (Uthus *et al.*, 1976; Savolainen, 1977; Pritchard *et al.*, 1977; Lamb *et al.*, 1979; Savolainen *et al.*, 1984).

In addition to increased hepatic lipid synthesis, one of the most consistent effects of ethanol on hepatic lipid metabolism is the inhibition of fatty acid oxidation. This has been documented in liver slices (Lieber and Schmid, 1961; Rebaucas and Isselbacher, 1961; Blomstrand *et al.*, 1973), perfused livers (Lieber *et al.*, 1967), isolated hepatocytes (Ontko, 1973), and *in vivo* (Blomstrand and Karger, 1973). Fatty acids are predominantly oxidized in the mitochondria through a process of β oxidation which leads to the formation of acetyl-CoA. This in turn is further oxidized to CO_2 in the citric acid cycle or, alternatively, utilized for the synthesis of ketone bodies and other products (Fig. 2). Initially, the impairment of fatty acid oxidation is linked to the inhibition of NAD-dependent steps of the citric acid cycle, due to the excessive generation of NADH from cytosolic ethanol and mitochondrial acetaldehyde oxidation (Forsander *et al.*, 1965a,b; Lieber *et al.*, 1967; Williamson *et al.*, 1969). The reducing equivalents generated by ethanol oxidation compete with those supplied by normal fuels such as fatty acids. The inhibition of β oxidation promotes accumulation of long-chain fatty acyl-CoA that can be used for the synthesis of glycerolipids and cholesteryl esters.

Following chronic ethanol consumption, the shift in redox state produced by ethanol oxidation is attenuated (Domschke *et al.*, 1974; Salaspuro *et al.*, 1981), and the acute effect of ethanol on fatty acid oxidation is decreased (Salaspuro *et al.*, 1981). However, in the perivenular zone of the hepatic lobule, which is exposed to relatively low concentrations of oxygen (French *et al.*, 1984), a greater redox shift is favored by an increased production due to ADH and a decreased oxidation of reducing equivalents (Jauhonen *et al.*, 1982; Baraona *et al.*, 1983). This may be one reason why ethanol-induced liver injury, including fibrogenesis, starts and predominates in this area.

In addition, chronic ethanol consumption leads to morphological and functional damage of the mitochondria associated with decreased oxidation of two-carbon fragments of fatty acids (Rubin *et al.*, 1972; Gordon, 1973). Thus, the development of mitochondrial injury converts an acute inhibitory effect of fatty acid oxidation, depending on the redox change, into a chronic one that persists even in the absence of ethanol.

b. Alcoholic Hyperlipemia. Both hypercholesterolemia and hypertriglyceridemia have been described as a common finding after ethanol abuse (Baraona, 1985). Alcoholic hyperlipemia is usually classified as type IV and V characterized by an increase in very low-density lipoproteins (VLDL) and chylomicrons. In patients with marked hypertriacylglyceridemia, plasma cholesterol is also found to be increased. Cholesterol is a component of all lipoprotein fractions, but most of it is transported in low-density lipoproteins (LDL) or β-lipoproteins and in high-density lipoproteins (HDL) or α-lipoproteins. The elevated serum lipids in the alcoholic originate from the liver, in which mechanisms such as microsomal enzyme induction have been turned on to handle the excess of fat by an increased secretion of lipoproteins into the circulation. However, during the progression to more severe alcoholic liver disease, lipoprotein secretion of the hepatocyte may decrease due to an ethanol-associated injury of the microtubular system. As a result, serum lipids may return to normal, and lipoproteins abnormal in function and structure may emerge in the circulation (Baraona, 1985).

The concept that moderate drinking might exert protective cardiovascular effects is based on the observation of increased levels of circulating HDL in experimental animals and in humans (Baraona and Lieber, 1970; Hulley and Gordon, 1981). This ethanol-induced increase in HDL was even suggested as a biological marker for alcoholism (Sanchez-Craig and Annis, 1981). However, HDL is a heterogeneous group of lipoproteins with two major subclasses, namely HDL_2, epidemiologically associated with a reduction in coronary heart disease, and HLD_3, which is not clearly related to arteriosclerosis. It has been shown that heavy alcohol abuse increases HDL_2 (Taskinen *et al.*, 1982), while moderate intake of ethanol leads to an elevation of HDL_3 (Haskell *et al.*, 1984). The mechanism by which alcohol increases HDL_3 is unknown, although it was speculated that HDL_3 derive mainly from nascent HDL released from the liver and that this increased production is caused by the ethanol-associated induction of microsomal enzymes (Lieber, 1984a).

4. Effect of Ethanol-Induced Redox Shift on Protein Metabolism

a. Plasma Proteins. The altered redox state due to ethanol oxidation by ADH influences the energy transfer potentially needed for protein synthesis and urea production. The findings with respect to the influence of ethanol on protein synthesis are controversial (Rothschild *et al.*, 1985). Studies using rat liver slices or isolated hepatocytes clearly demonstrate an inhibition of glycoprotein and albumin synthesis by acute and chronic ethanol administration (Tuma *et al.*, 1981; Sorrell *et al.*, 1983; Harbitz *et al.*, 1984). However, Moreland *et al.* (1981) found no effect of 50–100 mM ethanol on protein synthesis using isolated rat hepatocytes. When rats received ethanol acutely, there was no detectable *in vivo* effect on hepatic albumin synthesis, and it was concluded that the inhibitor effect on protein synthesis produced by ethanol *in vitro* reflects the inability of isolated liver preparations to handle the excess of reducing equivalents generated by ethanol oxidation (Baraona *et al.*, 1980). Finally, a rat albumin cDNA clone was used to evaluate the effect of chronic ethanol administration on hepatic albumin synthesis, and with this technique the hepatic protein synthesis machinery was found to be normal (Zern *et al.*, 1983). Data on the effect of ethanol on hepatic protein synthesis in humans are rare. Potter *et al.* (1985) demonstrated a decreased transferrin synthesis in patients with alcoholic cirrhosis, while in patients with alcoholic fatty liver transferrin turnover was found to be accelerated.

Again, it should be pointed out that the perivenular zone of the hepatic lobule, which is somewhat hypoxic already in the normal stage, may represent an area of exaggerated toxicity (French *et al.*, 1984) due to the striking increase of the ethanol-induced redox shift, and could be therefore a predominant location for impaired protein synthesis. (Rothschild *et al.*, 1985).

b. Collagen Metabolism. Collagen metabolism is closely linked to hepatic fibrogenesis. The fibrotic process of the liver is not only a response to inflammation and cell necrosis but can also be initiated by ethanol at the fatty liver stage without development of alcoholic hepatitis (Lieber, 1984b). Biochemically, as an initial step in fibrogenesis, an accumulation of hepatic collagen occurs. This accumulation of hepatic collagen is due either to accelerated ethanol-mediated collagen synthesis or to decreased collagen degradation or to both.

The two major determinants of collagen synthesis are the hepatic-free proline pool size and the activity of hepatic peptidylproline hydroxylase (PPH), the key enzyme in collagen synthesis. Both factors are influenced by chronic ethanol ingestion. An increased activity of hepatic PPH has been found in rats and in primates, and an increased incorporation of [^{14}C]proline into hepatic collagen in rat liver slices was demonstrated (Feinman and Lieber, 1972). A possible mechanism whereby ethanol ingestion may be linked to collagen formation is the elevation of tissue lactate, which was found to be associated with an increased activity of PPH *in vitro* (Green and Goldberg, 1964) and *in vivo* (Lindy *et al.*, 1971). Ethanol also increases the hepatic-free proline pool size (Hakkinen and Kulonen, 1975; Mezey and Potter, 1981), which has been incriminated in the regulation of collagen synthesis (Rojkind and DeLeon, 1970). In addition, chronic ethanol ingestion was associated with an enhanced hepatic uptake of proline, probably due to acetaldehyde (Mendenhall *et al.*, 1984). Elevated serum proline and hydroxyproline levels have been reported in patients with alcoholic cirrhosis (Mata *et al.*, 1975). Again, lactate may lead to this increase in proline (Kershenobich *et al.*, 1970) by the inhibition of proline oxidase (Kowaloff *et al.*, 1977). In cirrhotic patients the reduced mitochondrial state has been incriminated for the rise in blood lactate and proline (Cerra *et al.*, 1979). However, Shaw *et al.* (1984) found hyperprolinemia only infrequently in patients with alcoholic cirrhosis. Nevertheless, even in the absence of proline and lactate increases in the peripheral blood, the postulated mechanism could be important, since it is related to the alcohol-induced redox change in the liver, which was found selectively exacerbated in the perivenular zone where the ethanol-induced hepatic lesions first occur.

Indeed, perivenular fibrosis is an early histological marker which indicates the progression to more severe alcoholic liver injury when ethanol abuse is continued (Worner and Lieber, 1985). In a study by Nakano *et al.* (1982), 80% of patients with steatosis and additional perivenular fibrosis progressed to fibrosis or even cirrhosis within 2 years of followup, while only 10% of patients with only fatty liver exhibited an impairment of liver histology during this time interval. The ultrastructure of the perivenular lesion showed a good correlation between the thickness of the perivenular rim and the number of mesenchymal cells surrounding the venules. Myofibroblasts, which are known to play an important role in fibrogenesis (Hahn and Schuppan, 1985), represent the most common cell type in the perivenular area after alcohol ingestion (Nakano *et al.*, 1982). It is generally believed that fat-storing cells (Ito cells) can be transformed into transitional cells and finally into myofibroblasts (Mak and Lieber, 1984; Hahn and Schuppan, 1985). Thus, it seems of interest that collagen synthesis can be stimulated in cultured myofibroblasts (Savolainen *et al.*, 1984) and in fibroblasts (Holt *et al.*, 1984), both by lactate and acetaldehyde. Both intermediates are predominantly produced in the perivenular area as already discussed.

In contrast to collagen synthesis, the mechanisms of collagen degradation are even more complex. It was suggested that the activity of hepatic collagenase paradoxically increases during the early stage of alcoholic liver injury (Okazaki *et al.*, 1977), but subsequently decreases, contributing to hepatic collagen accumulation (Maruyama *et al.*, 1982). This increased activity of hepatic collagenase is associated with an enhanced turnover of collagen as demonstrated by Mezey and Potter (1981).

5. *Effect of Ethanol-Induced Redox Shift on Carbohydrate Metabolism*

Ethanol-induced hepatic redox changes decrease the intracellular concentrations of glucoplastic intermediates such as pyruvate and oxaloacetate, while lactate and malate increase (Fig. 2). Since the citric acid cycle with its concentrations of α-ketoglutarate and succinate is also slowed down, a reduced production of phosphoenolpyruvate occurs (Ishii *et al.*, 1978). As a result, hepatic gluconeogenesis is inhibited (Schüller *et al.*, 1985). This fact, as well as a depletion of hepatic glycogen stores associated with an inadequate intake of calories, may occasionally lead to hypoglycemia in the alcoholic. On the other hand, hyperglycemia may result when an ethanol-mediated stimulation of catecholamine release in the presence of sufficient glycogen predominates. Ethanol does not influence basal levels of insulin, but increases insulin release after stimulation (Gordon and Southren, 1977). Furthermore, ethanol also affects hepatic insulin receptors (Schüller *et al.*, 1985). Figure 2 summarizes the effect of ethanol on carbohydrate metabolism and its link to lipid metabolism.

The conversion of galactose to glucose is a very sensitive NAD^+-dependent reaction and is therefore easily inhibited by an increase in cellular NADH. The determination of galactose elimination rate is an excellent parameter for characterizing the ethanol-associated hepatic redox state.

6. *Effect of Ethanol-Induced Redox Shift on Steroid Metabolism*

Steroid metabolism in liver and gonads is predominantly shifted to reductive pathways after ethanol consumption. Since ethanol is also oxidized in Leydig cells via ADH, the occurrence of an increased NADH/NAD ratio leads to an inhibition of testosterone biosynthesis (Chiao *et al.*, 1981). Alcohol may further interfere with testicular vitamin A activation, which is essential for normal spermatogenesis (Van Thiel *et al.*, 1974). Similarly, acetaldehyde, either produced directly in the testes as a result of testicular metabolism of ethanol or by entering the testes from the plasma, may have deleterious effects on testicular mitochondria, organelles which are critical for steroidogenesis (Lester *et al.*, 1979). Thus, the conversion of cholesterol to pregnenolone is inhibited (Van Thiel and Gavaler, 1985). Furthermore, chronic ethanol ingestion leads to a hypothalamic–pituitary defect in gonadotropin secretion and to a decreased binding of gonadotropin to testicular tissue (Van Thiel and Gavaler, 1985).

On the other hand, testosterone is more rapidly metabolized by the liver due to microsomal enzyme induction of 5α-A-ring reductase (Rubin *et al.*, 1976). However, during progression to more severe hepatic injury, the activity of this enzyme decreases (Gordon *et al.*, 1979). As a result of the metabolic effects of

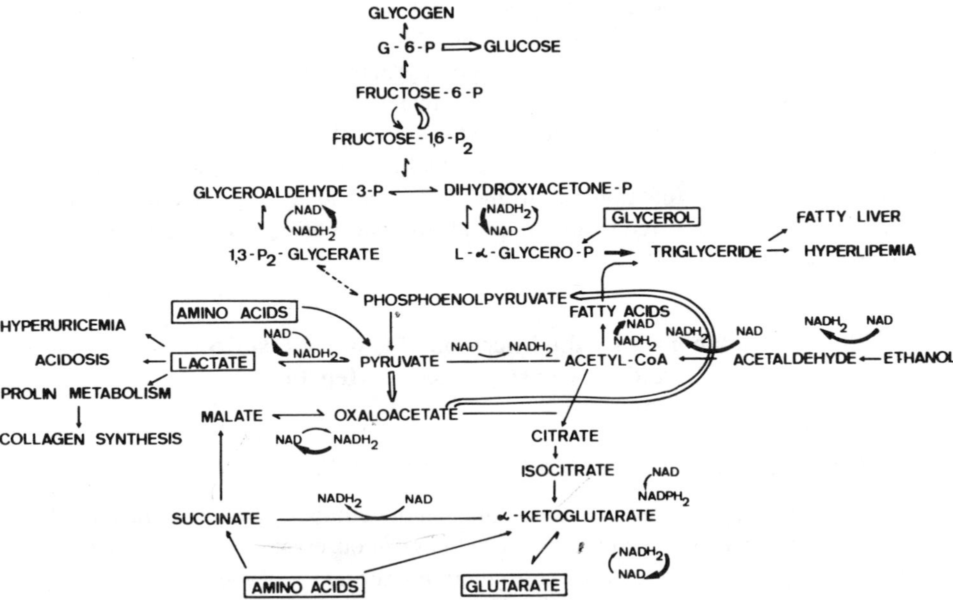

Fig. 2. Metabolic pathways of hepatic gluconeogenesis during fasting and its link to the metabolism of ethanol, lipids, uric acid, and collagen. The possible precursors of glucose are framed. The specific enzymatic steps on which the reversibility of glycolysis depends are indicated by open arrows. Ethanol oxidation and favored reactions due to the increased NADH/NAD ratio (caused by ethanol oxidation) are indicated by solid arrows.

ethanol on hepatic and extrahepatic testosterone metabolism, hypogonadism and hypotestosteronemia occur.

In addition, alcoholics also exhibit hyperestrogenization, which may be explained by an increased estrogen/testosterone ratio (Lester *et al.*, 1979). Ethanol also influences hepatic cytosolic estrogen receptors and hepatic production of sex steroid-binding globulin. All these alterations of steroid hormone metabolism by ethanol are responsible for the clinical appearance of feminization in the alcoholic patient. An excellent review of this topic has been given by Van Thiel and Gavaler (1985).

7.   *Ethanol and Porphyrin Metabolism*

Ethanol is an important precipitating and aggravating factor in human hepatic porphyrias. The mechanisms responsible for these interactions include an inhibition of uroporphyrinogen decarboxylase (UPD) in erythrocytes (McColl *et al.*, 1981) and an induction of δ-aminolevulinic acid synthase (ALAS) in the liver (Held, 1977; Lana and Steward, 1983). Therefore, ethanol interferes with a preexisting UPD defect in chronic hepatic porphyria and augments the inducibility of ALAS in acute hepatic porphyrias. In addition, ethanol also inhibits

ALA dehydratase (Moore *et al.*, 1971), coproporphyrinogen oxidase (CPO) (McColl *et al.*, 1981) and ferrochelatase (McColl *et al.*, 1981). Therefore, ethanol can produce secondary coproporphyrinuria and protoporphyrinemia (Doss, 1985). The mechanism by which ethanol inhibits the activity of these enzymes involved in porphyrin metabolism are complex and may include a shift of the mitochondrial redox state due to ethanol oxidation (CPO), an impairment of the mitochondrial function due to increased acetaldehyde production (CPO, ferrochelatase), and a reduction in pyridoxal phosphate, a cofactor for ferrochelatase (Doss, 1985).

B. Ethanol Metabolism by the Microsomal Ethanol-Oxidizing System (MEOS) and Its Consequences on Hepatic Intermediary Metabolism

1. The Microsomal Ethanol-Oxidizing System (MEOS)

The first indication of an interaction of ethanol with the microsomal fraction of the hepatocyte was provided by the morphological observation of a proliferation of the SER after chronic ethanol consumption (Iseri *et al.*, 1966). This increase in SER resembles that seen after the administration of a wide variety of xenobiotic compounds, including known hepatotoxins (Meldolesi, 1967), therapeutic agents (Conney, 1967), and food additives (Lane and Lieber, 1967). Most of these substances that induce a proliferation of the SER are metabolized in the microsomal fraction of the hepatocyte that comprises the SER. Thus, the observation that ethanol produces a proliferation of the SER raised the question of whether ethanol can be metabolized by microsomes. In addition, since ethanol metabolism cannot be completely blocked by the administration of pyrazole, a potent ADH inhibitor (Salaspuro *et al.*, 1975), another oxidative pathway of alcohol metabolism besides ADH had to be considered.

Orme-Johnson and Ziegler (1965) described a microsomal system capable of oxidizing methanol. However, its capacity to oxidize ethanol was extremely low, and it was capable of metabolizing long-chain aliphatic alcohols such as butanol. It was concluded that this system is different from the cytochrome *P*-450-dependent system and involves the H_2O_2-mediated ethanol peroxidation by catalase (Ziegler, 1972).

However, Lieber and DeCarli (1970a) were the first to describe a microsomal ethanol-oxidizing system (MEOS) with a high oxidation rate for ethanol. This system is a mixed-function oxidase with its typical requirement for NADPH and O_2, and it is relatively insensitive to catalase inhibition (Lieber and DeCarli, 1968, 1970b). This MEOS is also capable of oxidizing long-chain aliphatic alcohols (Teschke *et al.*, 1975), which are not substrates for catalase (Chance and Oshino, 1971). MEOS activity increases with increasing concentrations of alcohol, which is due to the higher K_m of MEOS compared to ADH (Thieden,

1971; Grunnet *et al.*, 1973; Matsuzaki *et al.*, 1981). The *in vitro* K_m of MEOS of 8–10 mM agrees well with the corresponding value of 9 mM for the pyrazole-insensitive pathway *in vivo* (Lieber and DeCarli, 1970a, 1972) and with a similar value in isolated hepatocytes (Matsuzaki *et al.*, 1981). It is now generally believed that MEOS plays a significant role in ethanol metabolism, especially at higher alcohol concentrations and after chronic consumption, while the rate of ethanol metabolism via catalase seems negligible (Lieber, 1984b, 1985).

Differentiation of MEOS from ADH was achieved by subcellular localization, pH optimum *in vitro,* cofactor requirement, and effects of inhibitors such as pyrazole (Lieber *et al.*, 1970; Lieber and DeCarli, 1973). In addition, MEOS was solubilized and separated from ADH and catalase activities by diethylaminoethyl cellulose column chromatography (Teschke *et al.*, 1972, 1974; Mezey *et al.*, 1973). More recently, the reconstitution of the ethanol-oxidizing activity with three microsomal components—cytochrome *P*-450, NADPH-cytochrome *c* reductase, and lecithin—was demonstrated (Ohnishi and Lieber, 1977; Winston and Cederbaum, 1983). Reductase-mediated ethanol oxidation was found to be less than oxidation catalyzed by ethanol-induced cytochrome *P*-450, but is equal to oxidation catalyzed by uninduced cytochrome *P*-450 (Ohnishi and Lieber, 1977). Superoxide dismutase inhibits the reductase-mediated reaction (Winston and Cederbaum, 1983), and there is evidence that the reductase operates via the hydroxyl radical mechanism (Bosterling and Trudel, 1981) and can therefore be expected to be dismutase-sensitive, whereas the ethanol-induced *P*-450 mechanism can be expected to be dismutase-insensitive. Thus, in noninduced cytochrome *P*-450 (Ingelman-Sundberg and Johansson, 1981), reductase-mediated inhibition by dismutase may be more apparent than in the more active ethanol-induced cytochrome *P*-450 (Ohnishi and Lieber, 1978).

MEOS activity is present not only in the liver but also in extrahepatic organs such as the small and large intestines (Seitz *et al.*, 1979, 1982) and the lungs (Pikkarainen *et al.*, 1981a). Although MEOS activity is much lower in these tissues compared to the liver, an increased acetaldehyde production via MEOS after chronic ethanol ingestion could be responsible for a variety of toxic effects also observed in extrahepatic tissue.

2. *Effect of Chronic Ethanol Ingestion of MEOS Activity*

Following chronic ethanol consumption, MEOS activity significantly increases (Lieber and DeCarli, 1970a). This is associated with an increase in various constituents of the SER such as phospholipids, cytochrome *P*-450 reductase, and cytochrome *P*-450 (Joly *et al.*, 1973; Ishii *et al.*, 1973; Comai and Gaylor, 1973; Sato *et al.*, 1978). Indeed, ethanol ingestion results in the occurrence of an ethanol-specific form of cytochrome *P*-450. This was supported by the shift in the cytochrome reduced spectrum maximum to higher wavelengths, by an increased cyanide affinity (Joly *et al.*, 1972; Comai and Gaylor, 1973; Hasumura *et al.*, 1975a), and by inhibitor studies (Ullrich *et al.*, 1975). More direct proof was obtained from studies with microsomal protein (Ohnishi and Lieber, 1977). The rise in cytochrome *P*-450 involved a hemoprotein different from those induced by phenobarbital and 3-methylcholanthrene treatment. The ethanol-induced form of cytochrome *P*-450 was found to exhibit different spectral and catalytic properties (Joly *et al.*, 1976, 1977). An ethanol-specific form of cytochrome *P*-450 has been revealed by gel electrophoresis in the rat (Ohnishi and Lieber, 1977) and in the deer mouse (Shigeta *et al.*, 1984), and subsequently this form of cytochrome *P*-450 was successfully purified from the rabbit (Koop *et al.*, 1982).

3. *Interaction of Ethanol with the Metabolism of Drugs, Toxins, and Procarcinogens*

a. Acute Effects of Ethanol. Since MEOS shares common components with microsomal mixed-function oxidases, interactions of ethanol with this system, especially with cytochrome *P*-450, is not surprising and may explain in large part the complicated effects of ethanol on drug metabolism, which have been recently reviewed (Hoyumpa and Schenker, 1982; Lieber, 1984b; Sato *et al.*, 1985; Seitz, 1985).

In the presence of ethanol, drug metabolism by microsomes is generally inhibited both *in vitro* and *in vivo. In vivo,* acute ethanol administration results in a prolongation of the half-life of various drugs such as meprobamate, pentobarbital (Rubin *et al.*, 1970a,b), diazepam (Hoyumpa *et al.*, 1980), lorazepam (Hoyumpa *et al.*, 1981), chlomethiazole (Hoyumpa and Schenker, 1982), tolbutamide (Carulli *et al.*, 1971), phenytoin, warfarin (Kater *et al.*, 1969a), and acetaminophen (Sato and Lieber, 1981). This inhibitory effect of ethanol has been implicated in the synergistic effect of alcohol and central nervous system depressants. In fact, chlordiazepoxide metabolism is impaired in the alcoholic (Whiting *et al.*, 1979; Desmond *et al.*, 1980), and Thomas *et al.* (1972) found elevated brain concentrations of pentobarbital in ethanol-treated rats. The metabolism of other drugs which are known to be metabolized by mixed-function oxidases, such as methadone (Borowsky and Lieber, 1978), phenothiazine (Milner and Landauer, 1971), and caffeine (Mitchell *et al.*, 1983), is also impaired in the presence of ethanol. In addition, systemic availability of drugs which undergo first-pass elimination, such as mephenytoin (Zysset *et al.*, 1980) and propoxyphene (Oguma and Levy, 1981), was found to be increased when the drug is taken orally in the presence of ethanol. *In vitro,* ethanol inhibits drug oxidation by microsomal enzymes such as aniline hydroxylase (Rubin *et al.*, 1970b), aminopyrine-*N*-demethylase (Rubin *et al.*, 1970b; Dicker and Cederbaum, 1983), ethylmorphine-*N*-demethylase (Borowsky and Lieber, 1978), and pentobarbital hydroxylase (Rubin *et al.*, 1970b). This inhibitory effect of ethanol has been explained by its interaction with cytochrome *P*-450. Ethanol produces a reverse type I binding spectrum when added to microsomes (Rubin *et al.*, 1971), suggesting the binding of ethanol to cytochrome *P*-450 or the dissociation of drugs from cytochrome *P*-450. In general, ethanol is a stronger inhibitor of microsomal metabolism of type II than type I binding drugs. Recent findings that ethanol-induced cytochrome *P*-450 has a high affinity for aniline hydroxylation as well as ethanol oxidation may be a possible explanation (Morgan *et al.*, 1982). In summary, the inhibitory effect of ethanol on drug metabolism has been primarily explained by an interaction on the cytochrome *P*-450 level. However, it has also been suggested that a decreased production of NADPH (Reinke *et al.*, 1980), as well as an increased release of corticosteroids after ethanol introduction, could be the cause for the inhibition of hexobarbital metabolism by alcohol (Chung and Brown, 1976).

In addition to its inhibitory effect on microsomal drug metabolism, ethanol can also alter nonmicrosomal metabolism of drugs. Thus, the inhibition of hepatic glucuronidation demonstrated for phenolphthalein, trichloroethanol, and diethyldithiocarbamate (a metabolite of disulfiram) is obviously due to the increased NADH/NAD ratio observed after alcohol ingestion (Moldeus *et al.*, 1978). The mechanism for the inhibition is a decreased formation of UDP-glucuronic acid, the donor for the conjugation reaction, from UDP-glucose, which is catalyzed by the NAD^+-dependent enzyme UDP-glucose dehydrogenase.

An increase in the acetylation of sulfanilamide was demonstrated in humans after the acute administration of ethanol (Olson and Morland, 1978). The enhanced cytosolic acetylation may be due to an increase in acetyl-CoA originating from acetate produced during ethanol oxidation.

Acute ethanol administration also inhibits hepatic nitrosamine metabolism by inhibiting competitively hepatic low-K_m dimethylnitrosamine (DMN) demethylase, the key enzyme responsible for the ultimate activation of DMN to a carcinogen (Tomera *et al.*, 1984). This inhibition of hepatic DMN metabolism by ethanol possibly prevents the first-pass elimination of nitrosamines by the liver (Swann *et al.*, 1984). As a result, more nitrosamines bypass the liver, and an increased exposure of nitrosamine-sensitive extrahepatic organs to the carcinogen occurs (Swann *et al.*, 1984). Thus, the administration of DMN and ethanol causes an increased methylation of esophageal DNA compared with the application of DMN alone. On the other hand, chronic ethanol ingestion increases the activity of hepatic (Garro *et al.*, 1981) and esophageal (Farinati *et al.*, 1985) DMN-demethylase as discussed in the next paragraph. It seems noteworthy that the esophageal enzyme has a much lower K_m for DMN compared to the liver (Swann *et al.*, 1984). The complex interaction of ethanol and nitrosamine metabolism could explain the cocarcinogenicity of ethanol in nitrosamine-induced carcinogenesis of the upper respiratory and alimentary tracts (Seitz, 1985), and this has been recently reviewed in detail (Seitz and Simanowski, 1986).

Inhibition of drug metabolism by ethanol is common, while the inhibition of ethanol metabolism by a drug is a rare event. For example, chloralhydrate, which is metabolized to trichlorethanol by ADH, may compete with ethanol for the same pathway and produce higher plasma concentrations of ethanol (Sellers *et al.*, 1972). Such an inhibition of ethanol oxidation has been also reported for the ADH blockers pyrazole (Salaspuro and Lindros, 1985) and chlorpromazine (Koff and Fitts, 1972). More recently, it was shown that the administration of the H_2-receptor antagonist cimetidine results in elevated ethanol serum concentrations in humans and rats (Seitz *et al.*, 1984a). However, the mechanism for this observation is still obscure.

b.   Chronic Effects of Ethanol. Chronic administration of ethanol in rats and humans increases the rate of plasma clearance of meprobamate (Misra *et al.*, 1971), phenobarbital (Misra *et al.*, 1971), tolbutamide (Carulli *et al.*, 1971), phenytoin, warfarin (Kater *et al.*, 1969b), and acetaminophen (Sato *et al.*, 1981). This increased rate persists for 4–9 weeks after cessation of alcohol consumption and is reproduced with the intake of large doses of ethanol (Iber, 1977). The enhanced metabolic disposal of antipyrine in alcoholic patients was found for up to 2 weeks after abstinence (Cushman *et al.*, 1982).

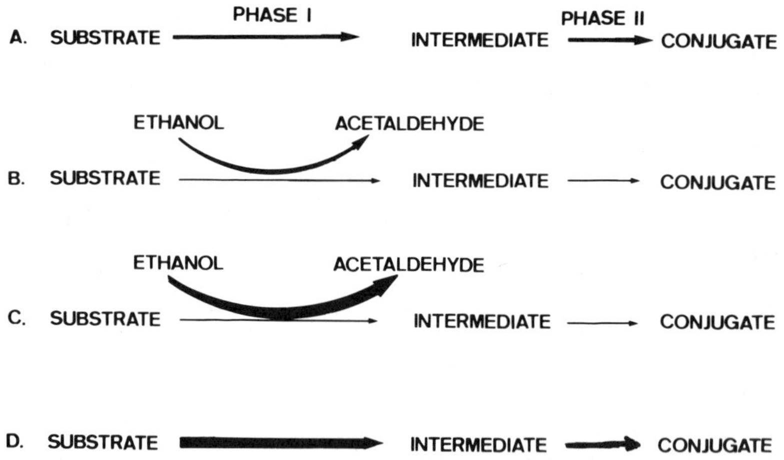

Fig. 3.   Interaction between microsomal metabolism of ethanol and xenobiotics. Phase I reaction is a mixed-function oxidase and depends on cytochrome *P*-450 (A). Phase II reaction mostly catalyzes the conjugation of glucuronic acid, glutathione, acetate, or sulfate to the intermediate to increase water solubility (A). In the presence of ethanol, phase I reaction of various drugs and xenobiotics is inhibited, since ethanol competes for cytochrome *P*-450 (B). Acute ethanol administration also inhibits glucuronidation (phase II), since the increased redox state decreases the availability of UDP-glucuronic acid (B). Chronic ethanol ingestion increases microsomal cytochrome *P*-450 and microsomal enzyme activity. Thus, in the presence of ethanol, microsomal ethanol oxidation is enhanced (C). Again, xenobiotic phase I reaction is inhibited. In addition, to decreased glucuronidation, glutathione conjugation is also impaired after chronic ethanol ingestion (C). Following withdrawal of ethanol, phase I and phase II reactions are enhanced (depending on the time interval between the last drink and xenobiotic exposure) due to microsomal enzyme induction (D).

TABLE I

Deleterious Effects of Microsomal Enzyme Induction by Ethanol

1. Enhanced microsomal ethanol oxidation and increased production of acetaldehyde
2. Increased oxygen consumption due to microsomal hypermetabolism
3. Increased microsomal production of hepatotoxic intermediates from drugs and environmental xenobiotics
4. Increased microsomal activation of procarcinogens
5. Increased microsomal metabolism of steroids including sex hormones
6. Increased microsomal degradation of vitamin A and production of toxic metabolites

Enhanced drug metabolism has also been observed *in vitro* after chronic ethanol consumption. Thus, the degradation of aniline (Rubin *et al.*, 1970a), pentobarbital (Rubin *et al.*, 1970a), and methadone (Borowsky and Lieber, 1978) was found to be accelerated. The mechanism by which chronic ethanol ingestion increases drug metabolism is based on the microsomal enzyme induction by alcohol (Fig. 3). Although chronic ethanol consumption leads to the appearance of an ethanol-specific form of cytochrome P-450, this cytochrome P-450 is also capable of binding a variety of xenobiotics, and therefore drug metabolism is accelerated when ethanol is absent from the body (Fig. 3).

4. *Toxicity Associated with Enhanced Microsomal Enzyme Activity following Chronic Ethanol Ingestion*

Although many microsomal changes after chronic ethanol consumption can be interpreted as adaptive alterations secondary to induction, some injurious consequences may occur. These are summarized in Table I. Drugs are not only metabolized faster, the accelerated metabolism can also result in the occurrence of toxic intermediates (Fig. 3). This is best known for halothane (Ishii *et al.*, 1983), cocaine (Smith *et al.*, 1981), and acetaminophen (Sato *et al.*, 1981).

Acetaminophen metabolism has been studied in detail, and it is irrefutable that chronic ethanol ingestion enhances acetaminophen-mediated hepatotoxicity by the increased microsomal production of toxic intermediates (Sato *et al.*, 1981, 1985). When the production of the reactive metabolite is sufficiently large to deplete hepatic glutathione, the reactive metabolites can no longer be detoxified by this pathway and bind to cellular protein, which produces hepatic injury (Sato *et al.*, 1981). There have been a number of case reports suggesting that alcoholics may have increased hepatic suscpetibility to an overdose of acetaminophen (Emby and Fraser, 1977). A similar enhancement of the hepatotoxicity of thioacetamide (Maling *et al.*, 1975), dimethylnitrosamine (Maling *et al.*, 1975), carbon tetrachloride (Hasumura *et al.*, 1974), and bromobenzene (Hetú *et al.*, 1983) after chronic ethanol consumption has been reported.

In contrast to chronic ethanol exposure, the simultaneous presence of ethanol and competing substrates may impair hepatic metabolism of the latter and may thereby increase its toxicity if the parent compound is toxic (Fig. 3). This is probably the case for xylene. Ingestion of a moderate dose of ethanol by volunteers prior to inhalation exposure to xylene doubles the blood xylene level (Riihimäki *et al.*, 1982).

Closely related to the alcohol–drug interaction is the enhanced activation of procarcinogens ultimately to carcinogens following chronic ethanol consumption in a variety of tissues. It has been reported that chronic ethanol ingestion increases microsomal procarcinogen-activating enzyme activities in the liver (Garro *et al.*, 1981; Seitz *et al.*, 1981b), in the gastrointestinal tract (Seitz *et al.*, 1981a), and in the lungs (Lieber *et al.*, 1979). An enhanced activation of environmental procarcinogens may at least in part contribute to the increased incidence of various cancers observed in the alcoholic (Lieber *et al.*, 1979; Seitz, 1985; Seitz and Simanowski, 1986).

Ethanol can also affect the hepatic microsomal metabolism of endogenous and exogenous steroids, as already discussed, and can alter the metabolism of structurally related vitamins such as vitamin A and D.

C. Increased Ethanol Metabolism following Chronic Consumption of Alcohol

Alcholics tolerate large amounts of alcoholic beverages, mainly because of central nervous system adaptation. In addition, alcoholics also develop metabolic tolerance, demonstrating an increased rate of ethanol metabolism (Kater *et al.*, 1969a; Ugarte *et al.*, 1972), which has also been demonstrated in animals (Feinman *et al.*, 1978; Pikkarainen and Lieber, 1980). This progressive acceleration of ethanol metabolism following chronic ingestion is different from the rise of ethanol metabolism seen after an acute dose of ethanol. The enhanced ethanol oxidation following acute ethanol administration, the so-called swift increase in alcohol metabolism, results from a stress-associated epinephrine discharge (Yuki and Thurman, 1980). The mechanism of the chronic acceleration is still subject to debate. Part of the effect is due to ADH-related changes in ethanol metabolism, and part is due to the microsomal oxidation of alcohol.

1. ADH-Related Increase in Ethanol Metabolism

It is now generally accepted that chronic ethanol ingestion does not affect hepatic ADH activity (Lieber, 1985). One of the mechanisms that could contribute to the acceleration of ADH-dependent ethanol metabolism after chronic ingestion of alcohol is an increased rate of NADH reoxidation due to an enhanced adenosine triphosphatase (ATPase) activity, which is susceptible to ouabain inhibition (Bernstein *et al.*, 1973). This increased mitochondrial ATPase activity is associated with a hypermetabolic state akin to hyperthyroidism (Bernstein *et al.*, 1973; Israel *et al.*, 1975a). It was reported that ouabain can completely block the additional ethanol oxidation rate observed after chronic consumption (Israel *et al.*, 1975a). This was found to be due to an inhibition of the mitochondrial Na,K-activated ATPase. In addition, oxygen consumption was found to be increased after chronic ethanol ingestion mimicking the effect of thyroxine (Bernstein *et al.*, 1975; Israel *et al.*, 1973, 1975b). It was therefore concluded that the condition observed after alcohol intake may be similar to the hepatic condition seen after treatment of animals with thyroid hormones, in which hypermetabolism also seems to be associated with an increased hydrolysis of ATP by Na,K-ATPase with a lowering of the phosphorylation potential (Ismail-Beigi and Edelman, 1971). This theory found additional support by the fact that alcohol-induced hepatic necrosis was suppressed when propylthiouracil, an antithyroid drug administered to rats (Israel *et al.*, 1975a).

However, not all investigators found an increased oxygen consumption after chronic ethanol intake (Cederbaum *et al.*, 1977; Gordon, 1977) and in fatty liver chronic ethanol ingestion was not found to be associated with increased hepatic ATPase activity (Gordon, 1977), and the increased rates of ethanol metabolism could not be abolished by ouabain (Cederbaum *et al.*, 1977). Yuki and Thurman (1980) have demonstrated that the ouabain effect is nonspecific and does not imply involvement of ATPase. Furthermore, Teschke *et al.* (1983) clearly demonstrated that in livers of alcoholics hyperthyroidism does not exist. On the basis of these data it is not surprising that the treatment of alcoholic hepatitis with the antithyroid drug propylthiouracil was found to be ineffective (Halle *et al.*, 1982), although early reports suggested this therapy because of the results obtained in the animal model (Orrego *et al.*, 1979). In conclusion, the theory of hepatic hypermetabolic state associated with an increased ATP catabolism due to ethanol is an attractive one to explain hypoxic liver damage in the rat. In humans, however, there is not much evidence for the existence of such metabolic conditions, as discussed recently (Szilagyi *et al.*, 1983).

2. *Non-ADH-Related Increase in Ethanol Metabolism*

As already discussed, following chronic ethanol consumption MEOS activity increases significantly, and this is associated with an increase of various components of the microsomal fraction of the hepatocyte. This microsomal enzyme induction leads to an accelerated ethanol metabolism and to a variety of side effects (Table I). It has been shown that the ADH inhibitor pyrazole was not capable of fully abolishing the acceleration of ethanol metabolism seen after chronic feeding (Salaspuro *et al.*, 1975). This raised the possibility of the involvement of non-ADH pathways in ethanol metabolism, especially at high ethanol concentrations at which ADH inhibitors only partially inhibit the accelerated metabolism (Matsuzaki *et al.*, 1981), while at low concentration an almost complete inhibition was reported (Thurman *et al.*, 1976). That chronic ethanol ingestion results in an increased activity in a hepatic non-ADH and noncatalase pathway was also shown in liver slices and isolated hepatocytes. Ethanol oxidation was enhanced by increasing the ethanol concentration employed *in vitro* from 10 to 30 mM, and this increase was even more pronounced in chronically ethanol-fed rats (Teschke *et al.*, 1977) and baboons (Pikkarainen and Lieber, 1980). Also, in humans, ethanol metabolism at high ethanol blood concentrations after chronic alcohol intake was significantly increased (Salaspuro and Lieber, 1978).

It has been reported that catalase activity increases (Carter and Isselbacher, 1971) or may not change (Hawkins *et al.*, 1966) after chronic ethanol ingestion. However, peroxidative ethanol metabolism in the liver is probably limited to the rate of H_2O_2 formation rather than by the amount of available catalase (Boveris *et al.*, 1972) (Fig. 1). Ethanol increases the activity of NADPH oxidase which can participate in H_2O_2 generation (Carter and Isselbacher, 1971; Lieber and DeCarli, 1970b). It is conceivable that this mechanism contributes to ethanol metabolism *in vivo* by furnishing the H_2O_2 needed for the oxidation mediated by the OH generated by the reductase (Ohnishi and Lieber, 1977; Winston and Cederbaum, 1983). In the presence of ethanol-induced cytochrome P-450, such mechanisms may be less important than the cytochrome P-450 (non-OH)-dependent oxidation of ethanol (Ohnishi and Lieber, 1977). At any rate, such a mechanism does not involve catalase, the role of which is probably limited to ethanol metabolism by H_2O_2 generated inside the peroxisomes. Chronic ethanol ingestion results also in a striking increase of NADPH-dependent oxidation of *n*-propanol and *n*-butanol (Teschke *et al.*, 1975), substances that fail to react peroxidatively with catalase H_2O_2.

Recently, it was convincingly illustrated that the capacity of MEOS is responsible for sustaining increased rates of ethanol metabolism in the deer mouse lacking ADH (Shigeta *et al.*, 1984). In conclusion, on the basis of all these experimental studies the adaptive increase in ethanol oxidation observed after chronic consumption of alcohol most likely involves the activity of MEOS, which plays a significant role in ethanol metabolism, especially at high alcohol blood concentrations and after chronic abuse.

D.   Acetaldehyde: A Toxic Metabolite of Ethanol Oxidation

1.   *Acetaldehyde Dehydrogenase (ALDH)*

Acetaldehyde is the first oxidation product of ethanol and under normal conditions it is oxidized further so rapidly that significant acetaldehyde concentrations can only be found in the liver. Aldehyde oxidase, xanthine oxidases, and aldehyde dehydrogenases are all capable of catalyzing aldehyde oxidation. However, the principal enzyme in acetaldehyde metabolism is acetaldehyde dehydrogenase (ALDH) (Fig. 4). Again, as already demonstrated for ADH, the ALDH reaction also increases the NADH/NAD ratio leading to an intramitochondrial accumulation of hydrogen. ALDH activity has been detected in various subcellular fractions of the hepatocyte such as mitochondria (Glenn and Vanko,

$$CH_3CHO + NAD^+ \xrightarrow[H_2O]{ALDH} HCH_3COO^- + NADH + H^+$$

Fig. 4. Metabolism of acetaldehyde by acetaldehyde dehydrogenase (ALDH).

1959), cytoplasm (Deitrich, 1966), and microsomes (Korsten *et al.*, 1975; Salaspuro and Lindros, 1985). Mitochondrial ALDH has a low K_m for acetaldehyde and is therefore responsible for the oxidation of most of the acetaldehyde present in the liver during ethanol oxidation (Lindros *et al.*, 1974). It should be mentioned that several molecular forms of ALDH do exist, although the exact number of human liver isoenzymes has not been fully established (Harada *et al.*, 1980; Agarwal *et al.*, 1981). These multiple forms of ALDH have certain physiological implications. About half of the Japanese population exhibits elevated blood acetaldehyde concentrations following alcohol ingestion (Mizoi *et al.*, 1979). This is associated with an acetaldehyde-induced catecholamine release, leading to tachycardia and facial flushing (Mizoi *et al.*, 1979; Inoue *et al.*, 1980). The reason for this observation is the inactivity of one of the ALDH isoenzymes because of a genetically determined defect in the synthesis of the enzyme molecule (Agarwal *et al.*, 1981; Ikawa *et al.*, 1983). In addition, ALDH activity can also be inhibited by a variety of chemicals including cyanamide and disulfiram (Kitson, 1977). The disulfiram alcohol reaction usually manifests itself in flushing of the face, throbbing headache, palpitations, dyspnea, hyperventilation, tachycardia, hypotension, vertigo, weakness, nausea, and vomiting (Salapuro and Lindros, 1985). Antidiabetic drugs of the sulfonylurea type also inhibit ALDH activity and may lead to similar symptoms when ethanol is ingested with the drug (Podgainy and Bressler, 1968). Other compounds known to induce alcohol-sensitizing reactions include the antioxidants and industrial agent *n*-butyraldoxime and the antibiotic metronidazole (Lal, 1969; Forsander, 1970). Disulfiram-like activity has also been reported after the use of alcohol concomitant with sulfonamides, chloramphenicol, griseofulvin, procarbazine, quinacrine, and tolazoline (Salaspuro and Lieber, 1985).

2. *Acetaldehyde Metabolism following Chronic Ethanol Ingestion*

Since hepatic concentrations of acetaldehyde depend on its production as well as on its degradation rate, three major alterations in the hepatic metabolism of ethanol and acetaldehyde may lead to elevated blood and tissue concentrations of acetaldehyde following chronic alcohol ingestion: (a) an increased production of acetaldehyde due to an enhanced ethanol oxidation; (b) a decreased degradation of acetaldehyde due to a decreased mitochondrial capacity to oxidize acetaldehyde; and (c) a decreased degradation of acetaldehyde due to a decreased activity of ALDH. Indeed, chronic ethanol consumption leads to elevated blood concentrations of acetaldehyde in humans (Korsten *et al.*, 1975; Lindros *et al.*,

1980; Palmer and Jenkins, 1982) and in baboons (Pikkarainen *et al.*, 1981b). In these reports blood acetaldehyde levels correlate positively with the rate of ethanol elimination, with the production rate of acetaldehyde, and, inversely, with liver mitochondrial ALDH activity. It has also been suggested that cytosolic ALDH plays a more important role in acetaldehyde metabolism in humans than is generally thought, and a reduction of cytosolic high-K_m ALDH has been reported in patients with alcoholic liver disease (Palmer and Jenkins, 1985). Although it was first thought that this reduction in enzyme activity is primarily a genetically determined defect in the alcoholic (Palmer and Jenkins, 1982; Thomas *et al.*, 1982), it seems now clear that the decreased activity of mitochondrial and cytosolic ALDH observed in the alcoholic is the result of chronic alcohol abuse (Jenkins *et al.*, 1984; Palmer and Jenkins, 1985). Since in human alcoholics acetaldehyde concentrations in hepatic venous blood vary between 2 and 165 μM after a moderate dose of ethanol (Nuutinen *et al.*, 1984), it seems obvious that hepatic low-K_m and not high-K_m ALDH plays the dominant role in acetaldehyde metabolism. Nuutunen *et al.* (1983) found a decrease of hepatic low-K_m ALDH in chronic alcoholics.

High-K_m ALDH is also present in erythrocytes, and it was demonstrated that this enzyme activity is depressed in the alcoholic (Agarwal *et al.*, 1982). Whether the determination of ALDH activity in the erythrocyte may serve as a biological marker for alcoholism remains to be determined (Agarwal *et al.*, 1982).

Chronic ethanol ingestion also results in a significant reduction in the mitochondrial capacity to oxidize acetaldehyde irrespective of the presence of substrate for NAD^+-linked dehydrogenase (Hasumura *et al.*, 1975b). This effect has been attributed at least in part to the reduced ability of mitochondria from ethanol-fed rats to reoxidize NADH (Cederbaum *et al.*, 1974). Subsequently, blood acetaldehyde has been suggested as a marker for a predisposition to alcoholism. Acetaldehyde blood concentrations have been found to be elevated in healthy male relatives of alcoholics compared to matched controls (Schuckitt and Rayes, 1979). However, the methodology of acetaldehyde determination in this study has been criticized (Eriksson, 1980).

3. *Toxicity of Acetaldehyde*

Acetaldehyde is both pharmacologically and chemically a very potent and reactive compound. Acetaldehyde releases vasoactive substances such as catecholamines, and this may be responsible for the systemic effects discussed above. Acetaldehyde may also condense with catecholamines and produce tetrahydroisoquinolines, which could serve as false neurotransmitters (Cohen, 1973). The organ toxicity of acetaldehyde is probably related to its capacity to form adducts with various tissue components. Thus, acetaldehyde binds to liver plasma membranes (Barry *et al.*, 1984) and to hepatic protein (Nomura and Lieber, 1981; Medina *et al.*, 1985). It was suggested that liver plasma membrane-bound acetaldehyde may activate the complement sequence and may initiate alcoholic liver injury (Barry and McGivan, 1985). Acetaldehyde also stimulates collagen and noncollagen protein production in human fibroblasts (Holt *et al.*, 1984). All these data emphasize the damaging effect of acetaldehyde on structure and function of the hepatocyte. However, studies by Nakatsukase *et al.* (1985) in which extremely high hepatic acetaldehyde concentrations were produced in the rat questioned the pathophysiological role of acetaldehyde in the development of alcoholic liver disease, since the livers of the animals were found to be histologically normal.

Chronic ethanol consumption results in morphological alterations of the mitochondria in animals and in humans (Lieber, 1985; Arai *et al.*, 1984). Loss of structure and giant mitochondria have been reported. These morphological alterations are partly accompanied by a loss of function (Gordon, 1973). Thus, chronic ethanol feeding in rats leads to a decrease in cytochromes *a* and *b* as well as in the activity of mitochondrial succinate dehydrogenase (Oudea *et al.*, 1970; Rubin *et al.*, 1970c). The reduced activity of ALDH observed after chronic ethanol intake may play an important role in the pathogenesis of mitochondrial damage (Palmer and Jenkins, 1985). This results in increasing hepatic concentrations of acetaldehyde, which further damages the mitochondria and initiates a vicious cycle. Besides acetaldehyde-mediated mitochondrial injury, direct alterations of the mitochondrial membrane by ethanol have been implicated in the functional alteration (Schanne *et al.*, 1981). However, Gordon *et al.* (1982) was not able to confirm this hypothesis, and French *et al.* (1983) demonstrated that the morphological and histological mitochondrial damage may not necessarily represent a progressive destructive effect of ethanol.

Another target of acetaldehyde are the hepatic microtubules. which decrease in number and become shorter and thicker after chronic alcohol abuse (Matsuda *et al.*, 1979). The result is a decrease in hepatic content of polymerized tubulin and an increase in free tubulin (Baraona *et al.*, 1984). The functional consequences are the same as after the application of colchicine or *Vinca* alkaloids, namely, an inhibition of protein secretion. Baraona *et al.* (1975) could demonstrate that hepatomegaly after alcohol ingestion is due not only to lipid accumulation but also to the accumulation of protein and water. Storage of lipoproteins leads to a significant enlargement of the Golgi apparatus (Matsuda *et al.*, 1979). The antimicrotubular activity is closely related to the presence of acetaldehyde. 4-Methylpyrazole, a potent ADH inhibitor, leads to a reduced production of acetaldehyde, and this abolishes the deleterious effect on the microtubules (Denk, 1985). On the other hand, the microtubular injury is enhanced by simultaneous administration of disulfiram, an ALDH inhibitor (Denk, 1985), which results in elevated acetaldehyde levels.

In this context it seems of interest that advanced ethanol-associated liver disease is indicated by a reduction of serum lipoproteins due to the ethanol-induced alteration of lipoprotein synthesis and secretion. Normal α- and pre-β-lipoproteins are absent in serum, and are replaced by functional and structural abnormal lipoproteins (Baraona, 1985). On the other hand, the consequence of the enlargement of the hepatocyte, the so-called ballooning, is a reduction in intercellular space associated with a decrease of Disse space and increased portal pressure (Orrego *et al.*, 1981). This mechanism, in addition to perivenular and perisinusoidal fibrosis, is another pathophysiological basis for the development of portal hypertension.

Acetaldehyde not only reacts with cell organelles, but also with a variety of intermediates such as mercaptans and L-cysteine which complex with acetaldehyde to form hemiacetals. Such binding with cysteine and glutathione may contribute to the depression of hepatic glutathione (Shaw *et al.*, 1981). Since glutathione offers one the possibility of scavenging toxic free radicals, a severe reduction of glutathione favors lipid peroxidation (Wendell and Thurman, 1979). It is well known that the MEOS is capable of producing lipid peroxides. In addition, increased activity of microsomal NADPH oxidase after chronic ethanol ingestion could result in an enhanced production of H_2O_2, also favoring lipid peroxidation (Lieber and DeCarli, 1970b).

In the rat, acute ethanol administration (3 gm/kg body weight) does not influence lipid peroxidation, while the same dose does produce lipid peroxidation after chronic alcohol feeding (Shaw *et al.*, 1981). This enhanced lipid peroxidation could be prevented by the administration of methionine, a precursor of glutathione. Decreased hepatic glutathione concentrations and an increased hepatic lipid peroxidation was also found in the baboon and in human liver biopsy specimens (Shaw *et al.*, 1983). It seems, however, probable that decreased glutathione concentrations per se are not sufficient to induce liver damage. As a second factor, an enhanced production of radicals, possibly resulting from microsomal induction, has to be considered.

III. NUTRITIONAL EFFECTS OF ETHANOL

On the basis of some animal experiments it was generally believed until the mid-1960s that liver disease of the alcoholic was due exclusively to malnutrition and not to direct toxic effects of ethanol itself (Best *et al.*, 1949). Characteristically, alcoholic cirrhosis was called "fatty nutritional cirrhosis." Meanwhile, however, ethanol was identified as the toxic agent, and even the dietary supplementation of choline, a potent lipotropic factor, cannot prevent alcholic liver disease in the baboon, but instead causes additional toxicity (Lieber *et al.*, 1985).

Alcoholics undoubtedly suffer from malnutrition for a variety of reasons. Alcohol has a high caloric value (1 gm supplies 7.1 calories), but alcoholic calories are so-called empty calories, since much of the energy is transferred into heat because of the ethanol-associated hypermetabolism as already discussed. Weight gain is significantly lower with ethanol than with isocaloric amounts of carbohydrates (Pirola and Lieber, 1972). Furthermore, alcoholic beverages are usually devoid of minerals, vitamins, and protein. Because alcohol fulfills much of the caloric requirement by providing a large fraction of the daily intake, it may result in a decreased intake of other nutrients and, in addition, indigestion and malabsorption may further contribute to secondary malnutrition.

A. Nutritional Effects of Alcohol-Associated Organ Damage

Apart from dietary intake and imbalance, the overall alcohol-mediated nutritional changes are determined by the associated organ damage. Alcoholic gastritis causes anorexia, retching, and vomiting. Intestinal alterations lead to difficulties in the absorption of specific nutrients including thiamin, folate, vitamin B_{12}, glucose, and amino acids (Mezey, 1985). In addition, diarrhea may occur probably because of the influence of alcohol on the cyclic AMP system in the large intestine (Seitz *et al.*, 1983). Pancreatic disease leads to steatorrhea with malabsorption of essential fatty acids, fat-soluble vitamins, and calcium (Singer and Goebell, 1985). Alcoholic liver disease leads to the failure of protein biosynthesis, amino acid imbalance, reduced zinc storage, enhanced metabolism, and failure to store vitamins A and B_6 (Sherlock, 1984).

As one consequence of protein malnutrition, cell-mediated immunity is depressed in alcoholic patients as shown by *in vitro* tests of suppressor cell function and by helper/suppressor cell ratios (Alexander *et al.*, 1983). Interestingly, triceps skinfold thickness and hypoalbuminemia correlate with skin test anergy (O'Keefe *et al.*, 1980). Alcoholics of good nutritional status also show poor responses to tetanus toxoid (Cherick *et al.*, 1959) and to hepatitis B vaccine (Degos *et al.*, 1983), indicating a reduced immunological response.

B. Effect of Ethanol on the Metabolism of Minerals and Vitamins

1. Iron and Zinc Metabolism

Acute ethanol administration may increase iron absorption from the intestine, probably due to the stimulation of gastric acid secretion or to folic acid deficiency (Mezey, 1985). In addition, ethanol or its metabolite acetaldehyde inhibits hematopoiesis, resulting in decreased iron utilization. These mechanisms could explain the increased hepatic iron stores observed in alcoholic liver disease which occasionally simulate hemochromatosis (Chapman *et al.*, 1983; LeSage *et al.*, 1983). However, serum iron levels are normal in most alcoholic patients, transferrin levels are low due to decreased hepatic synthesis, and iron stores are normal in patients without liver injury (Sherlock, 1984).

Chronic alcoholic patients exhibit low serum zinc levels as well as decreased concentrations of zinc in the liver and in the leukocytes, which is occasionally associated with clinical signs of zinc deficiency (McClain and Su, 1983; Sullivan and Lankford, 1965). Hyperzincuria and poor dietary intake may contribute toward zinc deficiency in alcoholics. In addition, intestinal zinc absorption was found to be impaired after chronic ethanol ingestion in animals (Antonson and Vanderhoof, 1983) and in humans (Dinsmore *et al.*, 1985), obviously due to alcohol itself, since Mills *et al.* (1983) found increased zinc absorption in patients with alcoholic cirrhosis but not currently consuming alcohol.

2. Vitamin Metabolism

a. Vitamin A. Symtpoms of vitamin A deficiency, including night blindness and hypogonadism, have been described in alcoholics (McClain *et al.*, 1979). Very low hepatic vitamin A levels have been found in patients with moderate alcoholic liver disease such as fatty liver in the presence of normal serum concentrations of vitamin A and retinol-binding protein (Leo *et al.*, 1982), and the reduction of vitamin A correlates with the degree of alcoholic liver injury in humans and in baboons (Leo *et al.*, 1983), and, a characteristic histological indication, the occurrence of multivesicular lysosomes has been reported. Vitamin A is metabolized by microsomal cytochrome P-450-dependent enzymes. Chronic ethanol ingestion increases this metabolism, which may result in a hepatic depletion of vitamin A (Sato and Lieber, 1982). In addition, enhanced vitamin A metabolism following chronic ethanol consumption probably results in the production of toxic vitamin A metabolites which may contribute to liver damage, exhibiting an increased number of lipocytes and myofibroblasts in the Disse's space, precursors of hepatic fibrosis (Leo *et al.*, 1982; Leo and Lieber, 1982, 1983; Lieber, 1984b). Therefore, although the alcoholic suffers from Vitamin A deficiency, supplementation of the vitamin seems crucial, since vitamin A in excess can initiate hepatic injury.

b. Vitamin B_1 (Thiamin). Approximately 30% of fairly well-nourished patients with alcoholic liver disease have thiamin deficiency as judged by low serum transketolase activity (Hoyumpa, 1983). The cause of thiamin deficiency is impaired intestinal absorption due to ethanol-induced alteration of the active transport system (Mezey, 1985).

c. Vitamin B_6 (Pyridoxine). The low serum concentrations of pyridoxine are probably due to ethanol and acetaldehyde acting on hepatic storage and metabolism of the vitamin (Bonjour, 1980), although liver disease by itself reduces serum pyridoxine concentrations. Pyridoxine deficiency may account for the appearance of ring sideroblasts in the bone marrow.

d. Folate and Vitamin B_{12}. Folate deficiency as shown by reduced serum and red cell concentrations is common in alcoholics (Leevy *et al.*, 1965). Alcohol ingestion accelerates the rate of decline of circulating folate and reduces the absorption and tissue uptake of folic acid (Mezey, 1985). In the monkey, decreased absorption of folic acid has been found after 12 months of ethanol feeding despite an adequate diet (Romero *et al.*, 1981). As a consequence of folate deficiency mild macrocytic anemia may be found, but the macrocytosis so common in alcoholics is related to a direct effect of ethanol on the bone marrow. Reduced folate, in turn, leads to malabsorption of thiamin, vitamin B_{12}, xylose, water, sodium, and folic acid itself.

Alcoholics rarely show deficiency of vitamin B_{12}, and, when present, the deficiency probably reflects interference by alcohol with vitamin B_{12} absorption (Leevy *et al.*, 1965; Sherlock, 1984).

e. Vitamin C (Ascorbic Acid). Low leukocyte levels of vitamin C as a measure of tissue stores are found in patients with alcoholic cirrhosis (McClain *et al.*, 1979). These levels correlate inversely with antipyrine half-life, suggesting that ascorbic acid deficiency interferes with drug metabolism (Sherlock, 1984).

f. Vitamin D. Alcoholics also exhibit low circulating concentrations of 25-hydroxyvitamin D. Ethanol as a microsomal enzyme inducer might increase the hepatic conversion of vitamin D to polar intermediates. Hydroxylation of vitamin D in the liver is probably not affected by alcohol (Sherlock, 1984).

ACKNOWLEDGMENTS

Original studies have been supported by the Deutsche Forschungsgemeinschaft (*Se* 333/-1,2,4-1,6-1,2).

REFERENCES

Agarwal, D. P., and Goedde, A. W. (1984). Alkohol metabolisierende Enzyme: Alkoholunverträglichkeit und Alkoholkrankheit. *In* "Klinische Genetik des Alkoholismus" (K. D. Zang, ed.), pp. 65–89. Kohlhammer Verlag, Stuggart.

Agarwal, D. P., Harada, S., and Goedde, A. W. (1981). Racial differences in biological sensitivity to ethanol: The role of alcohol dehydrogenase and aldehyde dehydrogenase isoenzymes. *Alcohol.: Clin. Exp. Res.* **5**, 12–16.

Agarwal, D. P., Tobar-Rojas, L., Meier-Tackmann, D., Harada, S., Schrappe, O., Kaschkat, G., and Goedde, H. W. (1982). Erythrocyte aldehyde dehydrogenase: A biochemical marker of alcoholism? *Alcohol.: Clin. Exp. Res.* **6**, 426–438.

Alexander, G. J. M., Nouri-Aria, K. T., Eddelston, A. L. W. F., and Williams, R. (1983). Contrasting relations between suppressor-cell function and suppressor cell number in chronic liver disease. *Lancet* **1**, 1291–1293.

Antonson, D. L., and Vanderhoof, J. A. (1983). Effect of chronic ethanol ingestion in zinc absorption in rat small intestine. *Dig. Dis. Sci.* **28**, 604–608.

Arai, M., Leo, M. A., Nakano, M., Gordon, E. R., and Lieber, C. S. (1984). Biochemical and morphological alterations of baboon hepatic mitochondria after chronic ethanol consumption. *Hepatology* **4**, 165–174.

Baraona, E. (1985). Ethanol and lipid metabolism. *In* "Alcohol Related Diseases in Gastroenterology" (H. K. Seitz and B. Kommerell, eds.), pp. 65–96. Springer-Verlag, Berlin and New York-Tokyo.

Baraona, E., and Lieber, C. S. (1970). Effect of chronic ethanol feeding of serum lipoprotein metabolism in the rat. *J. Clin. Invest.* **49**, 769–778.

Baraona, E., Leo, M. A., Borowski, S. A., and Lieber, C. S. (1975). Alcoholic hepatomegaly: Accumulation of protein in the liver. *Science* **190**, 794–795.

Baraona, E., Leo, M. A., Borowski, S. A., and Lieber, C. S. (1977). Pathogenesis of alcohol-induced accumulation of protein in the liver. *J. Clin. Invest.* **60**, 546–554.

Baraona, E., Pikkarainen, P., Salaspuro, M., Finkelman, F., and Lieber, C. S. (1980). Acute effects of ethanol on hepatic protein synthesis and secretion in the rat. *Gastroenterology* **79**, 104–111.

Baraona, E., Jauhonen, P., Miyakawa, H., and Lieber, C. S. (1983). Zonal redox changes as a cause of selective perivenular hepatotoxicity of ethanol. *Pharmacol., Biochem. Behav.* **18** Suppl. 1, 449–454.

Baraona, E., Finkelman, F., and Lieber, C. S. (1984). Reevaluation of the effects of alcohol consumption on rat liver microtubules. *Res. Commun. Chem. Pathol. Pharmacol.* **44**, 265–278.

Barry, R. E., and McGivan, J. D. (1985). Acetaldehyde alone may initiate hepatocellular damage in acute alcoholic liver disease. *Gut* **26**, 1065–1069.

Barry, R. E., McGivan, J. D., and Hayes, M. (1984). Acetaldehyde binds to liver cell membranes without affecting membrane function. *Gut* **25**, 412–416.

Bernstein, J., Videla, L., and Israel, Y. (1973). Metabolic alterations produced in the liver by chronic ethanol administration. Changes related to energetic parameters of the cell. *Biochem. J.* **134**, 515–522.

Bernstein, J., Videla, L., and Israel, Y. (1975). Hormonal influence in the development of the hypermetabolic state of the liver produced by chronic administration of ethanol. *J. Pharmacol. Exp. Ther.* **192**, 583–591.

Best, C. H., Hartroft, W. S., and Lucas, S. S. (1949). Liver damage produced by feeding alcohol or sugar and its prevention by choline. *Br. Med. J.* **2**, 1001–1006.

Björkhem, I. (1972). On the role of alcohol dehydrogenase in ω-oxidation of fatty acids. *Eur. J. Biochem.* **30**, 441–445.

Blomstrand, R., and Karger, L. (1973). The combustion of triolein-1-^{14}C and its inhibition by alcohol in man. *Life Sci.* **13**, 113–123.

Blomstrand, R., Karger, L., and Lantto, O. (1973). Studies on the ethanol-induced decrease of fatty acid oxidation in rat and human liver slices. *Life Sci.* **13**, 1131–1141.

Bode, J. C., Rust, S., and Bode, C. (1984). The effect of cimetidine treatment on ethanol formation in the human stomach. *Scand. J. Gastroenterol.* **19**, 853–856.

Bonjour, S. A. (1980). Vitamins and alcoholism. III. Vitamin B_6. *Int. J. Vitam. Nutr. Res.* **50**, 215–230.

Borowsky, S. A., and Lieber, C. S. (1978). Interaction of methadone and ethanol metabolism. *J. Pharmacol. Exp. Ther.* **207**, 123–129.

Bosterling, B., and Trudel, J. R. (1981). Association of cytochrome b_5 and cytochrome P-450 reductase with cytochrome P-450 in the membrane of reconstituted vesicles. *J. Biol. Chem.* **257**, 4783–4787.

Boveris, A., Oshino, N., and Chance, B. (1972). The cellular production of hydrogen peroxide. *Biochem. J.* **128**, 617–630.

Buehler, R., Hess, M., and von Wartburg, J. P. (1982). Immunistochemical localization of human liver alcohol dehydrogenase in liver tissue, cultured fibroblasts and HeLa cells. *Am. J. Pathol.* **108**, 89–99.

Burnett, D. A., and Sorrell, M. F. (1981). Alcoholic cirrhosis. *Clin. Gastroenterol.* **10**, 443–455.

Carter, E. A., and Isselbacher, K. J. (1971). The role of microsomes in the hepatic metabolism of ethanol. *Ann. N.Y. Acad. Sci.* **179**, 282–294.

Carulli, N., Maneti, F., Gallo, M., and Saviolo, G. F. (1971). Alcohol–drug interactions in man: Alcohol and tolbutamide. *Eur. J. Clin. Invest.* **1**, 421–424.

Cederbaum, I. A., Lieber, C. S., and Rubin, E. (1974). Effects of chronic ethanol treatment on mitochondrial functions. *Arch. Biochem. Biophys.* **165**, 560–569.

Cederbaum, I. A., Dicker, E., and Lieber, C. S. (1977). Factors contributing to the adaptive increase in ethanol metabolism due to chronic consumption of ethanol. *Alcohol.: Clin. Exp. Res.* **1**, 27–31.

Cerra, F. B., Caprioli, J., Siegel, J. H., McMenamy, R. R., and Border, J. R. (1979). Proline metabolism in sepsis, cirrhosis and general surgery: The peripheral energy deficit. *Ann. Surg.* **190**, 557–586.

Chance, B., and Oshino, N. (1971). Kinetics and mechanisms of catalase in peroxisomes of the mitochondrial fraction. *Biochem. J.* **122**, 225–233.

Chapman, R. W., Morgan, M. Y., Bell, R., and Sherlock, S. (1983). Hepatic iron uptake in alcoholic liver disease. *Gastroenterology* **84**, 143–147.

Cherrick, G. R., Pothier, L., Dufour, J. J., and Sherlock, S. (1959). Immunologic response to tetanus toxoid inoculation in patients with hepatic cirrhosis. *N. Engl. J. Med.* **261**, 340–342.

Chiao, Y. B., Johnson, A. B., Gavaler, J. S., and Van Thiel, D. H. (1981). Effect of chronic ethanol feeding on testicular content on enzymes required for testosterone genesis. *Alcohol.: Clin. Exp. Res.* **5**, 230–235.

Chung, H., and Brown, D. R. (1976). Mechanism of the effect of acute ethanol on hexobarbital metabolism. *Biochem. Pharmacol.* **25**, 1613–1616.

City of New York, Department of Health (1981). "Summary of Vital Statistics of the City of New York." Bureau of Health Statistics and Analysis.

Cohen, G. (1973). Tetraisoquinoline alkaloids: Uptake, storage and secretion by adrenal medulla and by adrenergic nerves. *Ann. N.Y. Acad. Sci.* **215**, 116–119.

Comai, K., and Gaylor, J. L. (1973). Existence and separation of three forms of cytochrome *P*-450 from rat liver microsomes. *J. Biol. Chem.* **248**, 4947–4955.

Conney, A. H. (1967). Pharmacological implications of microsomal enzyme induction. *Pharmacol. Rev.* **19**, 317–366.

Cushman, P., Barboriak, J. J., Liao, A., and Hoffman, N. E. (1982). Association between plasma high-density lipoprotein cholesterol and antipyrine metabolism in alcoholics. *Life Sci.* **30**, 1721–1724.

Daughaday, W. H., Lipicky, R. J., and Rasinski, D. C. (1962). Lactic acidosis as a cause of nonketotic acidosis in diabetic patients. *N. Engl. J. Med.* **267**, 1010–1014.

DeCarli, L. M., and Lieber, C. S. (1967). Fatty liver in the rat after prolonged intake of ethanol with a nutritionally adequate new liquid diet. *J. Nutr.* **91**, 331–336.

Degos, F., Brechot, C., and Nalmas, B. (1983). Hepatitis B vaccination and alcoholic cirrhosis. *Lancet* **2**, 1498.

Deitrich, R. A. (1966). Tissue and subcellular distribution of mammalian aldehyde oxidizing capacity. *Biochem. Pharmacol.* **15**, 1911–1922.

Denk, H. (1985). Ethanol, Mallory bodies, and microtubular system. *In* "Alcohol Related Diseases in Gastroenterology" (H. K. Seitz and B. Kommerell, eds.), pp. 154–171. Springer-Verlag, Berlin and New York.

Desmond, P. V., Pardwarthan, R. V., Schenker, S., and Hoyumpa, H. M. (1980). Short term ethanol administration impairs the elimination of chlordiazepoxide in man. *Eur. J. Clin. Pharmacol.* **18**, 275–278.

Dicker, E., and Cederbaum, A. I. (1983). Effect of ethanol and metabolic substrates on the oxidation of aminopyrine, formaldehyde and formate by isolated hepatocytes. *J. Pharmacol. Exp. Ther.* **227**, 687–693.

Dinsmore, W., Callender, M., McMaster, D., Todd, S. J., and Love, A. H. G. (1985). Zinc absorption in alcoholics using zinc-65. *Digestion* **32**, 238–242.

Domschke, S., Domschke, W., and Lieber, C. S. (1974). Hepatic redox state: Attenuation of the acute effects of ethanol induced by chronic ethanol consumption. *Life Sci.* **15**, 1327–1334.

Doss, M. O. (1985). Alcohol and porphyrin metabolism. *In* "Alcohol Related Diseases in Gastroenterology" (H. K. Seitz and B. Kommerell, eds.), pp. 232–252. Springer-Verlag, Berlin and New York.

Emby, D. J., and Fraser, B. N. (1977). Hepatotoxicity of paracetamol enhanced by ingestion of alcohol: Report of two cases. *S. Afr. Med. J.* **51**, 208–209.

Eriksson, C. J. P. (1980). Elevated blood acetaldehyde levels in alcoholics and their relatives: A reevaluation. *Science* **207**, 1383–1384.

Faller, J., and Fox, I. H. (1982). Ethanol-induced hyperuricemia evidence for increased urate production by activation of adenine nucleotide turnover. *N. Engl. J. Med.* **307**, 1598–1602.

Farinati, F., Zhou, Z., Bellah, J., Lieber, C. S., and Garro, A. J. (1985). Effect of chronic ethanol consumption on activation of nitrosopyrrolidine to a mutagen by rat upper alimentary tract, lung, and hepatic tissue. *Drug Metab. Dispos.* **13**, 210–214.

Feinman, L., and Lieber, C. S. (1972). Hepatic collagen metabolism: Effect of alcohol consumption in rats and baboons. *Science* **176**, 795.

Feinman, L., Baraona, E., Matzusaki, S., Korsten, M. A., and Lieber, C. S. (1978). Concentration dependence of ethanol metabolism in vivo in rats and man. *Alcohol.: Clin. Exp. Res.* **2**, 381–385.

Forsander, O. A. (1970). Influence of ethanol and butyraldoxime on liver metabolism. *Biochem. Pharmacol.* **19**, 2131–2136.

Forsander, O. A., Maenppa, P. H., and Salaspuro, M. P. (1965a). Influence of ethanol on the lactate/pyruvate and β-hydroxybutyrate/acetate ratios in rat liver experiments. *Acta Chem. Scand.* **19**, 1770–1771.

Forsander, O. A., Räihä, N., Salaspuro, M. P., and Mäenppä, P. (1965b). Influence of ethanol on the liver metabolism of fed and starved rats. *Biochem. J.* **94**, 259–265.

French, S. W. (1967). Effects of chronic ethanol feeding on rat liver phospholipids. *J. Nutr.* **91**, 292–298.

French, S. W., Ruebner, B. H., Mezey, E., Tamura, T., and Halsted, C. H. (1983). Effect of chronic ethanol feeding on hepatic mitochondria in the monkey. *Hepatology* **3**, 34–40.

French, S. W., Benson, N. C., and Sun, P. S. (1984). Centrolobular liver necrosis induced by hypoxia in chronic ethanol fed rats. *Hepatology* **4**, 912–917.

Garro, A. J., Seitz, H. K., and Lieber, C. S. (1981). Enhancement of dimethylnitrosamine metabolism and activation to a mutagen following chronic ethanol consumption. *Cancer Res.* **41**, 120–124.

Glenn, J. L., and Vanko, M. (1959). Choline and aldehyde oxidation by rat liver. *Arch. Biochem. Biophys.* **82**, 145–152.

Gordon, E. R. (1973). Mitochondrial functions in ethanol induced fatty liver. *J. Biol. Chem.* **248**, 8271–8280.

Gordon, E. R. (1977). ATP metabolism in an ethanol induced fatty liver. *Alcohol.: Clin. Exp. Res.* **1**, 21–25.

Gordon, E. R., Rochman, J., Arai, M., and Lieber, C. S. (1982). Lack of correlation between hepatic mitochondrial membrane structure and function in ethanol fed rats. *Science* **216**, 1319–1321.

Gordon, G. G., and Southren, A. L. (1977). Metabolic effects of alcohol on the endocrine system. *In* "Metabolic Aspects of Alcoholism" (C. S. Lieber, ed.), pp. 249–303. MTP Press, Lancaster.

Gordon, G. G., Vittek, J., Ho, R., Rosenthal, W. S., Southren, A. L., and Lieber, C. S. (1979). Effect of chronic alcohol use on hepatic testosterone 5α-A-ring reductase in the baboon and in the human being. *Gastroenterology* **77**, 110–114.

Green, H., and Goldberg, B. (1964). Collagen and cell protein synthesis by an established mammalian fibroblast line. *Nature (London)* **204**, 347–349.

Grunnet, N., Quistroff, B., and Thieden, H. I. D. (1973). Rate-limiting factors in ethanol concentration, fructose, pyruvate and pyrazole. *Eur. J. Biochem.* **40**, 275–282.

Hahn, E. G., and Schuppan, D. (1985). Ethanol and fibrogenesis in the liver. *In* "Alcohol Related Diseases in Gastroenterology" (H. K. Seitz and B. Kommerell, eds.), pp. 124–153. Springer-Verlag, Berlin and New York.

Hakkinen, H. M., and Kulonen, E. (1975). Effect of ethanol on the metabolism of alanine glutamic acid, and proline in the liver. *Biochem. Pharmacol.* **24**, 199–204.

Halle, P., Pare, P., Kapstein, E., Kanel, G., Redeker, A. G., and Reynolds, T. B. (1982). Double blind controlled trial of propylthiouracil in patients with severe acute alcoholic hepatitis. *Gastroenterology* **82**, 925–931.

Harada, S., Misawa, S., Agarwall, D. P., and Goedde, H. W. (1980). Liver alcohol dehydrogenase and aldehyde dehydrogenase in the Japanese: Isoenzyme variation and its possible role in alcohol intoxixation. *Am. J. Hum. Genet.* **32**, 8–15.

Harbitz, I., Wallin, B., Hauge, J. G., and Morland, J. (1984). Effect of ethanol metabolism on initiation of protein synthesis in rat hepatocyte. *Biochem. Pharmacol.* **33**, 3465–3470.

Haskell, W. L., Camargo, C., and Williams, P. T. (1984). The effect of cessation and resumption of moderate alcohol intake on serum high density lipoprotein subfractions: A controlled study. *N. Engl. J. Med.* **310**, 805–810.

Hasumura, Y., Teschke, R., and Lieber, C. S. (1974). Increased carbon tetrachloride hepatotoxicity and its mechanism, after chronic ethanol consumption. *Gastroenterology* **66**, 415–422.

Hasumura, Y., Teschke, R., and Lieber, C. S. (1975a). Hepatic microsomal ethanol oxidizing system (MEOS): Dissociation from reduced nicotinamide adenine dinucleotide phosphate-oxidase and possible role of form I cytochrome *P*-450. *J. Pharmacol. Exp. Ther.* **194**, 469–474.

Hasumura, Y., Teschke, R., and Lieber, C. S. (1975b). Acetaldehyde oxidation by hepatic mitochondria. Decrease after chronic ethanol consumption. *Science* **189**, 727–729.

Hawkins, R. D., Kalant, H., and Khanna, J. M. (1966). Effects of chronic intake of ethanol on rate of ethanol metabolism. *Can. J. Physiol. Pharmacol.* **44**, 241–257.

Held, H. (1977). Effect of alcohol on the heme and prophyrin synthesis interaction with phenobarbital and pyrazole. *Digestion* **15**, 136–146.

Hetú, C., Dumont, A., and Joly, J. G. (1983). Effect of chronic ethanol administration on bromobenzene liver toxicity in the rat. *Toxicol. Appl. Pharmacol.* **67**, 166–177.

Holt, K., Bennett, M., and Chojkier, M. (1984). Acetaldehyde stimulates collagen and noncollagen protein by human fibroblasts. *Hepatology* **5**, 843–848.

Hoyumpa, A. M. (1983). Alcohol and thiamine metabolism. *Alcohol.: Clin. Exp. Res.* **7**, 11–14.

Hoyumpa, A. M., and Schenker, S. (1982). Major drug interactions: Effect of liver disease, alcohol and malnutrition. *Annu. Rev. Med.* **33**, 113–149.

Hoyumpa, A. M., Desmond, P. V., Roberts. R. K., Nichols, S., Johnson, R. F., and Schenker, S. (1980). Effect of ethanol and benzodiazepine disposition in dogs. *J. Lab. Clin. Med.* **95**, 310–322.

Hoyumpa, A. M., Patwardhan, R., Maples, M., Desmon, P. V., Johnson, R. F., Sinclair, A. P., and Schenker, S. (1981). Effect of short term ethanol administration on lorazepam clearance. *Hepatology* **1**, 47–53.

Hulley, S. B., and Gordon, S. (1981). Alcohol and high density lipoprotein cholesterol. Causal inference from diverse study design. *Circulation* **64**, 57–63.

Iber, F. L. (1977). Drug metabolism in heavy consumers of ethyl alcohol. *Clin. Pharmacol. Ther.* **22**, 735–742.

Ikawa, M., Impraim, C. C., Wang, G., and Yoshida, A. (1983). Isolation and characterization of aldehyde dehydrogenase isoenzymes from usual and atypical human livers. *J. Biol. Chem.* **258**, 6282–6287.

Ingelman-Sundberg, M., and Johansson, I. (1981). The mechanism of cytochrome P-450-dependent oxidation of ethanol in reconstituted membrane vesicles. *J. Biol. Chem.* **256,** 6321.

Inoue, K., Rukunaga, M., and Yamasawa, K. (1980). Correlation between human erythrocyte aldehyde dehydrogenase activity and sensitivity to alcohol. *Pharmacol., Biochem. Behav.* **13.** 295–297.

Iseri, O. A., Lieber, C. S., and Gottlieb, L. S. (1966). The ultrastructure of fatty liver induced by prolonged ethanol ingestion. *Am. J. Pathol.* **48,** 535–555.

Ishii, H., Joly, J. G., and Lieber, C. S. (1973). Effect of ethanol on amount and enzyme activities of hepatic rough and smooth microsomal membranes. *Biochim. Biophys. Acta* **291,** 411–420.

Ishii, H., Okuno, F., Joly, J. G., and Tsuchiya, M. (1978). Alcohol induced changes of carbohydrate metabolism. *Leber, Magen, Darm* **8,** 247–254.

Ishii, H., Takagi, T., Okuno, F., Ebihara, Y., Taschiro, M., and Tsuchiya, M. (1983). Halothane-induced hepatic necrosis in ethanol pretreated rats. *In* "Biological Approach to Alcoholism" (C. S. Lieber, ed.), Res. Monogr. Vol. 11, pp. 152–159. U.S. Department of Health and Human Services, NIAAA, Maryland.

Ismail-Beigi, F., and Edelman, I. S. (1971). Mechanism of thyroid calorigenesis: Role of active sodium transport. *Proc. Natl. Acad. Sci. U.S.A.* **67,** 1071–1078.

Israel, Y., Videla, L., MacDonald, A., and Bernstein, J. (1973). Metabolic alterations produced in the liver by chronic ethanol administration. Comparison between the effect produced by ethanol and by thyroid hormones. *Biochem. J.* **134,** 523–529.

Israel, Y., Videla, L., Fernandes-Videla, V., and Bernstein, J. (1975a). Effect of chronic ethanol treatment and thyroxine administration on ethanol metabolism and liver oxidative capacity. *J. Pharmacol. Exp. Ther.* **192,** 565–574.

Israel, Y., Kalant, H., Orrego, H., Khanna, J. M., Videla, L., and Phillips, J. M. (1975b). Experimental alcohol-induced hepatic necrosis: Suppression by propylthiouracil. *Proc. Natl. Acad. Sci. U.S.A.* **72,** 1137–1141.

Jauhonen, P., Baraona, E., Miyakawa, H., and Lieber, C. S. (1982). Mechanisms for selective centrilobular hepatotoxicity of ethanol. *Alcohol.: Clin. Exp. Res.* **6,** 350–357.

Jenkins, W. J., Cakebread, K., and Palmer, K. R. (1984). Effect of ethanol consumption on hepatic aldehyde dehydrogenase activity in alcoholic patients. *Lancet* **1,** 1048–1049.

Joly, J. G., Ishii, H., and Lieber, C. S. (1972). Microsomal cyanide-binding cytochrome: Its role in hepatic ethanol oxidation. *Gastro enterology* **62,** 174.

Joly, J. G., Ishii, H., Teschke, R., Hasumura, Y., and Lieber, C. S. (1973). Effect of chronic ethanol feeding on the activities and submicrosomal distribution of reduced nicotinamide adenine dinucleotide phosphate (NADPH)-cytochrome P-450 reductase and demethylase for aminopyrine and ethylmorphine. *Biochem. Pharmacol.* **22,** 1532–1535.

Joly, J. G., Hetu, C., Mavier, P., and Villeneuve, J. P. (1976). Mechanisms of induction of hepatic drug-metabolizing enzymes by ethanol. I. Limited role of microsomal phospholipids. *Biochem. Pharmacol.* **25,** 1995–2001.

Joly, J. G., Villeneuve, J. P., and Mavier, P. (1977). Chronic ethanol administration induces a form of cytochrome P-450 with specific spectral and catalytic properties. *Alcohol.: Clin. Exp. Res.* **1,** 17–20.

Jorfeldt, L., and Juhlin-Dannfelt, A. (1978). The influence of ethanol on splanchnic and skeletal muscle metabolism in man. *Metab., Clin. Exp.* **27,** 97–106.

Jörnvall, H., and Pietruszko, R. (1972). Structural studies of alcohol dehydrogenase from human liver. *Eur. J. Biochem.* **25,** 283–290.

Kater, R. M. H., Carulli, M., and Iber, F. L. (1969a). Differences in the rate of ethanol metabolism in recently drinking alcoholic and non-alcoholic subjects. *Am. J. Clin. Nutr.* **22,** 1608–1617.

Kater, R. M. H., Roggin, G., Tobon, F., Zieve, F., and Iber, F. L. (1969b). Increased rate of clearance of drugs from the circulation of alcoholics. *Am. J. Med. Sci.* **258,** 35–39.

Kershenobich, D., Fierro, F. J., and Rojkind, M. (1970). The relationship between free pool of proline and collagen content in human liver cirrhosis. *J. Clin. Invest.* **49,** 2246–2249.

Kitson, T. M. (1977). The disulfiram–ethanol reaction. *J. Stud. Alcohol* **38,** 96–113.

Koff, R. S., and Fitts, J. J. (1972). Chlorpromazine inhibition of ethanol metabolism without prevention of fatty liver. *Biochem. Med.* **6,** 77–81.

Koop, D. R., Morgan, E. T., Tarr, G. E., and Coon, M. J. (1982). Purification and characterisation of a unique isoenzyme of cytochrome *P*-450 from liver microsomes of ethanol treated rabbits. *J. Biol. Chem.* **257,** 8472–8480.

Korsten, M. A., Matsusaki, S., Feinman, L., and Lieber, C. S. (1975). High blood acetaldehyde levels after ethanol administration. *N. Engl. J. Med.* **292,** 386–389.

Kowaloff, E. M., Phang, J. M., Granger, A. S., and Downing, S. J. (1977). Regulation of proline oxidase activity by lactate. *Proc. Natl. Acad. Sci. U.S.A.* **74,** 5368–5371.

Krebs, H. A. (1968). Effect of ethanol on gluconeogenesis in the prefused rat liver. *Konf. Ges. Biol. Chem., 3rd, 1967,* pp. 216–224.

Krebs, H. A., and Perkins, I. R. (1970). The physiological role of liver alcohol dehydrogenase. *Biochem. J.* **118,** 635–644.

Kreisberg, R. A., Owen, W. C., and Siegal, A. M. (1971). Ethanol induced hyperlactacidemia: Inhibition of lactate utilization. *J. Clin. Invest.* **50,** 166–174.

Lal, S. (1969). Metronidazole in the treatment of alcoholism: A clinical trial and review of the literature. *J. Stud. Alcohol* **30,** 140–151.

Lamb, R. G., Wood, C. K., and Fallon, H. J. (1979). The effect of acute and chronic ethanol intake on hepatic glycerolipid biosynthesis in the hamster. *J. Clin. Invest.* **63,** 14–20.

Lana, S. E., and Steward, M. E. (1983). Alcohol mediated effects on the level of cytochrome *P*-450 and heme biosynthesis in cultured rat hepatocytes. *Biochim. Biophys. Acta* **755,** 313–317.

Lane, B. P., and Lieber, C. S. (1967). Effect of butylated hydroxyanisole on the ultrastructure of rat hepatocyte. *Lab. Invest.* **16,** 341–348.

Leevy, C. M., Baker, H., and Tenhove, W. (1965). B-complex vitamins in liver disease of the alcoholic. *Am. J. Clin. Nutr.* **16,** 339–346.

Lefevre, A. F., Adler, H., and Lieber, C. S. (1970). Effect of ethanol on ketone metabolism. *J. Clin. Invest.* **49,** 1775–1782.

Leo, M. A., and Lieber, C. S. (1982). Hepatic vitamin A depletion in alcoholic liver injury. *N. Engl. J. Med.* **307,** 597–601.

Leo, M. A., and Lieber, C. S. (1983). Hepatic fibrosis after long-term administration of ethanol and moderate vitamin A supplementation in the rat. *Hepatology* **3,** 1–11.

Leo, M. A., Arai, M., Sato, M., and Lieber, C. S. (1982). Hepatotoxicity of vitamin A and ethanol in the rat. *Gastroenterology* **82,** 194–205.

Leo, M. A., Sato, M., and Lieber, C. S. (1983). Effect of hepatic vitamin A depletion on the liver in humans and rats. *Gastroenterology* **84,** 562–572.

LeSage, G. D., Baldus, W. P., Fairbanks, V. F., Baggenstoss, A. H., McCall, J. T., Moore, S. B., Taswell, H. F., and Gordon, H. (1983). Hemochromatosis: Genetic or alcohol-induced? *Gastroenterology* **84,** 1471–1477.

Lester, R., Eagon, P. K., and Van Thiel, D. H. (1979). Feminization of the alcoholic: The estrogen/testosterone ratio (E/T). *Gastroenterology* **76,** 415–417.

Levitt, M. D., Doizaki, W., and Levine, A. S. (1982). Hypothesis: Metabolic activity of the colonic bacteria influences organ injury from ethanol. *Hepatology* **2,** 598–600.

Lieber, C. S. (1984a). To drink (moderately) or not to drink? *N. Engl. J. Med.* **310,** 846–848.

Lieber, C. S. (1984b). Alcohol and the liver: Update 1984. *Hepatology* **4,** 1243–1260.

Lieber, C. S. (1985). Ethanol metabolism and pathophysiology of alcoholic liver disease. *In* "Alcohol Related Diseases in Gastroenterology" (H. K. Seitz and B. Kommerell, eds.), pp. 19–47. Springer-Verlag, Berlin and New York.

Lieber, C. S., and DeCarli, L. M. (1968). Ethanol oxidation by hepatic microsomes: Adaptive increase after ethanol feeding. *Science* **162,** 917–918.

Lieber, C. S., and DeCarli, L. M. (1970a). Hepatic microsomal ethanol oxidizing system: In vitro characteristics and adaptive properties in vivo. *J. Biol. Chem.* **245,** 2505–2512.

Lieber, C. S., and DeCarli, L. M. (1970b). Reduced nicotinamide adenine dinucleotide phosphate oxidase activity enhanced by chronic ethanol consumption. *Science* **170,** 78–80.

Lieber, C. S., and DeCarli, L. M. (1970c). Quantitative relationship between the amount of dietary fat and the severity of the alcoholic fatty liver. *Am. J. Clin. Nutr.* **23,** 474–478.

Lieber, C. S., and DeCarli, L. M. (1972). The role of hepatic microsomal ethanol oxidizing system (MEOS) for ethanol metabolism in vivo. *J. Pharmacol. Exp. Ther.* **181,** 279–287.

Lieber, C. S., and DeCarli, L. M. (1973). The significance and characterization of hepatic microsomal ethanol oxidation in the liver. *Drug Metab. Dispos.* **1,** 428–440.

Lieber, C. S., and DeCarli, L. M. (1974). An experimental model of alcohol feeding and liver injury in the baboon. *J. Med. Primatol.* **3,** 153–163.

Lieber, C. S., and DeCarli, L. M. (1982). The feeding of alcohol in liquid diets: Two decades of application and 1982 update. *Alcohol.: Clin. Exp. Res.* **6,** 523–531.

Lieber, C. S., and Schmid, R. (1961). The effect of ethanol on fatty acid metabolism: Stimulation of hepatic fatty acid synthesis in vitro. *J. Clin. Invest.* **40,** 394–399.

Lieber, C. S., and Spritz, N. (1966). Effect of prolonged ethanol intake in man: Role of dietary, adipose and endogenously synthesized fatty acids in the pathogenesis of alcoholic fatty liver. *J. Clin. Invest.* **45,** 1400–1411.

Lieber, C. S., Jones, D. P., and DeCarli, L. M. (1965). Effect of prolonged ethanol intake on production of fatty liver despite adequate diets. *J. Clin. Invest.* **44,** 1009–1021.

Lieber, C. S., Leevy, C. M., Stein, S. W., Georg, W. S., Cherrick, G. R., Abelmann, W. H., and Davidson, C. S. (1962). Effect of ethanol on plasma free fatty acids in man. *J. Lab. Clin. Med.* **59,** 826–832.

Lieber, C. S., Lefevre, A., Spritz, N., Feinmal, L., and DeCarli, L. M. (1967). Difference in hepatic metabolism of long and medium chain fatty acids: Role of fatty acid chain length in the production of alcoholic fatty liver. *J. Clin. Invest.* **46,** 1451–1460.

Lieber, C. S., Rubin, E., and DeCarli, L. M. (1970). Hepatic microsomal ethanol oxidizing system (MEOS): Differentiation from alcohol dehydrogenase and NADPH oxidase. *Biochem. Biophys. Res. Commun.* **40,** 858–865.

Lieber, C. S., Seitz, H. K., Garro, A. J., and Worner, T. M. (1979). Alcohol related diseases and carcinogenesis. *Cancer Res.* **39,** 2363–2886.

Lieber, C. S., Leo, M. A., Mak, K. M., DeCarli, L. M., and Sato, S. (1985). Choline fails to prevent liver fibrosis in ethanol fed baboons but causes toxicity. *Hepatology* **5,** 561–572.

Lindros, K. O., Oshino, N., Parilla, R., and Williamson, J. R. (1974). Characteristics of ethanol acetaldehyde oxidation on flavine and pyridine nucleotide fluorescence changes in perfused rat liver. *J. Biol. Chem.* **249,** 7956–7963.

Lindros, K. O., Stowell, A., Pikkarainen, P., and Salaspuro, M. (1980). Elevated blood acetaldehyde in alcoholics with accelerated ethanol elimination. *Pharmacol., Biochem. Behav.* **13,** 119–124.

Lindy, S., Petersen, F. B., Turt, H., and Uitto, J. (1971). Lactate, lactate dehydrogenase and protocollagen proline hydroxylase in rat skin autografts. *Hoppe-Seyler's Z. Physiol. Chem.* **352,** 1113–1118.

Lundquist, F., Tygstrup, N., Winkler, K., and Jensen, B. (1965). Glycerol metabolism in the human liver. *Science* **151,** 616–617.

McClain, C. J., and Su, L. C. (1983). Zinc deficiency in the alcoholic: A review. *Alcohol.: Clin. Exp. Res.* **7,** 5–10.

McClain, C. J., VanThie, D. H., and Parker, S. (1979). Alteration in zinc, vitamin A and retinol-binding protein in chronic alcoholics: A possible mechanism for night blindness and hypogonadism. *Alcohol.: Clin. Exp. Res.* **3,** 135–141.

McColl, K. E. L., Moore, M. R., Thompson, G. G., and Goldberg, A. (1981). Abnormal heme biosynthesis in chronic alcoholics. *Eur. J. Clin. Invest.* **10,** 461–468.

McManus, I. R., Contag, A. O., and Olson, R. E. (1966). Studies on the identification and origin of ethanol in mammalian tissues. *J. Biol. Chem.* **241,** 349–356.

Maddrey, W. C., and Boyer, J. L. (1973). The acute and chronic effects of ethanol administration on bile secretion in the rat. *J. Lab. Clin. Med.* **82,** 215–225.

Mak, K. M., and Lieber, C. S. (1984). Alcoholic liver injury in baboons: Transformation of lipocytes to transitional cells. *Gastroenterology* **87,** 188–200.

Maling, H. M., Stripp, B., Sipes, I. G., Highman, B., Saul, W., and Williams, M. A. (1975). Enhanced hepatotoxicity of carbon tetrachloride, thioacetamide and dimethylnitrosamine by pretreatment of rats with ethanol and some comparison with potentiation by isopropanol. *Toxicol. Appl. Pharmacol.* **33,** 291–308.

Marin, G. A., Ward, N. L., and Fischer, R. (1973). Effect of ethanol on pancreatic and biliary secretion in humans. *Am. J. Dig. Dis.* **18,** 825–833.

Marin, G. A., Karjoo, M., Ward, N. L., and Rosato, E. (1975). Effects of alcohol biliary lipids in the presence of a chronic biliary fistula. *Surg., Gynecol. Obstet.* **141,** 352–356.

Maruyama, K., Feinman, L., Fainsilber, Z., Nakano, M., Okazaki, I., and Lieber, C. S. (1982). Measurement of mammalian collagenase in alcohol fed baboons and patients with alcoholic liver disease: Decrease in activity with development of cirrhosis. *In* "Proceedings of the Conference on Connective Tissue of the Normal and Fibrotic Human Liver" (J. Rauterbaerg, ed.), pp. 196–198. Thieme, Stuttgart.

Mata, J. M., Kershenobich, D., Villareal, E., and Rojkind, M. (1975). Serum free proline and free hydroxyproline in patients with chronic liver disease. *Gastroenterology* **68,** 1265–1269.

Matsuda, Y., Baraona, E., Salaspuro, M., and Lieber, C. S. (1979). Effects of ethanol on liver microtubules and Golgi apparatus. *Lab. Invest.* **41,** 455–463.

Matsuzaki, S., Gordon, E., and Lieber, C. S. (1981). Increased ADH independent ethanol oxidation at high ethanol concentrations in isolated rat hepatocytes: The effect of chronic ethanol feeding. *J. Pharmacol. Exp. Ther.* **217,** 133–137.

Medina, V. A., Donohue, T. M., Sorrell, M. F., and Tuma, D. J. (1985). Covalent binding of acetaldehyde to hepatic proteins during ethanol oxidation. *J. Lab. Clin. Med.* **105,** 5–10.

Mendenhall, C. L., Bradford, R. H., and Furman, R. H. (1969). Effects of ethanol on glycerolipid metabolism in rat liver. *Biochim. Biophys. Acta* **187,** 501–509.

Mendenhall, C. L., Chedid, A., and Kromme, C. (1984). Altered proline uptake by mouse liver cells after chronic exposure to ethanol and its metabolites. *Gut* **25,** 138–144.

Meldolesi, J. (1967). On the significance of the hypertrophy of the smooth endoplasmic reticulum in liver cells after administration of drugs. *Biochem. Pharmacol.* **16,** 125–131.

Mezey, E. (1985). Effect of ethanol on intestinal morphology, metabolism and function. *In* "Alcohol Related Diseases in Gastroenterology" (H. K. Seitz and B. Kommerell, eds.), pp. 342–360. Springer-Verlag, Berlin and New York.

Mezey, E., and Potter, J. J. (1981). Effect of ethanol on hepatic proline-metabolizing enzymes in the rat. *J. Lab. Clin. Med.* **98,** 776–783.

Mezey, E., Potter, J. J., and Reed, W. D. (1973). Ethanol oxidation by components of liver microsomes rich in cytochrome *P*-450. *J. Biol. Chem.* **248,** 1183–1187.

Mills, P. R., Fell, G. S., and Bessent, R. G. (1983). A study of zinc metabolism in alcoholic cirrhosis. *Clin. Sci.* **64,** 527–535.

Milner, G., and Landauer, A. A. (1971). Alcohol, thioridazine and chlorpromazine effects on skills related to driving behaviour. *Br. J. Psychiatry* **118,** 351–352.

Misra, P. S., Lefevre, A., Ishii, H., Rubin, E., and Lieber, C. S. (1971). Increase of ethanol, meprobamate and pentobarbital metabolism after chronic ethanol administration in man and in rats. *Am. J. Med.* **51,** 346–351.

Mitchell, M. C., Hoyumpa, A. M., Schenker, S., Johnson, R. F., Nichols, S., and Patwardhan, R. V. (1983). Inhibition of caffeine elimination by short term ethanol administration. *J. Lab. Clin. Med.* **101,** 826–834.

Mizoi, Y., Ijiri, I., Tatsuno, Y., Kijima, T., Fujiwara, S., and Adachi, J. (1979). Relationship between facial flushing and blood acetaldehyde levels after alcohol intake. *Pharmacol., Biochem. Behav.* **10**, 303–311.

Moldeus, P., Andersson, B., and Norling, A. (1978). Interaction of ethanol oxidation with glucuronidation in isolated hepatocytes. *Biochem. Pharmacol.* **27**, 2583–2588.

Moore, M. R., Beattie, A. D., Thompson, G. G., and Goldberg, A. (1971). Depression of aminolevulinic acid dehydratase activity by ethanol in man and in rats. *Clin. Sci.* **40**, 81–88.

Moreland, J., Rothschild, M. A., Oratz, M., Mongelli, J., Donor, D., and Schreiber, S. S. (1981). Protein secretion in suspension of isolated rat hepatocytes: No influence of acute ethanol administration. *Gastroenterology* **80**, 159–165.

Morgan, E. T., Koop, D. R.,and Coon, M. J. (1982). Catalytic activity of cytochrome *P*-450 isoenzyme 3a isolated from liver microsomes of ethanol treated rabbits. *J. Biol. Chem.* **257**, 13951–13957.

Nakano, M., Worner, T. M., and Lieber, C. S. (1982). Perivenular fibrosis in alcoholic liver injury: Ultrastructure and histologic progression. *Gastroenterology* **83**, 777–785.

Nakatsukasa, H., Watanabe, A., Kobayashi, M., Hobara, N., Fujiwara, M., Yamauchi, Y., Shiota, T., Higashi, T., and Nagashima, N. (1985). Effect of high hepatic acetaldehyde levels following simultaneous administration of ethanol and cyanamide on liver function in rats. *Res. Exp. Med.* **185**, 221–225.

Nikkilä, E. A., and Ojala, K. (1963). Role of hepatic L-glycerophosphate and triglyceride synthesis in the production of fatty liver by ethanol. *Proc. Soc. Exp. Biol. Med.* **113**, 814–817.

Nomura, F., and Lieber, C. S. (1981). Binding of acetaldehyde to rat liver microsomes: Enhancement after chronic ethanol consumption. *Biochem. Biophys. Res. Commun.* **100**, 131–137.

Nuutinen, H., Lindros, K. O., and Salaspuro, M. (1983). Determinants of blood acetaldehyde levels during ethanol oxidation in chronic alcoholics. *Alcohol.: Clin. Exp. Res.* **7**, 163–168.

Nuutinen, H., Salaspuro, M., Valle, M., and Lindros, K. O. (1984). Blood acetaldehyde concentration gradient between hepatic and antecubital venous blood in ethanol intoxicated alcoholics and controls. *Eur. J. Clin. Invest.* **14**, 306–311.

Oguma, T., and Levy, G. (1981). Acute effects of ethanol on hepatic first pass elimination of propoxyphene in rats. *J. Pharmacol. Exp. Ther.* **219**, 7–13.

Ohnishi, K., and Lieber, C. S. (1977). Reconstitution of the microsomal ethanol oxidizing system (MEOS): Qualitative and quantitative changes of cytochrome *P*-450 after chronic ethanol consumption. *J. Biol. Chem.* **252**, 7124–7131.

Ohnishi, K., and Lieber, C. S. (1978). Respective role of superoxide and hydroxyl radical in the activity of the reconstituted microsomal ethanol oxidizing system. *Arch. Biochem. Biophys.* **191**, 798–803.

Okazaki, I., Feinman, L., and Lieber, C. S. (1977). Hepatic mammalian collagenase: Development of an assay and demonstration of increased activity after ethanol consumption. *Gastroenterology* **73**, 1236.

O'Keefe, S. J., El-Zayadi, A. R., Carraherte, T. E., Davis, M., and Williams, R. (1980). Malnutrition and immunocompetence in patients with liver disease. *Lancet* **2**, 615–616.

Okuda, K., and Takigawa, N. (1970). Rat liver 5-cholestane-3,7,12,26-tetrol dehydrogenase as a liver alcohol dehydrogenase. *Biochim. Biophys. Acta* **22**, 141–148.

Olson, H., and Morland, J. (1978). Ethanol induced increase in drug acetylation in man and isolated rat liver cells. *Br. Med. J.* **2**, 1260–1262.

Ontko, J. A. (1973). Effect of ethanol on the metabolism of free fatty acids in isolated liver cells. *J. Lipid Res.* **14**, 78–85.

Orme-Johnson, W. H., and Ziegler, D. M. (1965). Alcohol mixed function oxidase activity of mammalian liver microsomes. *Biochem. Biophys. Res. Commun.* **21**, 78–82.

Orrego, H., Kalant, H., Israel, Y., Blake, J., Medline, A., Rankin, J. G., Armstrong, A., and Kapur, B. (1979). Effect of short term therapy with propylthiouracil in patients with alcoholic liver disease. *Gastroenterology* **76**, 106–115.

Orrego, H., Blendis, L. M., Crossley, I. R., Medline, A., MacDonald, A., Ritchie, S., and Israel, Y. (1981). Correlation of intrahepatic pressure with collagen in the Disse space and hepatomegaly in humans and in the rat. *Gastroenterology* **80**. 546–566.

Oudea, M. C., Launay, A. N., Queneherve, S., and Oudea, P. (1970). The hepatic lesions produced in the rat by chronic alcohol intoxication. Histological, ultrastructural and biochemical observations. *Rev. Etud. Clin. Biol.* **15**, 748–764.

Palmer, K. R., and Jenkins, W. J. (1982). Impaired acetaldehyde oxidation in alcoholics. *Gut* **23**, 729–733.

Palmer, K. R., and Jenkins, W. J. (1985). Aldehyde dehydrogenase in alcoholic subjects. *Hepatology* **5**, 260–263.

Paronetto, F. (1985). Ethanol and the immune system. *In* "Alcohol Related Diseases in Gastroenterology" (H. K. Seitz and B. Kommerell, eds.), pp. 269–281. Springer-Verlag, Berlin and New York.

Pequignot, G., and Tuyns, A. J. (1980). Compared toxicity of ethanol on various organs. *In* "Alcohol and the Gastrointestinal Tract" (C. Stock and H. Sarles, eds.), pp. 17–32. INSERM, Paris.

Pestalozzi, D. M., Buehler, R., von Wartburg, J. P., and Hess, M. (1983). Immunohistochemical localisation of alcohol dehydrogenase in the human gastrointestinal tract. *Gastroenterology* **85**, 1011–1016.

Pikkarainen, P., and Lieber, C. S. (1980). Concentration dependency of ethanol elimination rates in baboons: Effect of chronic alcohol consumption. *Alcohol.: Clin. Exp. Res.* **4**, 40–43.

Pikkarainen, P., Baraona, E., Jauhonen, P., Seitz, H. K., and Lieber, C. S. (1981a). Contribution of oropharynx microflora and of lung microsomes to acetaldehyde in expired air after ethanol ingestion. *J. Lab. Clin. Med.* **97**, 631–636.

Pikkarainen, P., Gordon, E., Lebsack, M. E., and Lieber, C. S. (1981b). Determinants of plasma free acetaldehyde levels during oxidation of ethanol. *Biochem. Pharmacol.* **30**, 799–802.

Pirola, R., and Lieber, C. S. (1972). The energy cost of the metabolism of drugs including ethanol. *Pharmacology* **7**, 185–196.

Podgainy, H., and Bressler, R. (1968). Biochemical basis of the sulfonylurea-induced Antabuse syndrome. *Diabetes* **17**, 679–683.

Popper, H., and Lieber, C. S. (1980). Histogenesis of alcoholic fibrosis and cirrhosis in the baboon. *Am. J. Pathol.* **98**, 695–716.

Potter, B. J., Chapman, W. G., Nunes, R. M., Sorrentino, D., and Sherlock, S. (1985). Transferrin metabolism in alcoholic liver disease. *Hepatology* **5**, 714–721.

Pritchard, P. H., Bowley, M., Burditt, S. L., Cooling, J., Glenny, H. P., Lawson, N., Sturton, R. G., and Brindley, D. N. (1977). The effect of acute ethanol feeding and of chronic Benfluorex administration on the activities of some enzymes of glycerolipid synthesis in rat liver and adipose tissue. *Biochem. J.* **166**, 639–642.

Rebaucas, G., and Isselbacher, K. J. (1961). Studies on the pathogenesis of the ethanol induced fatty liver. I. Synthesis of fatty acids by the liver. *J. Clin. Invest.* **40**, 1355–1361.

Reinke, L. A., Kauffman, F. C., Belinsky, S. A., and Thurman, G. R. (1980). Interaction between ethanol metabolism and mixed function oxidation in perfused rat liver: Inhibition of p-nitroanisole O-demethylation. *J. Pharmacol. Exp. Ther.* **213**, 70–78.

Riihimäki, V., Savolainen, K., and Pfaffli, P. (1982). Metabolic interaction between m-xylene and ethanol. *Arch. Toxicol.* **49**, 253–263.

Rojkind, M., and DeLeon, L. D. (1970). Collagen biosynthesis in cirrhotic rat slices. A regulatory mechanism. *Biochim. Biophys. Acta* **217**, 512–522.

Romero, J. J., Tamura, T., and Halsted, C. H. (1981). Intestinal absorption of ^{3}H-folic acid in the chronic alcoholic monkey. *Gastroenterology* **80**, 99–102.

Rothschild, M. A., Oratz, M., and Schreiber, S. S. (1985). Alcohol effects on albumin synthesis. *In* "Alcohol Related Diseases in Gastroenterology" (H. K. Seitz and B. Kommerell, eds.), pp. 96–105. Springer-Verlag, Berlin and New York.

Rubin, E., Gang, H., Misra, P. S., and Lieber, C. S. (1970a). Inhibition of drug metabolism by acute ethanol intoxication: A hepatic microsomal mechanism. *Am. J. Med.* **49,** 801–806.

Rubin, E., Bacchin, P., Gang, H., and Lieber, C. S. (1970b). Induction and inhibition of hepatic microsomal and mitochondrial enzymes by ethanol. *Lab. Invest.* **22,** 569–580.

Rubin, E., Beattie, D. S., and Lieber, C. S. (1970c). Effects of ethanol on the biogenesis of mitochondrial membranes and associated mitochondrial functions. *Lab. Invest.* **23,** 620–627.

Rubin, E., Lieber, C. S., Alvarez, A. P., Levine, W., and Kuntzman, R. (1971). Ethanol binding to hepatic microsomes—its increase by ethanol consumption. *Biochem. Pharmacol.* **20,** 229–231.

Rubin, E., Beattie, D. S., Toth, A., and Lieber, C. S. (1972). Structural and functional effects of ethanol on hepatic mitochondria. *Fed. Proc., Fed. Am. Soc. Exp. Biol.* **31,** 131–140.

Rubin, E., Lieber, C. S., Altman, K., Gordon, G. G., and Southren, A. L. (1976). Prolonged ethanol consumption increases testosterone metabolism in the liver. *Science* **191,** 563–564.

Salaspuro, M., and Lieber, C. S. (1978). Non-uniformity of blood ethanol elimination: Its exaggeration after chronic consumption. *Ann. Clin. Res.* **10,** 294–297.

Salaspuro, M., and Lindros, K. O. (1985). Metabolism and toxicity of acetaldehyde. *In* "Alcohol Related Diseases in Gastroenterology (H. K. Seitz and B. Kommerell, eds.), pp. 106–123. Springer-Verlag, Berlin and New York.

Salaspuro, M., Lindros, K. O., and Pikkarainen, P. (1975). Ethanol and galactose metabolism as influenced by 4-methylpyrazole in alcoholics with and without nutritional deficiencies. Preliminary report of a new approach to pathogenesis and treatment in alcoholic liver disease. *Ann. Clin. Res.* **7,** 269–272.

Salaspuro, M., Shaw, S., Jayatilleke, E., Ross, W. A., and Lieber, C. S. (1981). Attenuation of the ethanol induced redox change after chronic alcohol consumption in baboons: Metabolic consequences in vitro and in vivo. *Hepatology* **1,** 33–38.

Sanchez-Craig, M., and Annis, H. M. (1981). Gamma-glutamyltranspeptidase and high density lipoprotein cholesterol in male problem drinkers: Advantages of a composite index for predicting alcohol consumption. *Alcohol.: Clin. Exp. Res.* **5,** 540–544.

Sato, C., and Lieber, C. S. (1981). Mechanism for the preventive effect of ethanol on acetaminophen-induced hepatotoxicity. *J. Pharmacol. Exp. Ther.* **218,** 811–815.

Sato, C., Matsuda, Y., and Lieber, C. S. (1981). Increased hepatotoxicity of acetaminophen after chronic ethanol consumption in the rat. *Gastroenterology* **80,** 140–148.

Sato, C., Hasumura, Y., and Takeuchi, J. (1985). Interaction of ethanol with drugs and xenobiotics. *In* "Alcohol Related Diseases in Gastroenterology" (H. K. Seitz and B. Kommerell, eds.), pp. 172–184. Springer-Verlag, Berlin and New York.

Sato, M., and Lieber, C. S. (1982). Increased metabolism of retinoic acid after chronic ethanol consumption in rat liver microsomes *Arch.Biochem. Biophys.* **213,** 557–564.

Sato, N., Kamada, T., Shiohiri, M., Hayashi, N., Matsomura, T., Abe, M., and Hagihara, B. (1978). The levels of the mitochondrial and microsomal cytochromes in drinkers' livers. *Clin. Chim. Acta* **87,** 347–351.

Savolainen, M. J. (1977). Stimulation of hepatic phosphatidate phosphohydrolase activity by a single dose of ethanol. *Biochem. Biophys. Res. Commun.* **75,** 511–518.

Savolainen, M. J., Baraona, E., Pikkarainen, P., and Lieber, C. S. (1984). Decreased hepatic triacylglycerol synthesizing capacity during progression of alcoholic liver damage in the baboon. *J. Lipid Res.* **25,** 813–820.

Schanne, F. A. X., Zucker, A. H., Farber, J. L., and Rubin, E. (1981). Alcohol dependent liver cell necrosis in vitro: A new model. *Science* **212,** 338–340.

Schuckitt, M. A., and Rayes, V. (1979). Ethanol ingestion: Differences intlood acetaldehyde concentrations in relatives of alcoholics and controls. *Science* **203,** 54–55.

Schüller, A., Moscat, J., Diez, E., Fernandez-Checa, J. C., Gavilanes, F. G., and Municio, A. M.

(1985). Functional properties of isolated hepatocytes from ethanol treated rat liver. *Hepatology* **5,** 677–682.

Seitz, H. K. (1985). Ethanol and carcinogenesis. *In* "Alcohol Related Diseases in Gastroenterology" (H. K. Seitz and B. Kommerell, eds.), pp. 196–212. Springer-Verlag, Berlin and New York.

Seitz, H. K. (1985). Alcohol effects on drug nutrients interactions. *Drug Nutr. Interact.* **4,** 143–163.

Seitz, H. K., and Simanowski, U. A. (1986). Ethanol and carcinogenesis of the alimentary tract. *Alcohol.: Clin. Exp. Res.* (in press).

Seitz, H. K., Korsten, M. A., and Lieber, C. S. (1979). Ethanol oxidation by intestinal microsomes: Increased activity after chronic ethanol administration. *Life Sci.* **25,** 1443–1448.

Seitz, H. K., Garro, A. J., and Lieber, C. S. (1981a). Enhanced pulmonary and intestinal activation of procarcinogens to mutagens after chronic ethanol consumption in the rat. *Eur. J. Clin. Invest.* **11,** 33–38.

Seitz, H. K., Garro, A. J., and Lieber, C. S. (1981b). Sex dependent effect of chronic ethanol consumption in rats on hepatic microsome mediated mutagenicity of benzo[a]pyrene. *Cancer Lett.* **13,** 97–102.

Seitz, H. K., Bösche, J., Czygan, P., Veith, S., and Kommerell, B. (1982). Microsomal ethanol oxidation in the colonic mucosa of the rat: Effect of chronic ethanol ingestion. *Arch. Pharmacol.* **320,** 81–84.

Seitz, H. K., Simon, B., Czygan, P., and Kommerell, B. (1983). Colonic cyclic AMP metabolism following chronic ethanol consumption in the rat: Effect of hormonal secretagoques. *Pharmacol., Biochem. Behav.* **18,** 337–340.

Seitz, H. K., Veith, S., Czygan, P., Bösche, J., Simon, B., Gugler, R., and Kommerell, B. (1984a). In vivo interactions between H_2-receptor antagonists and ethanol metabolism in man and in rats. *Hepatology* **4,** 1231–1234.

Seitz, H. K., Czygan, P., Waldherr, R., Veith, S., Raedsch, R., Kässmodel, H., and Kommerell, B. (1984b). Enhancement of 1,2-dimethylhydrazine-induced rectal carcinogenesis following chronic ethanol consumption in the rat. *Gastroenterology* **86,** 886–891.

Sellers, E. M., Lang, M., and Koch-Weser, J. (1972). Interaction of chloral hydrate and ethanol in man. *Clin. Pharmacol. Ther.* **13,** 37–42.

Shaw, S., Jayatilleke, E., Ross, W. A., Gordon, E., and Lieber, C. S. (1981). Ethanol induced lipid peroxidation: potentiation by chronic alcohol feeding and attenuation by methionine. *J. Lab. Clin. Med.* **98,** 417–425.

Shaw, S., Rubin, K. P., and Lieber, C. S. (1983). Depressed hepatic glutathione and increased diene conjugates in alcoholic liver disease: Evidence of lipid peroxidation. *Dig. Dis. Sci.* **28,** 585–589.

Shaw, S., Worner, T. M., and Lieber, C. S. (1984). Frequency of hyperprolinemia in alcoholic liver cirrhosis: Relationship to blood acetate. *Hepatology* **4,** 295–299.

Sherlock, S. (1984). Nutrition and the alcoholic. *Lancet* **1,** 436–439.

Shigeta, Y., Nomura, F., Iida, S., Leo, M. A., Felder, M. R., and Lieber, C. S. (1984). Ethanol metabolism in vivo by the microsomal ethanol oxidizing system in deermice lacking alcohol dehydrogenase (ADH). *Biochem. Pharmacol.* **33,** 807–814.

Singer, M. V., and Goebell, H. (1985). Acute and chronic actions of alcohol on pancreatic exocrine secretion in humans and animals. *In* "Alcohol Related Diseases in Gastroenterology" (H. K. Seitz and B. Kommerell, eds.), pp. 376–415. Springer-Verlag, Berlin and New York.

Smith, A. C., Freeman, R. W., and Harbison, R. D. (1981). Ethanol enhancement of cocaine-induced hepatotoxicity. *Biochem. Pharmacol.* **30,** 453–458.

Smith, M., Hopkinson, D. A., and Harris, H. (1972). Alcohol dehydrogenase isoenzyme in adult human stomach and liver: Evidence for activity of the ADH_3 locus. *Ann. Hum. Genet.* **35,** 243–253.

Sorrell, M. F., Nauss, J. M., Donohue, T. M., and Tuma, D. J. (1983). Effects of chronic ethanol administration on hepatic glycoprotein secretion in the rat. *Gastroenterology* **84,** 580–586.

Spencer, R. P., Brody, K. R., and Lutters, B. M. (1964). Some effects of ethanol on the gastrointestinal tract. *Am. J. Dig. Dis.* **9,** 599–604.

Sullivan, J. F., and Lankford, H. G. (1965). Zinc metabolism and chronic alcoholism. *Am. J. Clin. Nutr.* **17,** 57–63.

Sussman, K. E., Alfrey, A., and Kirsch, W. M. (1970). Chronic lactic acidosis in an adult. *Am. J. Med.* **48,** 104–112.

Swann, P. F., Coe, A. M., and Mace, R. (1984). Ethanol and dimethylnitrosamine metabolism and disposition in the rat. Possible relevance to the influence of ethanol on human cancer incidence. *Carcinogenesis (London)* **5,** 1337–1343.

Szilagyi, A., Lerman, S., and Resnick, R. H. (1983). Ethanol, thyroid hormones and acute liver injury: Is there a relationship? *Hepatology* **3,** 593–600.

Taraschi, T. F., and Rubin, E. (1985). Ethanol and biological membranes: Experimental studies and theoretical considerations. *In* "Alcohol Related Diseases in Gastroenterology (H. K. Seitz and B. Kommerell, eds.), pp. 213–231. Springer-Verlag, Berlin and New York.

Taskinen, M. R., Välimäki, M., Nikkilä, E. A., Kuusi, T., Ehnholm, C., and Ylikahri, R. (1982). High density lipoprotein subfractions and postherparin plasma lipases in alcoholic men before and after ethanol withdrawal. *Metab., Clin. Exp.* **31,** 1168–1174.

Teschke, R., Hasumura, Y., Joly, J. G., Ishii, H., and Lieber, C. S. (1972). Microsomal ethanol-oxidizing system (MEOS): Purification and properties of a rat liver system free of catalase and alcohol dehydrogenase. *Biochem. Biophys. Res. Commun.* **49,** 1187–1193.

Teschke, R., Hasumura, Y., and Lieber, C. S. (1974). Hepatic microsomal ethanol oxidizing system: solubilization, isolation and characterization. *Arch. Biochem. Biophys.* **163,** 404–415.

Teschke, R., Hasumura, Y., and Lieber, C. S. (1975). Hepatic microsomal ethanol oxidizing system. Affinity for methanol, ethanol and propanol. *J. Biol. Chem.* **250,** 7379–7404.

Teschke, R., Matsusaki, S., Ohnishi, K., DeCarli, L. M., and Lieber, C. S. (1977). Microsomal ethanol oxidizing system (MEOS): Current status of its characterization and its role. *Alcohol.: Clin. Exp. Res.* **1,** 7–15.

Teschke, R., Moreno, F., Heinen, E., Herrmann, J., Krüskemper, H. L., and Strohmeyer, G. (1983). Hepatic thyroid hormone levels following chronic alcohol consumption: Direct experimental evidence in rats against the existence of a hyperthyroid hepatic state. *Hepatology* **3,** 469–474.

Thieden, H. I. D. (1971). The effect of ethanol concentration on ethanol oxidation rate in rat liver slices. *Acta Chem. Scand.* **25,** 3421–3427.

Thomas, B. H., Coldwell, B. B., Solomanraj, G., Zeitz, W., and Trenholm, H. L. (1972). Effect of ethanol on the fate of pentobarbital in the rat. *Biochem. Pharmacol.* **21,** 2605–2614.

Thomas, M., Halsall, S., and Peters, T. J. (1982). Role of hepatic acetaldehyde dehydrogenase in alcoholism: Demonstration of persistent reduction of cytosolic activity in abstaining patients. *Lancet* **1,** 1057–1059.

Thurman, R. G., McKenna, W. R., and Caffrey, T. B. (1976). Pathways responsible for the adaptive increase in ethanol utilization following chronic treatment with ethanol: Inhibitior studies with the hemoglobin-free perfused rat liver. *Mol. Pharmacol.* **12,** 156–166.

Tipton, K. F., McCrodden, J. M., Weir, D. G., and Ward, K. (1983). Isoenzymes of human liver alcohol dehydrogenase and aldehyde dehydrogenase in alcoholic and non-alcoholic subjects. *Alcohol Alcohol.* **18,** 219–225.

Tomera, J. F., Skipper, P. L., Wishnok, J. S., Tannenbaum, S. R., and Brunengraber, H. (1984). Inhibition of *N*-nitrosodimethylamine metabolism by ethanol and other inhibitors in the isolated perfused rat liver. *Carcinogenesis (London)* **5,** 113–116.

Tuma, D. J., Jennett, R. B., and Sorrell, M. F. (1981). Effect of ethanol on the synthesis and secretion of hepatic secretory glycoproteins and albumin. *Hepatology* **1,** 590, 598.

Ugarte, G., Pereda, I., Pino, M. E., and Iturriaga, H. (1972). Influence of alcohol intake, length of abstinence, and meprobamate on the rate of ethanol metabolism in man. *Q. J. Stud. Alcohol* **33**, 698–705.

Ullrich, V., Weber, P., and Wollenberg, P. (1975). Tetrahydrofuran—an inhibitor for ethanol induced liver microsomal cytochrome *P*-450. *Biochem. Biophys Res. Commun.* **64**, 808–813.

Uthus, E. O., Skurdal, D. N., and Cornatzer, W. E. (1976). Effect of ethanol on choline phosphotransferase and phosphatidyl ethanolamine methyltransferase activities in liver microsomes. *Lipids* **11**, 641–644.

Van Thiel, D. H., and Gavaler, J. S. (1985). Ethanol and the endocrine system. *In* "Alcohol Related Diseases in Gastroenterology" (H. K. Seitz and B. Kommerell, eds.), pp. 324–341. Springer-Verlag, Berlin and New York.

Van Thiel, D. H., Gavaler, J. S., and Lester, R. (1974). Ethanol inhibition of vitamin A metabolism in the testes, possible mechanism for sterility in alcoholics. *Science* **186**, 941–942.

Vasdev, S. C., Subrahmanyam, D., Chakravarti, R. N., and Wahi, P. L. (1974). Effect of chronic ethanol feeding on the major lipids of red blood cells, liver, heart of the rhesus monkey. *Biochim. Biophys. Acta* **369**, 323–330.

Veech, R. L., Guynn, R., and Veloso, D. (1972). The time course of the effects of ethanol on the redox and phosphorylation states of rat liver. *Biochem. J.* **127**, 387–397.

von Wartburg, J. P., Papenberg, J., and Aebi, H. (1965). An atypical human alcohol dehydrogenase *Can. J. Biochem.* **43**, 889–898.

Wendell, G., and Thurman, R. G. (1979). Effect of ethanol concentration on rates of ethanol elimination in normal and alcohol treated rats in vivo. *Biochem. Pharmacol.* **28**, 273–279.

Whiting, B., Lawrence, J. R., Skellern, G. C., and Meier, J. (1979). Effect of acute alcohol intoxication on the metabolism and plasma kinetics of chlordiazepoxide. *Br. J. Clin. Pharmacol.* **7**, 95–100.

Williamson, J. R., Scholz, R., Browning, E. T., Thurman, R. G., and Fukami, M. K. (1969). Metabolic effects of ethanol in perfused rat liver. *J. Biol. Chem.* **244**, 5044–5054.

Winston, G. W., and Cederbaum, A. I. (1983). NADPH-dependent production of oxy radicals by purified components of the rat liver mixed function oxidase system. *J. Biol. Chem.* **258**, 1514–1519.

Worner, T. M., and Lieber, C. S. (1985). Perivenular fibrosis as a precursor lesion of cirrhosis. *JAMA, J. Am. Med. Assoc.* **254**, 627–630.

Yuki, T., and Thurman, R. G. (1980). The swift increase in alcohol metabolism. Time course of the increase in hepatic oxygen uptake and involvement of glycolysis. *Biochem. J.* **186**, 119–126.

Zern, M. A., Chakraborty, P. R., Ruiz-Opazo, N., Yap, S. H., and Shafritz, D. A. (1983). Development and use of a rat albumin cDNA clone to evaluate the effect of chronic ethanol administration on hepatic protein synthesis. *Hepatology* **3**, 317–322.

Ziegler, D. M. (1972). Discussion. *In* "Microsomes and Drug Oxidation" (R. W. Estabrook, J. L. Gilette, and K. C. Liebman, eds.), pp. 458–460. Williams & Wilkins, Baltimore, Maryland.

Zysset, T., Preisig, R., and Bircher, J. (1980). Increased systemic availability of drugs during acute ethanol intoxication: Studies with mephenytoin in the dog. *J. Pharmacol. Exp. Ther.* **213**, 173–178.

4

Effects of Malnutrition on Drug Metabolism and Toxicity in Humans

Kamala Krishnaswamy

I. INTRODUCTION

Because of advances in the science of nutrition, a nutritionist must understand the modulation of toxic effects by interactions of diet, metabolism, disposition of

NUTRITIONAL TOXICOLOGY, VOL. II

Copyright © 1987 by Academic Press, Inc.
All rights of reproduction in any form reserved.

toxicants, and nutritional status. A combined knowledge of both nutrition and toxicology can contribute to better therapy and selective protection against toxic agents. For nutritionists and other health professionals, nutrition–drug interactions have become an important area of responsibility. The impacts of diet, especially the naturally occurring forms of human malnutrition, on disposition, metabolism, and toxicity of drugs are described in this chapter.

Safe and effective therapeutics require precise judgment of dosages based on knowledge of factors affecting the pharmacological and toxicological actions of drugs. Drug research in the present decade places emphasis on individualization of drug therapy, because the body burden and actions of chemicals and drugs are governed by absorption, distribution, binding, receptor sensitivity, tissue uptake, metabolism, and excretion. These various processes are influenced by both endogenous and exogenous factors (Vesell, 1977; Dollery *et al.*, 1979). In developing countries, the genetic profile, body weight, diet, and the environment are four major variables which have a direct bearing on appropriate drug dosage (Krishnaswamy and Teoh, 1980).

Nutrient–drug interactions thus are an important group of reactions which have a direct bearing on the outcome of drug therapy as well as on the nutritional condition of individuals. These interactions are complex and still not completely understood. Diet–drug interactions can be due to physical, chemical, physiological, or pathological interactions between drugs, nutrients, and the human body.

The influence of malnutrition in humans on the bioprocesses which govern the disposition and action of drugs needs much further research. Information on pharmacokinetics, adverse drug reactions, and drug efficacy in marginal and severe malnutrition is very incomplete. Attempts are now being made to gain knowledge in this area in order to provide more specifically appropriate drug therapy.

II. HUMAN MALNUTRITION

The major nutritional disorders which are widely prevalent in all developing countries are protein–energy malnutrition (PEM), vitamin A deficiency, iron deficiency, anemia, vitamin B-complex deficiency, and iodine deficiency (Table I). The development of nutritional problems in any population is determined by dietary inadequacy, its duration, and the presence or absence of superadded insults such as infections.

Nutritional deficiencies affect all age groups, but the repercussions are strongest in children and pregnant or lactating women. Malnutrition of an individual can begin soon after conception; these prenatal effects are now the subject of much research.

TABLE I

Common Deficiency Disorders in Developing Countries

---

1. Protein–energy malnutrition (PEM)
   Severe forms—kwashiorkor, marasmus, nutritional edema
   Moderate forms—growth retardation, nutritional dwarfism
2. Vitamin A deficiency
   Xerophthalmia, keratomalacia, blindness
3. Anemia
   Iron, folacin, vitamin B_{12} deficiencies
4. B-Complex and vitamin C deficiencies
   Beriberi, ariboflavinosis, pellagra, pyridoxine deficiency, scurvy
5. Mineral and trace element deficiencies
   Deficiencies of calcium, magnesium, potassium, zinc, copper, selenium, and iodine

---

A. Protein–Energy Malnutrition

According to the Food and Agriculture Organization (1978), around 15–20% of the world's population has dietary energy intakes below the critical level (120% of the basal metabolic rate), and PEM of varying severity is encountered throughout all sections of many populations. PEM is a collective term: marasmus, kwashiorkor, and adult nutritional edema are the major clinical forms. PEM is not a disease of sudden onset. It is a continuous and insidious transition from normalcy to a fully developed clinical disease. In many communities, subjects are encountered at all stages of clinical manifestation. Kwashiorkor and marasmus are seen in up to 5% of the population in many countries. Mild and moderate forms detected as varying degrees of growth retardation have much higher incidence (Gopalan and Srikantia, 1979).

Until recently, it was widely believed that PEM was primarily due to protein deficiency. It is now clear that with habitual diets of cereals and legumes, energy deficiency is more common than protein deficiency (Sukhatme, 1970; Gopalan and Narasinga Rao, 1971). If the energy deficit is great enough, however, any protein consumed will be used primarily for energy metabolism. This use of protein can result in conditioned protein deficiency.

B. Anemia

Anemia is a global problem, and its prevalence among children, women of reproductive age, and adults with intestinal infestations is very high. Intestinal parasites can cause much iron loss and thus are a major factor in nutritional anemia. In addition to inadequate intake of iron, folate deficiency also causes anemia. Poor bioavailability, as well as inadequate quantity of dietary iron, contributes to iron deficiency.

C. Other Vitamin and Mineral Deficiencies

Vitamin A deficiency has a global distribution and is one of the important etiological factors in preventable blindness. Vitamin C deficiency and the vitamin B-complex deficiency diseases, such as those associated with deficiencies of thiamin, riboflavin, niacin, and pyridoxine, still occur. The prevalence of subclinical vitamin deficiencies is very high. Deficiencies of copper, zinc, and selenium occur in some populations.

Intestinal function, endocrine functions, body composition, intellectual performance, work capacity, and immune responses are adversely affected by malnutrition. Concomitant deficiencies of two or more nutrients often further contributes to both functional and structural disorders. Many deficiencies occur simultaneously and involve a number of organs, tissues. and physiological processes. The clinical and pathological manifestations are complex, overlapping, and variable.

III. DIETARY EFFECTS ON DRUG ABSORPTION

Drugs are most frequently administered by the oral route. The absorption of drugs, therefore, is a primary source of variability in plasma drug levels and systemic responses, reflecting onset, intensity, and duration of action (Melander and McLean, 1983; Toothaker and Welling. 1980). Factors which influence drug absorption, such as pH in the stomach and intestinal lumen, gastric emptying time, intestinal transit time, surface area of gastrointestinal mucosa, intestinal (splanchnic) blood flow, gut bacteria, and gut wall metabolism of drugs, can be altered either by dietary composition or by nutrient deficiency disorders. The pathophysiological changes due to PEM, infections and infestations, and mineral or vitamin deficiencies can impair absorption of drugs. Further, malabsorption syndromes and nonspecific enteropathies may contribute to changes in drug absorption. In such situations, malabsorption of nutrients has received more research and clinical attention that the altered absorption of drugs (Krishnaswamy, 1983, 1985). Concomitant ingestion of food can also influence certain pharmaceutical variables, such as drug disintegration and dissolution.

Food delays and sometimes reduces the absorption of several antibiotics, such as penicillin, ampicillin, oxacillin, and some preparations of erythromycin. Tetracycline absorption can be reduced by calcium-containing food items such as milk and cheese and by iron supplement preparations. Availability of antitubercular drugs, such as isoniazid and rifampicin, is significantly reduced by food. Dietary protein, carbohydrate, and fat may differ in their effects on drug absorption (Melander, 1978).

Food intake is also known to enhance absorption of drugs such as β-blockers, hydralazine, hydrochlorothiazide, nitrofurantoin, propoxyphene, chloroquine, diazepam, lithium, anticonvulsants (phenytoin and carbamazepine), and anti-fungal agents (griseofulvin). Presystemic clearance of drugs depends on the chemical nature of the drug. Lipophilic bases are cleared better than lipophilic acids, and food markedly reduces clearance and thus enhances bioavailability of lipophilic bases (e.g., β-blockers) (Melander and McLean, 1983).

Nutrient deficiencies can alter gastrointestinal structure and function, thereby altering drug absorption. The absorptive efficiencies of nutrients such as fat, peptides, vitamin A, iron, and vitamin B_{12} are decreased in malnutrition. Absorption of tetracycline (Raghuram and Krishnaswamy, 1981a) and rifampicin (Polasa *et al.*, 1984) is significantly reduced in malnutrition. Absorption of chloramphenicol (Mehta *et al.*, 1981a) and anticonvulsants (Banu *et al.*, 1984) is delayed but effects on total absorption are not clear. Availability by parenteral administration of drugs such as cefoxitin, penicillin, streptomycin, and tobramycin is normal in malnourished children and adults (Krishnaswamy, 1982), indicating that transport and tissue uptake are normal in these persons. Utilization of water-soluble parenteral substances is likely to be normal, whereas that of fat-soluble pharmaceutical preparations (e.g., vitamin A) may be reduced (Reddy and Srikantia, 1966).

Nutrients administered as medicaments can also be affected by food, particularly by interactions in the lumen resulting in decreased absorption of both nutrient and drug, for example, tetracycline and iron. Nonnutrient dietary substances can modify gut bacteria or gut wall metabolism of drugs, thus altering drug bioavailability and potency (Conney *et al.*, 1976). The net effect of food–drug interactions on drug bioavailability cannot always be predicted because of the multiple mechanisms and the varying physicochemical properties of drugs. Specific information is needed on each food–drug combination to allow accurate conclusions and predictions.

IV. DRUG–PROTEIN BINDING AND DRUG DISTRIBUTION

Plasma is a complex solution containing different proteins, of which albumin, α_1-acid glycoprotein, lipoproteins, and globulins transport endogenous compounds (e.g., hormones) and exogenous compounds (e.g., drugs and other xenobiotics). Many drugs are bound to plasma proteins, principally to albumin and globulins. The extent of binding varies and depends on the chemical nature of the drug, its affinity to a particular plasma protein, and the concentration of that protein. Albumin is quantitatively the most important binding protein in plasma, although basic drugs bind mostly to α_1-acid glycoprotein.

Several conditions of impaired function, such as liver disease, renal disorders, endocrine disorders, stress, and aging, are known to alter albumin synthesis and concentration in plasma. Nutrients, particularly protein and energy, will directly

POLYTECHNIC OF NORTH LONDON
LIBRARY & INFORMATION SERVICE

influence the plasma protein profile and also the rate of tissue protein synthesis and turnover. Drug–protein binding, therefore, may be expected to be differently altered in varying grades of malnutrition. It may be expected also to change in relation to endogenous nutrient-related substances like fatty acids, bilirubin, tryptophan, uric acid, steroid hormones, and thyroxine, which also bind to albumin. A significant reduction in binding of several drugs has been documented in malnutrition in both adults and children (Buchanan, 1977; Krishnaswamy, 1983). Qualitative and quantitative changes in food intake can directly influence not only synthesis of protein and albumin levels but also alter levels of fatty acids, amino acids, and hormones.

The practical clinical significance of drug–protein binding is uncertain. The sensitivity of organ clearance of a drug to changes in binding depend on efficiency of clearance of the unbound fraction (Rowland, 1984). For drugs with a low single-pass extraction ratio in the liver, a decrease in binding will significantly increase the clearance. Gugler *et al.* (1975) found such a direct relationship between free-drug concentration and plasma clearance of phenytoin. Our observations on phenylbutazone, rifampicin, and doxycycline in undernourished subjects are similar (Krishnaswamy *et al.*, 1981; Raghuram and Krishnaswamy, 1982; Polasa *et al.*, 1984). If the free-drug concentration increases, however, the drug response will be enhanced only for drugs without restrictive clearance, such as propranolol.

Drug distribution subsequent to tissue equilibration usually is assessed by the apparent volume of distribution, and this index varies from drug to drug, depending on the combination of tissues and body fluids in which the drug equilibrates. Drug distribution, therefore, may be altered by a change in the unbound fraction in the tissues and by alteration in tissue binding (Wilkinson, 1984). The volume of distribution for the free fraction will be altered significantly by binding only for drugs with small volumes of distribution. Such changes for drugs with large volumes of distribution are rare, unless binding to tissue is altered also. Our studies on tetracycline in malnutrition indicate that tissue uptake, and perhaps tissue binding, is significantly reduced (Raghuram and Krishnaswamy, 1981b).

Body protein and fat are directly influenced by nutrients. There are no direct data on tissue binding of drugs in human malnutrition. Pharmacokinetic data in obesity are available for only a limited number of drugs. Drug distribution, especially for fat-soluble drugs, is significantly altered in obesity (Abernethy and Greenblatt, 1982).

V. RENAL ELIMINATION OF DRUGS

Urinary excretion is the primary route of elimination for water-soluble drugs and their metabolites. They are handled by filtration, selective reabsorption, and secretion. Drug excretion by the kidney is closely connected to other pharmacokinetic parameters. There are conflicting reports on kidney function, particularly glomerular filtration, renal blood flow, and tubular function, in malnutrition (Krishnaswamy, 1978a). It is generally assumed that only the free drug is available for metabolism and filtration. The urinary excretion of drugs and their metabolites depends on the rate of delivery of substances to the kidney, that is, on the renal blood flow. Drugs that are reabsorbed have pH-dependent excretion patterns. Only a few drugs are actively absorbed by the tubules, whereas others are secreted by the tubules. Tubular secretion is not limited by drug–protein binding (Hewitt and Hook, 1983). Additionally, uptake and sequestration within lysosomes can affect drug clearance.

Recent studies indicate that protein intake influences glomerular filtration and endogenous creatinine clearance (Bosch *et al.*, 1983). Diet-induced changes in urine pH and ionization of drugs also alter drug reabsorption. Severe malnutrition decreases elimination of drugs such as tetracycline (Raghuram and Krishnaswamy, 1981b), cefoxitin, gentamycin, penicillin, and tobramycin (Buchanan, 1984), drugs excreted mainly through the kidneys. In contrast, mild or moderate undernutrition without kidney damage causes more rapid drug elimination. Much additional research is needed to quantitate renal function and drug excretion in different types and grades of malnutrition.

VI. BIOTRANSFORMATION OF DRUGS

Metabolism of drugs may result in detoxification or in increased pharmacological or toxicological potency. Metabolism is by a group of enzyme systems with wide substrate specificity. The reactions usually are classified as phase I (oxidation, reduction, hydrolysis, etc.) and phase II (conjugation), and are catalyzed by enzymes located primarily in the liver and secondarily in the intestinal mucosa, skin, lungs, kidneys, placenta, and other organs. Oxidation by the cytochrome *P*-450-dependent mixed-function oxidase (MFO) system is the most common phase I reaction. The phase I reactions introduce or expose a functional group. Common examples of phase I reactions are hydroxylation, epoxidations, and oxidative demethylation. Products of phase I metabolism, or some compounds directly without phase I transformation, are conjugated by certain endogenous reactants to produce the phase II products. Methylation, acetylation, sulfation, glucuronic acid conjugation, and glutathione transfer (leading to mercapturic acid formation) are common phase II reactions.

Metabolism is a major determinant of drug clearance and, therefore, of concentration and action. In addition to drugs and other foreign compounds, endogenous substances such as steroids, cholesterol, cortisol, and vitamin D are substrates for both phase I and phase II enzyme systems.

A. Nutrient Functions in Biotransformations

Most nutrients participate, either directly or indirectly, in the functioning of enzyme systems involved in biotransformation of drugs. The experimental nutrition literature is replete with evidence that nutritional constraints alter drug metabolism (Campbell and Hayes, 1974; Campbell, 1977; Kato, 1977; Hathcock and Coon, 1978; Basu, 1980; Parke and Ioannides, 1981). These metabolic effects are dependent on species, strain, stress conditions, age, sex, the type, degree, and duration of malnutrition, and the particular drug being investigated. In general, all specific deficiencies except those of thiamin and iron decrease metabolism of most drugs. Oxidative metabolism most often is diminished in starvation, but for uncertain reasons the opposite is sometimes true. Conjugation reactions usually are increased in starvation.

B. Comparison of Animal and Human Studies

Although animal experiments provide background for human studies, extrapolations must be made with great caution. Because drug metabolism can vary quite widely between species, the possibility of great differences in the responses of humans and animals cannot be ignored. Whenever feasible and practical, inferences about nutritional effects on drug metabolism in humans should be based on human observations.

Preclinical toxicity studies are done in animals before a drug is used in clinical trials with human volunteers. All phases of these clinical trials must be completed, with appropriate results, before a drug can be introduced into the market.

The difference in animal and human response to drugs in various malnourished states is very important because of the complex and concurrent nature of human nutritional deficiencies and the common occurrence of complications such as infections and exposure to other substances in human patients. Drug responses in the malnourished are an intimate expression of the interplay of factors such as genetics, nutrient deficiencies, environmental contamination, and infectious disease.

C. Human Studies

Recently, studies to quantitate drug metabolism in human malnutrition have been made using prototype drugs or certain drugs already in clinical use. These studies have utilized both children and adults with the full range of severity of PEM, anorexia nervosa, anemia, and deficiencies of zinc and ascorbic acid. Metabolic experiments to evaluate the roles of macronutrients such as protein, carbohydrate, and fat also have been conducted.

D. Drug Metabolism in Malnourished Children

Most studies have involved children with severe forms of malnutrition, such as marasmus and kwashiorkor, with 40% or greater weight deficits. Almost all the results indicate that oxidative metabolism of drugs, as indicated by antipyrine clearance, is significantly impaired in such children; this becomes normal on nutritional rehabilitation (Buchanan, 1978; Buchanan *et al.*, 1979, 1980b; Homeida *et al.*, 1979; Narang *et al.*, 1979). Drug conjugations also have been reported to decrease in severe malnutrition (Mehta *et al.*, 1975, 1981b). Acetanilide metabolism is impaired in children with kwashiorkor (Buchanan *et al.*, 1980a). Metabolism of chloroquine, salicylate, sulfadiazine, and acetaminophen (paracetamol) metabolism are all adversely affected in children with severe malnutrition (Wharton and McChesney, 1970; Monckeberg *et al.*, 1978; Mehta, 1983). Toxic reactions to tetrachloroethylene suggest that metabolism is decreased in kwashiorkor (Balmer *et al.*, 1970). Reports on isoniazid metabolism in children are inconsistent and controversial (Akbani *et al.*, 1977; Buchanan *et al.*, 1979).

E. Drug Metabolism in Malnourished Adults

Studies in adults with mild and moderate forms of undernutrition who have been exposed to other environmental factors indicate that oxidative metabolism of drugs is usually enhanced but is sometimes normal, whereas metabolism and clearance of drugs is impaired in severe forms of malnutrition such as nutritional edema (Krishnaswamy and Naidu, 1977: Adithan *et al.*, 1979; Krishnaswamy *et al.*, 1981: Raghuram and Krishnaswamy, 1982; Polasa *et al.*, 1984; Tupule and Krishnaswamy, 1983). Similar observations have been made in children. Clearance of drugs such as antipyrine, phenylbutazone, doxycycline, rifampicin, and chloroquine are faster in mildly and moderately undernourished adults, whereas drugs accumulate in adults with severe malnutrition (Krishnaswamy, 1978b). Acetylation of sulfadiazine (Shastri and Krishnaswamy, 1979) and metabolism of salicylate (Shastri, 1984) are faster and normal, respectively, in malnourished adults.

Metabolic clearance rate of antipyrine has been reported recently to be different in adults with primary energy deficiency, compared with those having primary protein deficiency. The results indicate a marked decrease in antipyrine clearance in protein deficiency and no significant alteration in energy deficiency (Tranvouez *et al.*, 1985).

Metabolism of contraceptive steroids is faster in undernourished women (Nair *et al.*, 1979; Prasad *et al.*, 1979). The α-hydroxylation of steroids is invariably faster in patients with malnutrition resulting from anorexia nervosa (Fishman and Bradlow, 1978).

Our recent observations *in vitro* of hepatic enzymes, benzo[*a*]pyrene hydroxylase and γ-glutamyl transpeptidase (GGT) activities in undernourished adults indicate that both are induced (Ramesh *et al.*, 1985). Antipyrine clearance *in vivo* and benzo[*a*]pyrene hydroxylation *in vitro* are well correlated (Kalamegham *et al.*, 1979). Thus, clearance of drugs which undergo metabolism and excretion can be monitored adequately by observation of clearance of appropriate drugs.

When adaptation to nutritional deprivation fails, clinical syndromes such as kwashiorkor and marasmus in children and nutritional edema in adults may develop (Waterlow, 1975; Metcoff, 1975; Jaya Rao, 1982). An important role of hormones appears to be in the process of adaptation. In mild and moderate malnutrition where adaptation is adequate, the free-cortisol concentration is higher (S. R. Smith *et al.*, 1975), and this increased hormone level may be responsible for induction of MFO activity. However, when malnutrition is severe and adaptation is inadequate, negative nitrogen balance occurs and both oxidation and conjugation reactions may decrease.

F. Specific Dietary Influences on Drug Metabolism

The effects of macronutrient intake on drug metabolism and clearance have been studied in human volunteers. Isocaloric substitution of protein for carbohydrate to levels well above the protein requirement stimulates clearance of theophylline and antipyrine (Alvares *et al.*, 1976; Anderson *et al.*, 1979, 1982). Studies with animals indicate that tryptophan serves as an inducer of the MFO system, in addition to its role as an essential amino acid (Sidransky, 1985), suggesting that high protein intake may have its effect through induction rather than a strictly nutritional effect.

Our study on varying human protein and energy intakes indicates that inadequate energy (60% of recommended) diminishes drug clearance, whereas somewhat milder deficits (65–70% of recommended) do not alter drug kinetics significantly. Reliance of carbohydrate energy in the absence of adequate protein intake, however, diminishes drug clearance even if the total energy intake is adequate; that is, protein deficiency decreases drug metabolism even if energy intake is adequate (Krishnaswamy *et al.*, 1984). Caucasian vegetarians and nonvegetarians have indistinguishable drug kinetics when there are no differences in amount of protein intake (Brodie *et al.*, 1980a). Asian vegetarians, however, have comparatively lower clearance of drug than similar nonvegetarians (Mucklow *et al.*, 1980). It is possible that difference in protein quality between the diets of vegetarian Caucasians and Asians might account for this discrepancy. Fat does not seem to have a significant effect, at least within the range of human intake.

In addition to the effects of PEM, the effects of iron, ascorbic acid, zinc, and folate deficiencies on drug metabolism in adults have been documented (see review in Krishnaswamy, 1982). Phenazone clearance is faster in subjects with low hemoglobin resulting from iron deficiency. Zinc deficiency in adults is associated with decreased clearance of this drug. Phenytoin levels decrease with folic acid supplementation due to increased formation and excretion of hydroxylated metabolites of the drug. Similarly, ascorbic acid supplementation increases antipyrine clearance, and ascorbate deficiency decreases metabolism of drugs (Holloway and Peterson, 1984).

G. Inducers and Inhibitors in Food

Naturally occurring nonnutrients such as indoles, flavones, and isothiocyanates are potent inducers found in many foods (Conney *et al.*, 1980). Consumption of vegetables of the *Brassica* genus stimulates drug clearance (Pantuck *et al.*, 1979), as does dietary charcoal-broiled beef (Conney *et al.*, 1976). These effects appear to be directly related to induction of the MFO system, but the identity of the inducers depends on the particular food: indoles occur in *Brassica* vegetables and polyaromatic hydrocarbons occur in charcoal-broiled beef.

Although the effects of nonnutrient dietary factors on drug metabolism are reasonably well documented, data are inadequate to substantiate the view that dietary inducers or inhibitors significantly alter either therapeutic or toxic effects of drugs. This clinical impact seems plausible but requires observational proof.

The multiple effects of nutrients and nonnutrients in the diet can produce wide differences in drug metabolism and clearance. Positive and negative influences may interact, and any prediction of the net effect requires detailed knowledge of the kinds and amounts of foods consumed.

VII. DRUG RECEPTORS AND PHARMACODYNAMIC RESPONSES

Pharmacodynamic alterations can occur in the presence of disease without altered drug concentrations if drug receptors in the target organ are changed in number or sensitivity. The therapeutic requirement for a drug may be quantitatively different in malnutrition due to tissue receptor changes. Organ susceptibility to damage may vary also with type and degree of malnutrition. Objective methods of evaluation are inadequate, and consequently there are very few data on drug receptors and pharmacodynamics in malnutrition. Studies with experimental animals, however, indicate that steroid receptors are increased in undernutrition (Nair *et al.*, 1981).

The hypotensive response to propranolol seems to be less in Kenyan subjects than others, particularly in the presence of severe undernutrition (Obel and Vere, 1978). Our observation on protein binding of propranolol in undernutrition suggests that the free-drug concentrations are lower due to concomitant increases in levels of α_1-acid glycoprotein (Jagadeesan and Krishnaswamy, 1984). This may explain the subnormal therapeutic response in these patients.

Studies on children indicate that plasma theophylline levels are higher and clinical response is greater with a very low protein intake (3% of diet) (Feldman *et al.*, 1980). To the contrary, studies in animals suggest that nutritional status is an important determinant of drug toxicity (McLean *et al.*, 1980). Anthracycline chemotherapy has been associated with cardiomyopathy more in malnourished than in normal children (Obama *et al.*, 1983). Conversely, hepatic injury due to acetaminophen has been shown to be low in anorexia nervosa patients (Newmann and Bargman, 1979). In malnutrition secondary to alcoholism, however, acetaminophen toxicity is distinctly higher because alcohol induces acetaminophen activation. Hypoalbuminemia often is associated with toxic reactions to drugs (Greenblatt and Koch-Weser, 1974; Boston Collaborative Surveillance Program, 1973).

The relationship of carcinogen metabolism and the subsequent reaction of the activated metabolite with DNA to the development of cancer is not yet clearly defined. Studies of mild to moderate undernutrition in adults (Ramesh *et al.*, 1985) indicate that the MFO system activities often are induced to a high level and, therefore, the slightly undernourished may be at greater risk of cancer. The toxicological significance of induction probably differs with type of substrate and nature of inducer.

Although genetic background is an important determinant of fetal outcome, the impact of nutritional status in women taking drugs cannot be ignored. The frequency of congenital malformations is much higher than normal in women using phenytoin, and several studies have suggested that the teratogenicity may be caused by interference with folic acid metabolism (Monson *et al.*, 1973; Richens, 1976). Flynn *et al.* (1981) have shown an association between low plasma zinc in pregnant alcoholic woemn and the number of birth defects in their children.

The alterations of drug kinetics by nutritional processes can result either in increased or decreased bioavailability and steady state of drugs, thus modifying the therapeutic and toxic responses. The clinical implications of such alterations, however, are not clearly established, but in malnutrition toxicity due to drugs or their metabolites is likely to be higher.

TABLE II

Major Drug-Induced Clinical Entities Related to Nutritional Deficiencies

1. Anorexia, nausea, steatorrhea
2. Decrease in body weight and growth rate
3. Neurological abnormalities (e.g., personality changes, peripheral neuropathy, convulsions)
4. Anemia (megaloblastic and sideroblastic types)
5. Bone disorders (osteoporosis and osteomalacia)

VIII.   DRUG-INDUCED NUTRITIONAL DISORDERS

One of the major types of drug toxicity is drug-induced nutritional deficiency, an effect especially likely in already moderately nourished persons (Table II). A number of collaborative and coordinative programs are required to detect or anticipate adverse effects of drugs on nutritional status and function. Such studies, for obvious reasons, are lacking in developing countries and are not as common as needed elsewhere.

Drugs induce nutrient deficiencies by numerous different mechanisms, including effects on intake, absorption, binding, transport, metabolism, function, and excretion of nutrients (Table III) (Hathcock, 1985; Roe, 1984a,b). These can result in inadequate nutrient uptake, storage depletion, or metabolic antagonism. The structure, chemistry, pharmacology, and treatment regime of a drug dictates whether it will produce nutritional antagonism. Additionally, physiological factors such as genetic profile, previous nutritional status, and disease further influence the biological vulnerability and precipitation of deficiencies.

Several groups of drugs induce anorexia, cause nausea, or inhibit absorption of nutrients (Levitsky, 1984). Amphetamine, an antinarcoleptic agent, is known for its anorectic and related weight-reducing properties; also, it has a serious abuse potential. Several other synthetic derivatives with similar structures are available and have similar effects on appetite but less abuse potential. Caffeine, other methylxanthines, and nicotine also adversely affect appetite and result in weight loss. Nicotine seems to enhance metabolic rate, in addition to suppressing appetite. Drugs which induce nausea, such as digitalis, some cancer chemotherapeutic agents, some sedatives, and a few tranquilizers also reduce net food intake and thus impair nutritional status.

Some drugs interfere with absorption of nutrients, although nutrient consumption may remain normal. Maldigestion and malabsorption of nutrients are produced by inhibition of digestive enzymes, damage to the mucosal brush border, or interference with mucosal transport mechanisms by drugs. The micronutrients, for stoichiometric reasons, are more susceptible than the macronutrients to these mechanisms. Agents that commonly produce these effects include antacids, laxatives, appetite suppressants, diuretics, antibiotics, col-

TABLE III

Mechanisms of Drug-Induced Nutritional Disorders

1. Anorexia
2. Decreased absorption, due to alteration in enzymes, mucosal damage, precipitation, chelation, or adsorption
3. Metabolic abnormalities (e.g., induction or inhibition of enzymes, and antimetabolite actions including inhibition of active-form synthesis and functional antagonism)
4. Increased elimination, including renal, hepatic, and intestinal effects

chicine, cholestyramine, alcohol, fiber, and other bulking agents, antitubercular drugs, and anticonvulsants (Roe, 1984a).

Some drugs are antimetabolites of nutrients through direct interference with function or through inhibition or formation of the active metabolite of the nutrient. Also, inducers and inhibitors of drug-metabolizing enzymes can alter formation of coenzymes or specific functions and result in deficits of nutrient function. Nutrients affected by such processes include vitamins A, D, and K, folate, and pyridoxine; drugs producing such effects include antitubercular drugs (isoniazid, rifampicin, pyrizinamide, etc.), anticonvulsants (diphenylhydantoin and phenobarbital), folate antagonists (methotrexate, pyrimethamine, and trimethoprim), oral contraceptive steroids, and corticosteroids (Roe, 1984a).

A number of drugs promote elimination of nutrients, usually minerals and vitamins (Roe, 1984a,b). Antibiotics, isoniazid, penicillamine, diuretics, and hypolipidemic drugs are commonly responsible for such actions. Nutrient loss due to microhemorrhage resulting from chronic heavy use of aspirin can cause very significant loss of iron because iron absorption and reabsorption are inefficient. The etiological factors that determine drug-induced nutritional deficiency syndromes may be sequential and interactive. A drug may have multiple mechanisms of nutritional antagonism and the ultimate result will depend on the interaction of many factors.

IX. DRUG-INDUCED DEFICIENCIES OF WATER-SOLUBLE VITAMINS

Vitamin deficiencies are very important clinically in developing countries, and the use of certain drugs can further exacerbate the situation. Certain groups are especially vulnerable, for example, pregnant women, alcoholics, and the aged.

Drug-induced or drug-exacerbated folate deficiency is quite common. Food folate is a mixture of mono- and polyglutamates and is actively absorbed in the upper small intestine. Because of the high requirement during growth and development, or other periods of intense metabolic activity, folate deficiency is more often found in pregnant or lactating women or children, rather than in adult men and nonpregnant or nonlactating women (Roe, 1984a). Anticonvulsants, antifolates, hypolipidemic agents, sulfa drugs, oral contraceptives, and alcohol compromise folate status (Table IV). Fetal malformations, megaloblastic anemia, megaloblastic changes in epithelial cells, reduction in blood folate, and urinary folate excretion occur in patients who were treated with one or more of these drugs (Roe, 1984a). Anticonvulsants, antifolates, and oral contraceptives have clinically more important impacts on folate function than do other drugs, probably because of the multiplicity of mechanisms these have for folate antagonism (Reynolds, 1974). Supplementation with folate to meet the increased needs has been recommended regardless of the risk of decreasing the therapeutic efficacy

TABLE IV

Drugs Leading to Folate Deficiency

Methotrexate	Cholestyramine
Pyrimethamine	Phenytoin
Trimethoprim	Sulfasalazine
Triamterene	Alcohol
Contraceptive steroids	

of the drug. Cases of megaloblastic anemia have occurred with methotrexate, pyrimethamine, trimethoprim, and triamterene treatment. Our studies in adult men and women on anticonvulsant therapy (unpublished) also indicate a relative deficiency of folate, although the red cell levels are not greatly compromised.

Thiamin, riboflavin, niacin, pyridoxine, and vitamin B_{12} status can be adversely affected by certain drugs. Considerable attention has been given to pyridoxine, whereas relatively little information exists on these other vitamins. Much of the research and clinical observation on thiamin and riboflavin are related to oral contraceptives. Diuretics such as furosemide can lead to thiamin deficiency (Yui *et al.*, 1980), and recent reports indicate that tranquilizers (chlorpromazine) and tricyclics in experimental animals can lead to riboflavin depletion (Pellicone *et al.*, 1983). Studies of patients are needed to establish the clinical significance of such effects.

Antitubercular drugs, hydralazine, D-penicillamine, and levodopa can produce pyridoxine deficiency (Table V). The common symptoms in such cases are peripheral neuropathy, behavioral changes, and mental changes. Generalized convulsions are rare, but few cases of pyridoxine deficiency anemia have been reported (McCurdy and Donohoe, 1966). In developing countries, pyridoxine deficiency during isoniazid therapy usually occurs in persons who are slow acetylators of drugs: they are treated with 2–4 mg of pyridoxine per day. Isoniazid forms a hydrazone complex with pyridoxine and pyridoxal phosphate; the complex is excreted in the urine. The complex itself may have a direct toxic effect on neural tissue (Gershoff, 1976). Isoniazid also is a competitive inhibitor of pyridoxal phosphate-requiring enzymes (Bhagvan and Brin, 1983). Pellagra can be produced by this drug in patients with marginal intakes of niacin.

TABLE V

Drugs Leading to Pyridoxine Deficiency

Isoniazid	Penicillamine
Cycloserine	Hydrazines
Levodopa	Alcohol
Contraceptive steroids	

X. DRUG-INDUCED DEFICIENCIES OF FAT-SOLUBLE VITAMINS

Drugs which interfere with fat digestion or absorption and some drugs which induce drug-metabolizing enzymes can cause deficiencies of the fat-soluble vitamins. Abuse of cathartics can lead to deficiencies of vitamins A and D. Neomycin and cholestyramine can decrease serum vitamin A levels (Levine, 1967; West and Lloyd, 1975). Indeed, all drugs that sequester bile salts can induce malabsorption of fat and fat-soluble vitamins. Widespread use of this type of hypolipidemic drug, however, has not resulted in highly prevalent deficiencies of the fat-soluble vitamins. Deficiencies of vitamins D, E, and K are not common, and the vitamin A deficiency problem is primarily attributable to dietary inadequacy.

Enzyme inducers or inhibitors such as anticonvulsants and antitubercular agents can result in a variety of disorders of vitamin D function and, conseuqently, of mineral and bone metabolism. The major clinical and biochemical manifestations are hypocalcemia, hypophosphatemia, increased alkaline phosphatase activity, decreased levels of 25-hydroxyvitamin D and 1,25-dihydroxyvitamin D, a mild increase in levels of parathyroid hormone, radiological evidence of decreased bone mass, increased incidence of bone fractures, and histological and radiological evidence of osteomalacia (Hahn and Avioli, 1984).

Vitamin D_3 is produced in the epidermis by UV irradiation of 7-dehydrocholesterol and then is transported to the liver for the first step of activation. The metabolite 1,25-dihydroxyvitamin D, produced by 25-hydroxylation in the liver followed by 1-hydroxylation in the kidney, is the active hormonal form of the vitamin; it promotes absorption of calcium and phosphorus from the intestine (DeLuca, 1980). Both hydroxylations are catalyzed by cytochrome *P*-450-dependent MFO systems.

Most of the drugs which induce alterations in bone metabolism also induce hepatic MFO enzymes. Induction of the MFO system appears responsible for increased steroid metabolism, including that of vitamin D. Polar metabolites are formed and plasma concentration of the 25-hydroxy form of vitamin D is decreased (Hahn *et al.*, 1972). Furthermore, phenytoin has direct detrimental effects on mineral transport mechanisms and collagen synthesis. Clinical reports on anticonvulsant-induced osteomalacia are numerous. Recent techniques of assessing vitamin D and bone mineral status permit demonstration of mild but significant toxic effects produced by these drugs, even in the absence of definite radiological evidence. Such effects by antitubercular drugs, however, are not well documented. Our recent studies in a group of low-socioeconomic-status individuals on combination therapy of isoniazid and rifampicin or isoniazid and other drugs show radiodensitometric and biochemical changes indicative of osteopenia (Krishnaswamy *et al.*, 1987). A single case report on rifampicin-induced osteomalacia has been made (Shah *et al.*, 1981). Studies of anticonvul-

TABLE VI

Mechanisms of Drug-Induced Vitamin D Deficiency

1. Decreased absorption of vitamin D
2. Induction of mixed-function oxidases
3. Alteration of 1,25-hydroxylase activity
4. Inhibition of renal cell membrane transport and intestinal transport of calcium ions
5. Inhibition of collagen synthesis
6. Inhibition of osteoclast activity

sant-treated epileptics indicate that to avoid negative calcium balance, an increase in vitamin D intake is essential (Peterson *et al.*, 1976). Recent evidence indicates that even antitubercular drugs such as isoniazid and rifampicin alter vitamin D metabolism and thereby result in osteopenia (Brodie *et al.*, 1980b, 1982). Overall, several mechanisms are involved in drug-induced vitamin D deficiency (Table VI).

Vitamin K deficiency sometimes occurs in neonates born to mothers treated with anticonvulsant drugs, one of the coumarin anticoagulants, or cholestyramine. These drugs accelerate vitamin K metabolism, interfere with absorption, and inhibit synthesis of vitamin K-dependent clotting factors, respectively. Prolonged bleeding is the common manifestation of vitamin K deficiency.

XI. ANTINUTRIENT EFFECTS OF CONTRACEPTIVE STEROIDS

Several studies have described significant alterations in vitamin metabolism and function in users of oral contraceptive steroids (OCS), particularly the combination pills (Prasad *et al.*, 1975; J. L. Smith *et al.*, 1975; Briggs, 1976; Bamji, 1978). These effects have been studied in women in widely different nutritional conditions. Folate, pyridoxine, riboflavin, and vitamin A are especially sensitive to the OCS.

After the initial report by Shojania *et al.* (1968) that users of OCS have altered folate status, much confusion developed regarding the net impact of these agents on folate function. Polyglutamate forms of folate have impaired absorption in OCS users who are deficient in dietary folate. In contrast, polyglutamate forms of folate are utilized normally in other women. OCS also may cause increased excretion of absorbed folate. Experiments with animals indicate that OCS alter utilization by increasing the cellular requirements for folate (Lakshmaiah and Bamji, 1979; Da Costa and Rothenberg, 1974). Recent studies in malnourished women indicate that vitamin deficiencies do not become worse with OCS use, particularly when low-dose preparations are used (Bamji, 1985). Although megaloblastic anemia has been reported in OCS users, several other factors such as inadequate intake and unrelated malabsorption may have a more important role than OCS use.

Abnormal tryptophan metabolism characterized by a block in the tryptophan to niacin pathway, due to very low kynurinase activity, has been observed consistently in OCS users (Briggs, 1976). The changes observed have been attributed also to changes in tryptophan oxygenase (Braidman and Rose, 1971). High doses of pyridoxine improve the mental depression associated with OCS use (Adams *et al.*, 1973).

Thiamin status apparently is not affected by OCS use, whereas most studies show that riboflavin status is significantly impaired (Bamji, 1978). More recent studies indicate that low-dose preparations do not significantly further impair vitamin functions in a population which is already deficient in vitamins (Bamji, 1985).

Use of synthetic steroids results in increased plasma vitamin A levels because of increased retinol-binding protein concentrations (Bamji *et al.*, 1979). The nutritional consequences of such effects, in terms of depletion of liver stores in malnourished persons, could have clinical consequences during subsequent dietary deficiency. The practical significance of this effect, if any, is not known.

OCS produce abnormalities in the glucose tolerance test and result in abnormal lipid profiles in Western women who are relatively well nourished and have comparatively high fat intakes. Nevertheless, a multicentric study in India by the World Health Organization has yielded results that are inconclusive. Significant impairment in glucose tolerance was observed in well-nourished and undernourished women, but the lipid profile did not alter as much in the undernourished women (Bamji, 1985).

Mineral depletion due to drug therapy can result from either malabsorption or excessive losses in bile or urine. Antacids, laxatives, diuretics, chelating agents, antibiotics, anticonvulsants, and steroids may cause depletion and deficiency of calcium, magnesium, phosphorus, sodium, potassium, iron, zinc, and copper. Clinical manifestations may be precipitated, particularly with multiple-drug combinations. Some of the nutritional deficiencies account for adverse drug reactions, such as fatigue, anemia, bone pain, convulsions, tetany, and abnormal therapeutic response to the main mode of therapy, that are encountered during drug therapy.

XII. CONCLUSIONS

The interactions of genetics, a wide variety of environmental factors operating at different levels, and the complex problem of malnutrition of varying types and severity must be properly interpreted. A large number of factors can interact, and there are no universal rules for drawing conclusions about drug–nutrient interactions. It must be determined whether, under the particular circumstances, drug metabolism actually is altered, and then arrive at the clinical implications for drug therapy. Conversely, the toxicity and antinutritional effects of drugs will depend strongly on two important variables: type of drug, and both type and degree of malnutrition. It is important to evaluate nutritional status prior to drug therapy in order to institute proper dosage regimes which are likely to provide maximum efficacy with a minimum of side effects.

Drug-induced nutritional disorders, especially in populations where dietary inadequacy is a permanent feature, need special attention and appropriate nutritional management. It is necessary to monitor plasma concentrations of drugs in the malnourished and to assess nutritional status in patients on chronic drug therapy. Toxicity of drugs and other xenobiotics is likely to be higher in malnourished persons. Pharmacologists, pharmacists, nutritionists, and physicians must understand drug–nutrient interactions, because many practical problems related to health are direct consequences of such interactions.

REFERENCES

Abernethy, D. R., and Greenblatt, D. J. (1982). Pharmacokinetics of drugs in obesity. *Clin. Pharmacokinet.* **7**, 108–124.

Adams, P. W., Rose, D. P., Folkard, J. *et al.* (1973). Effect of pyridoxine hydrochloride upon depression associated with oral contraceptives. *Lancet* **1**, 897–904.

Adithan, C., Gandhi, I. S., and Chandrasekar, S. (1979). Pharmacokinetics of phenylbutazone in undernutrition. *Indian J. Pharmacol.* **10**, 301–308.

Akbani, Y., Bolme, P., Lindbald, B. S., and Rahimtoola, R. J. (1977). Control of streptomycin and isoniazid in malnourished children treated for tuberculosis. *Acta Paediatr. Scand.* **66**, 237–240.

Alvares, A. P., Anderson, K. E., Conney, A. H., and Kappas, A. (1976). Interactions between nutritional factors and drug biotransformations in man. *Proc. Natl. Acad. Sci. U.S.A.* **73**, 2501–2504.

Anderson, K. E., Conney, A. H., and Kappas, A. (1979). Nutrition and oxidative metabolism in man: Relative influence of dietary lipids, carbohydrates and protein. *Clin. Pharmacol. Ther.* **26**, 493–501.

Anderson, K. E., Conney, A. H., and Kappas, A. (1982). Nutritional influences on chemical biotransformation in humans. *Nutr. Rep. Int.* **40**, 161–171.

Balmer, S., Howells, G., and Wharton, B. (1970). The effects of tetrachlorethylene in children with kwashiorkor and hookworm infestation. *J. Trop. Pediatr.* **16**, 20–23.

Bamji, M. S. (1978). Implication of oral contraceptive use on vitamin nutritional status. *Indian J. Med. Res.* **68**, Suppl., 80–87.

Bamji, M. S. (1985). Oral contraceptives and nutrient interactions. *Indian Council. Med. Res. Bull.* **15**, 85–89.

Bamji, M. S., Prema, K., Ramalakshmi, B. A. *et al.* (1979). Oral contraceptive use and vitamin nutritional status of malnourished women—effect of continuous and intermittent supplements. *J. Steroid Biochem.* **11**, 487–491.

Banu, G., Sharma, D. B., and Raina, R. K. (1984). Pharmacokinetics of phenytoin in protein energy malnutrition. *Indian J. Pharmacol.* **17**, 77–78.

Basu, T. K. (1980). Nutritional status drug therapy. *In* "Clinical Implications of Drug Use" (T. K. Basu, ed.), Vol. 1, pp. 61–72. CRC Press, Boca Raton, Florida.

Bhagvan, H. N., and Brin, M. (1983). Drug vitamin B_6 interaction. *In* "Nutrition and Drugs" (M. Winick, ed.), pp. 1–12. Wiley, New York.

Bosch, J., Saccaggi, A., Lauer, A., Ronco, C. *et al.* (1983). Renal function reserve in humans: Effect of protein intake on glomerular filtration rate. *Am. J. Med.* **75**, 943–949.

Boston Collaborative Drug Surveillance Program (1973). Diphenylhydantoin side effects and serum albumin level. *Clin. Pharmacol. Ther.* **529**, 1973.

Braidman, I, P., and Rose, D. P. (1971). Effects of sex hormones on three glucocorticoid inducible enzymes concerned with aminoacid metabolism in liver. *Endocrinology (Baltimore)* **89**, 1250–1255.

Briggs, M. (1976). Biochemical effects of oral contraceptives. *Adv. Steroid Biochem. Pharmacol.* **5**, 65–160.

Brodie, M. J., Boobis, A. R., Toverud, E. L. *et al.* (1980a). Drug metabolism in vegetarians. *Br. J. Clin. Pharmacol.* **9**, 523–525.

Brodie, M. J., Boobis, A. R., Hillyard, C. J. *et al.* (1980b). Effect of isoniazid on vitamin D metabolism and hepatic monooxygenase activity. *Clin. Pharmacol. Ther.* **30**, 363–367.

Brodie, M. J., Boobis, A. R., Hillyard, C. J. *et al.* (1982). Effect of rifampicin and isoniazid on vitamin D metabolism. *Clin. Pharmacol. Ther.* **32**, 525–530.

Buchanan, N. (1977). Drug protein binding and protein energy malnutrition. *S. Afr. Med. J.* **52**, 733–737.

Buchanan, N. (1978). Drug kinetics in protein energy malnutrition. *S. Afr. Med. J.* **53**, 327–330.

Buchanan, N. (1984). Effect of protein energy malnutrition on drug metabolism in man. *World Rev. Nutr. Diet.* **43**, 129–139.

Buchanan, N., Eyeberg, C., and Davis, M. D. (1979). Antipyrine phearmacokinetics and D-glucaric acid excretion in kwashiorkor. *Am. J. Clin. Nutr.* **32**, 2439–2442.

Buchanan, N., Davis, M. D., Henderson, D. M. *et al.* (1980a). Acetanilide pharmacokinetics in kwashiorkor. *Br. J. Clin. Pharmacol.* **9**, 525–526.

Buchanan, N., Davis, M., Danhaf, M., and Breimer, D. D. (1980b). Antipyrine metabolite formation in children in the acute phase of malnutrition and after recovery. *Br. J. Clin. Pharmacol.* **9**, 623–627.

Campbell, T. C. (1977). Nutrition and drug metabolising enzymes. *Clin. Pharmacol. Ther.* **22**, 699–706.

Campbell, T. C., and Hayes, T. R. (1974). Role of nutrition in drug metabolising system. *Pharmacol. Rev.* **26**, 171–197.

Conney, A. H., Pantuck, E. J., Hsiao, K. C. *et al.* (1976). Enhanced phenacetin metabolism in human subjects fed charcoal-broiled beef. *Clin. Pharmacol. Ther.* **20**, 633–642.

Conney, A. H., Buening, M. K., Pantuck, E. J. *et al.* (1980). Regulation of human drug metabolism by dietary factors. *Ciba Found. Symp.* **76**, 147–167.

Da Costa, M., and Rothenberg, S. P. (1974). Appearance of a folate binder in leukocytes and serum of women who are pregnant or taking oral contraceptives. *J. Lab. Clin. Med.* **83**, 207–214.

DeLuca, H. F. (1980). Some new concepts emanating from a study of the metabolism and function of vitamin D. *Nutr. Rev.* **38**, 169–182.

Dollery, C. T., Fraser, H. S., Mucklow, J. C., and Bulpitt, J. (1979). Contribution of environmental factors to variability in human drug metabolism. *Drug Metab. Rev.* **9**, 207–220.

Feldman, C. H., Hutchinson, V. E., Pipenger, C. E. *et al.* (1980). Effect of dietary protein and carbohydrate on theophylline metabolism in children. *Pediatrics* **66**, 956–962.

Fishman, J., and Bradlow, H. L. (1978). Effect of malnutrition on the metabolism of sex hormones in man. *Clin. Pharmacol. Ther.* **22**, 721–728.

Flynn, A., Martier, S. S., Sokol, R. J. *et al.* (1981). Zinc status of pregnant alcoholic women—a determinant of foetal outcome. *Lancet* **1**, 572–575.

Food and Agricultural Organization (1978). "The Fourth World Food Survey," pp. 47–65. FAO, Rome.

Gershoff, S. N. (1976). Vitamin B_6. *In* "Present Knowledge in Nutrition," pp. 141–166. Nutr. Found. Inc., New York.

Gopalan, C., and Narasinga Rao, B. S. (1971). Nutritional constraints on growth and development in current Indian dietaries. *Indian J. Med. Res.* **39,** Suppl., 111–122.

Gopalan, C., and Srikantia, S. G. (1979). Nutrition and diseases. *In* "Nutrition and World Food Problem" (M. Rechceigl, Jr., ed)., Vol. 6, pp. 134–163. Karger, Basel.

Greenblatt, D. J., and Koch-Weser, J. (1974). Clinical toxicity of chlordiazepoxide and diazepam in relation to serum albumin concentrations. A report from the Boston Collaborative Drug Surveillance Program. *Eur. J. Clin. Pharmacol.* **7,** 259.

Gugler, R., Shoeman, D. W., Hoffman, D. H. *et al.* (1975). Pharmacokinetics of drugs in patients with nephrotic syndrome. *J. Clin. Invest.* **55,** 1182–1186.

Hahn, T. J., and Avioli, L. V. (1984). Anticonvulsant drug-induced mineral disorders. *In* "Drugs and Nutrients" (D. A. Roe and T. C. Campbell, eds.), pp. 409–427. Dekker, New York.

Hahn, T. J., Hendin, B. A., Scharp, C. R., and Haddad, J. G. (1972). Effect of chronic anticonvulsant therapy on serum 25-hydroxycholecalciferol levels in adults. *N. Engl. J. Med.* **287,** 900–904.

Hathcock, J. N., and Coon, J., eds (1978). "Nutrition and Drug Interactions." Academic Press, New York.

Hathcock, J. N. (1985). Metabolic mechanisms of drug-nutrient interactions. *Fed. Proc., Fed. Am. Soc. Exp. Biol.* **44,** 124–129.

Hewitt, W. R., and Hook, J. B. (1983). The renal excretion of drugs. *Prog. Drug Metabo.* **7,** 11–56.

Holloway, D. E., and Peterson, F. J. (1984). Ascorbic acid in drug metabolism. *In* "Drugs and Nutrients" (D. A. Roe and T. C. Campbell, eds.), Dekker, New York.

Homeida, M., Karrar, Z. A., and Roberts, C. J. C. (1979). Drug metabolism in malnourished children: A study with antipyrine. *Arch. Dis. Child.* **54,** 299–302.

Jagadeesan, V., and Krishnaswamy, K. (1984). Drug binding in under-nourished: A study of the binding of propranolol to α_1 acid glycoproteins. *Eur. J. Clin. Pharmacol.* **27,** 657–659.

Jaya Rao, K. S. (1982). Endocrines in protein energy malnutrition. *World Rev. Nutr. Diet.* **39,** 53–84.

Kalamegham, R., Krishnaswamy, K., Krishnamurthy, S., and Bhargava, R. N. K. (1979). Metabolism of drugs and carcinogens in man: Antipyrine elimination as an indicator. *Clin. Pharmacol. Ther.* **25,** 67–73.

Kato, R. (1977). Drug metabolism under pathological and abnormal physiological status in animals and man. *Xenobiotica* **7,** 25–92.

Krishnaswamy, K. (1978a). Drug metabolism and pharmacokinetics in malnutrition. *Clin. Pharmacokinet.* **3,** 216–240.

Krishnaswamy, K. (1978b). Nutrition and drug metabolism. *Indian J. Med. Res.* **68,** 109–120.

Krishnaswamy, K. (1982). Pharmacokinetics and drug disposition in the under-nourished/malnourished subjects. *In* "Pharmacy in the Third World" (T. Maguire, ed.), pp. 92–126. International Pharmaceutical Students Federation, Belfast.

Krishnaswamy, K. (1983). Drug metabolism and pharmacokinetics in malnutrition. *Trends Pharmacol. Sci.* **4,** 295–299.

Krishnaswamy, K. (1985). The effect of nutritional status on drug action. *Pharm. Int.* **6,** 41–44.

Krishnaswamy, K., and Naidu, A. N. (1977). Microsomal enzymes in malnutrition as determined by plasma half life of antipyrine. *Br. Med. J.* **1,** 538–540.

Krishnaswamy, K., and Teoh, P. C. (1980). *In* "Drug Treatment" (G. S. Avery, ed.), pp. 1175–1209. Adis Press, Sydney, Australia.

Krishnaswamy, K., Ushasri, V., and Naidu, A. N. (1981). The effect of malnutrition on the pharmacokinetics of phenylbutazone. *Clin. Pharmacokinet.* **6,** 152–159.

Krishnaswamy, K., Kalamegham, R., and Naidu, A. N. (1984). Dietary influences on the kinetics of antipyrine and aminopyrine in human subjects. *Br. J. Clin. Pharmacol.* **17,** 139–146.

Krishnaswamy, K., Raghuramulu, N., and Murthy, K. J. R. (1987). INH, Rifampicin and osteopenia (to be published).

Lakshmaiah, N., and Bamji, M. S. (1979). Effect of oral contraceptives on folate economy: A study in female rats. *Horm. Metab. Res.* **11,** 64–67.

Levine, R. A. (1967). Effect of dietary gluten upon neomycin-induced malabsorption. *Gastroenterology* **52,** 685–690.

Levitsky, D. A. (1984). Drugs, appetite and body weight. *In* "Drugs and Nutrients" (D. A. Roe and T. C. Campbell, eds.), pp. 375–408. Dekker, New York.

McCurdy, P. R., and Donohoe, R. F. (1966). Pyridoxine responsive anaemia conditioned by isonicotinic acid hydrazide. *Blood* **27,** 352–362.

McLean, A. E. M., Witts, D. J., and Jane, D. (1980). The influence of nutrition and inducers on mechanisms of toxicity in humans and animals. *Ciba Found. Symp.* **76,** 275–288.

Mehta, S. (1983). Drug disposition in children with protein energy malnutrition. *J. Pediatr. Gastroenterol. Nutr.* **2,** 407–417.

Mehta, S., Kalsi, H. K., Jayaraman, S., and Mathur, V. S. (1975). Chloramphenicol metabolism in children with protein calorie malnutrition. *Am. J. Clin. Nutr.* **28,** 977–981.

Mehta, S., Nair, C. K., Sharma, B., and Mathur, V. S. (1981a). Bioavailability and pharmacokinetics of chloramphenicol palmitate in malnourished children. *Indian J. Med. Res.* **74,** 244–250.

Mehta, S., Nair, C. K., Sharma, B., and Mathur, V. S. (1981b). Steady state of chloramphenicol in malnourished children. *Indian J. Med. Res.* **73,** 538–542.

Melander, A. (1978). Influence of food on the bioavailability of drugs. *Clin. Pharmacokinet.* **3,** 337–351.

Melander, A., and McLean, A. (1983). Influence of food intake on pre-systemic clearance of drugs. *Clin. Pharmacokinet.* **8,** 286–296.

Metcoff, J. (1975). Cellular energy metabolism. *In* "Protein Calorie Malnutrition" (R. E. Olson, ed.), pp. 65–84. Academic Press, London.

Monckeberg, F., Bravo, M., and Gonzdez, O. (1978). Drug metabolism and infantile undernutrition. *In* "Nutrition and Drug Interrelations" (J. N. Hathcock and J. Coon, eds.), pp. 399–408. Academic Press, New York.

Monson, R. R., Rosenberd, L., Hartz, S. C. *et al.* (1973). Diphenylhydantoin and related congenital malformations. *N. Engl. J. Med.* **289,** 1049–1052.

Mucklow, J. C., Rawlins, M. D., Brodie, M. J. *et al.* (1980). Drug oxidation in Asian vegetarians. *Lancet* **2,** 151.

Nair, K. M., Sivakumar, B., Prema, K., and Rao, B. S. N. (1979). Pharmacokinetics of levonorgestrel in Indian women belonging to low socio-economic group. *Contraception* **20:** 303–317.

Nair, K. M., Sivakumar, B., and Narasinga Rao, B. S. (1981). Effect of food restriction on pharmacokinetics of levonorgestrel in rabbits. *Contraception* **23,** 549–561.

Narang, R. K., Mehta, S., and Mathur, V. S. (1979). Pharmacokinetics study of antipyrine in malnourished children. *Am. J. Clin. Nutr.* **30,** 1979–1982.

Newmann, T. J., and Bargman, G. J. (1979). Acetaminophen toxicity and malnutrition. *Am. J. Gastroenterol.* **72,** 647–650.

Obama, M., Cangir, A., and Van Eys, J. (1983). Nutritional status and anthracycline cardiotoxicity in children. *South. Med. J.* **76,** 577–578.

Obel, A. O. K., and Vere, D. W. (1978). Antipyrine and propranolol disposition in malnutrition. *East Afr. Med. J.* **55,** 20.

Pantuck, E. J., Pantuck, C. B., Garland, W. A., and Min, B. H. (1979). Effect of dietary brussels sprouts and cabbage on human drug metabolism. *Clin. Pharmacol. Ther.* **25,** 88–95.

Parke, D. V., and Ioannides, C. (1981). The role of nutrition in toxicology. *Ann. Rev. Nutr.* **1,** 207–234.

Pellicone, N., Pinto, J., Huang, Y. P., and Rivlin, R. (1983). Accelerated development of riboflavin deficiency by treatment with chlorpromazine. *Biochem. Pharmacol.* **32**, 2949–2953.

Peterson, P., Gray, P., and Tolman, K. G. (1976). Calcium balance in drug induced osteomalacia response to vitamin D. *Clin. Pharmacol. Ther.* **19**, 63–67.

Polasa, K., Murthy, K. J. R., and Krishnaswamy, K. (1984). Rifampicin kinetics in undernutrition. *Br. J. Clin. Pharmacol.* **17**, 481–484.

Prasad, A. S., Oberleas, D., Lei, K. Y. *et al.* (1975). Effects of oral contraceptive agents on nutrients. *Am. J. Clin. Nutr.* **28**, 371.

Prasad, K. V. S., Rao, B. S. N., Sivakumar, B., and Prema, K. (1979). Pharmacokinetics of norethindrone in Indian women. *Contraception* **20**, 77–90.

Raghuram, T. C., and Krishnaswamy, K. (1981a). Tetracycline absorption in malnutrition. *Drug-Nutr. Interact.* **1**, 23–25.

Raghuram, T. C., and Krishnaswamy, K. (1981b). Tetracycline kinetics in undernourished subjects. *Int. J. Clin. Pharmacol., Ther. Toxicol.* **19**, 409–413.

Raghuram, T. C., and Krishnaswamy, K. (1982). Pharmacokinetics and plasma steady state levels of doxycycline in undernutrition. *Br. J. Clin. Pharmacol.* **14**, 785–789.

Ramesh, R., Kalamegham, R., Chary, A. K., and Krishnaswamy, K. (1985). Hepatic drug metabolising enzymes in undernourished man. *Toxicology* **37**, 259–266.

Reddy, V., and Srikantia, S. G. (1966). Serum Vitamin A in kwashiorkor. *Am. J. Clin. Nutr.* **18**, 105–109.

Reynolds, E. H. (1974). Iatrogenic nutritional effects of anticonvulsants. *Proc. Nutr. Soc.* **33**, 225–229.

Richens, A. (1976). "Drug Treatment of Epilepsy," pp. 127–129. Henry Kimpton, London.

Roe, D. A. (1984a). Risk factors in drug-induced nutritional deficiency. *In* "Drugs and Nutrients" (D. A. Roe and T. C. Campbell, eds.), pp. 505–523. Dekker, New York.

Roe, D. A. (1984b). Food, formulae and drug effect on the disposition of nutrients. *World Rev. Nutr. Diet.* **43**, 80–94.

Rowland, M. (1984). Protein binding and drug clearance. *Clin. Pharmacokinet.* **9**, Suppl., 11–17.

Shah, S. C., Sharma, R. K., Chitle, H., and Chitle, A. R. (1981). Rifampicin induced osteomalacia. *Tubercle* **62**, 207–209.

Shastri, R. A. (1984). Salicylic acid kinetics in undernutrition. *World Rev. Nutr. Diet.* **43**, 192–197.

Shastri, R. A., and Krishnaswamy, K. (1979). Metabolism of sulphadiazine in malnutrition. *Br. J. Clin. Pharmacol.* **7**, 69–73.

Shojania, A. M., Hornady, G., and Barnes, P. H. (1968). Oral contraceptives and serum folate levels. *Lancet* **1**, 1376–1377.

Sidransky, H. (1985). Tryptophan. *In* "Nutritional Pathology" (H. Sidransky, ed.), pp. 1–62. Dekker, New York.

Smith, J. L., Goldsmith, G. H., and Lawrence, J. D. (1975). Effect of oral contraceptive steroids on vitamin and lipid levels in serum. *Am. J. Clin. Nutr.* **28**, 371–376.

Smith, S. R., Beldose, J., and Chhetri, M. K. (1975). Cortisol metabolism and the pituitary adrenal-axis in adults with protein calorie malnutrition. *J. Clin. Endocrinol. Metab.* **40**, 43–52.

Sukhatme, P. V. (1970). Incidence of protein deficiency in relation to different diets in India. *Br. J. Nutr.* **24**, 477–487.

Theuer, R. C. (1972). Effect of oral contraceptive agents on vitamins and mineral needs, a review. *J. Reprod. Med.* **8**, 13–19.

Toothaker, R. D., and Welling, P. G. (1980). The effect of food and drug bioavailability. *Annu. Rev. Pharmacol. Toxicol.* **20**, 173–199.

Tranvouez, J. L., Lerebours, E., Chrétin, P. *et al.* (1985). Hepatic antipyrine metabolism in malnourished patients: Influence of the type of malnutrition and course of the nutritional rehabilitation. *Am. J. Clin. Nutr.* **41**, 1257–1269.

Tulpule, A., and Krishnaswamy, K. (1983). Chloroquine kinetics in the undernourished. *Eur. J. Clin. Pharmacol.* **24**, 273–276.

Vesell, E. S. (1977). Genetic and environmental factors affecting drug disposition in man. *Clin. Pharmacol. Ther.* **22,** 659–679.

Waterlow, J. K. (1975). Adaptation of low protein intake. *In* "Protein Calorie Malnutrition" (R. E. Olson, ed.), pp. 23–24. Academic Press, London.

West, J., and Lloyd, J. K. (1975). The effect of cholestyramine on intestinal absorption. *Gut* **16,** 93–98.

Wharton, B. P., and McChesney, E. W. (1970). Chloroquine metabolism in kwashiorkor. *J. Trop. Pediatr.* **16,** 130–132.

Wilkinson, G. R. (1984). Plasma binding, distribution and elimination. *In* "Drugs and Nutrients" (D. A. Roe and T. C. Campbell, eds.), pp. 21–49. Dekker, New York.

Yui, Y., Itokowa, Y., and Kawai, C. (1980). Furosemide induced thiamine deficiency. *Cardiovasc. Res.* **14,** 537–540.

5

Nutritional Influences on Chromatin:

Toxicological Implications

C. Elizabeth Castro

I. INTRODUCTION

Nutritional toxicology examines the interaction of nutrients and nutritional processes with drug metabolism and action. It is a complex interaction as the amount, type, and timing of consumed foods affect drug absorption, distribution, metabolism, and excretion (Hathcock, 1985). ''Drug'' is a nonspecific term in this sense and may better be considered as any xenobiotic, an agent not naturally found in the biological system under study. However, an agent that is naturally a part of a biological system may occur in nonphysiological quantities and assume the characteristics and designation of a xenobiotic.

129

Copyright © 1987 by Academic Press, Inc.
All rights of reproduction in any form reserved.

Toxicology is itself a comprehensive science as it envelops the processes of mutagenesis, carcinogenesis, teratogenesis, cellular damage and necrosis, and allergic hypersensitivity. These diverse biological processes are conceptually related, however, in that they exhibit fundamental molecular mechanisms of toxic action. One fundamental aspect in common is the sequential phases of toxic action which include the exposure phase, the toxicokinetic phase, and the toxicodynamic phase (Ariëns and Simonis, 1982). The latter two stages as they occur in the eukaryotic cell nucleus will be emphasized in this chapter. The toxicokinetic aspect includes toxigen metabolism and is exemplified in Fig. 1 as detoxifying enzymes of the nuclear matrix or nuclear envelope. An inclusive discussion of the detoxifying capability of the nucleus is beyond the scope of this chapter and, where appropriate, the reader will be directed to more in-depth reviews. A focal point in this discussion will be the toxicodynamic phase, that in which a reactive toxigen interacts with the target tissue. The site of action will be limited to nuclear chromatin, which has been shown to be responsive to nutritional state. The structure or configuration of chromatin within the nucelus is a key feature in its accessibility to toxigens and is also a determinant in gene expression (Fig. 1).

This chapter emphasizes the interaction of nutrient intake with DNA and chromatin, and how such interactions may affect the process of toxicogenesis in the nucleus. Recent observations that variation in nutrient intake alters the fine structure (Klaude and von der Decken, 1985; Castro, 1983) and the global configuration of chromatin (Castro *et al.*, 1986b; Stankiewicz *et al.*, 1983; Castro and Sevall, 1980) have focused attention on underlying nutrient–genome

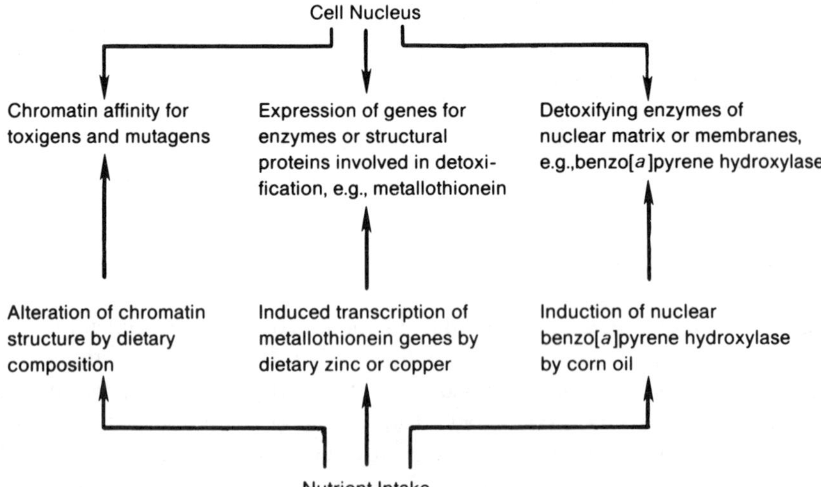

Fig. 1. Examples of nutritional influence on the multifunctional role of the nucleus in toxicogenesis.

interactions. Another series of observations which demonstrate nuclear metabolism of xenobiotics (Baker *et al.*, 1983; Hennig *et al.*, 1983; Yoshizawa *et al.*, 1981; Holder *et al.*, 1981; Romano *et al.*, 1983) has heightened interest in the role of the nucleus in toxicogenesis. The proximity of reactive molecules to the genome makes these findings particularly noteworthy, especially since it is well documented that the microsomal counterparts of the nuclear metabolizing enzymes are influenced by diet.

One goal of nutritional toxicology is to identify nutrient effects on genome structure which would alter the susceptibility to toxigen binding. One of several molecular mechanisms of toxic action is modification of DNA by reactive electrophiles. An aspect to consider is that DNA and chromatin are not passive, static molecules; rather, there is dynamic activity along the DNA fiber in the form of replication, transcription, recombination, and repair. There exist multiple points of action where nutrient intake could influence the structure and direction of the genome and consequently the degree of toxigen binding. For this reason, a basic understanding of fundamental nutrient–genome interactions is necessary.

II. AFFINITY OF TOXIGENS TOWARD NUCLEAR CHROMATIN

The negatively charged DNA molecule is a potential target site for the binding of a great array of electrophilic, reactive compounds. In addition to covalent binding by reactive electrophiles, intercalation of DNA and noncovalent, hydrophobic interactions may modify DNA structure. Polycyclic aromatic hydrocarbons are a class of molecules including benzo[*a*]pyrene (B[*a*]P), 7,12-dimethylbenz[*a*]anthracene, 2-acetylaminofluorene (2-AAF), aflatoxin B_1, (AFB$_1$), 2-aminoanthracene, for which detailed metabolic studies have lead to a clearer understanding of electrophile–DNA interaction. N-Hydroxylation of the primary aromatic amines generates reactive electrophiles that covalently bind to DNA and initiate mutagenesis and carcinogenesis (Frederick *et al.*, 1982; Mitchell, 1985; Radomski, 1979; Mita *et al.*, 1981; Miller and Miller, 1981; Miller *et al.*, 1964; Kriek and Westra, 1979). An excellent correlation has been found between carcinogenicity and the quantitative covalent binding of chemicals to DNA (Brookes and Lawley, 1964; Lutz, 1979).

The most striking correlation between DNA binding and cancer is seen between hepatocarcinogenesis and DNA adducts (Lutz, 1979). In many instances, the predominant metabolite of a hepatocarcinogen forming DNA adducts is known. A secondary metabolite of B[*a*]P, 7β,8α-dihydroxy-9α,10α-epoxy-7,8,9,10-tetrahydro-B[*a*]P, is highly mutagenic and readily binds covalently with DNA (Huberman *et al.*, 1976; Jeffrey *et al.*, 1977). After the dietary administration of AFB$_1$, analysis of nucleic acid bases by high-performance liquid chromatography showed that the principal AFB$_1$ metabolite which forms

DNA adducts in liver is 8,9-dihydro-8-(N^7-guanyl)-9-hydroxyaflatoxin B$_1$ (Kensler *et al.*, 1985). A study of the intranuclear distribution of initial and prolonged DNA adducts induced *in vivo* after injections of another hepatocarcinogen, 2-AAF, showed that all regions of DNA loops are equally susceptible to adduct formation (Gupta *et al.*, 1985). Supercoiled DNA loops are a higher order packaging structure of eukaryotic chromatin (Castro and Sevall, 1983, for review). After an initial dose of 2-AAF, two acetylated [*N*-acetyl-*N*-(deoxyguanosin-8-yl)-2-aminofluorene and 3-(deoxyguanosin-N^2-yl)-2-AAF] adducts and one deacetylated [*N*-(deoxyguanosin-8-yl)-2-aminofluorene] adduct were found to be randomly distributed along the genome. However, a nonrandom persistence of the deacylated adduct in the regions where DNA loops are anchored by the nuclear matrix suggest that marked regional differences in adduct repair may influence chemically induced hepatocarcinogenesis (Gupta *et al.*, 1985). How nutrient intake affects higher order DNA structure, such as supercoiled loops, is discussed in a preceding section.

In addition to activated carcinogens which interact with DNA, some alkylating antitumor agents also interact with DNA and consequently exhibit genotoxic properties. One of these agents, cyclophosphamide, is metabolized to a nor-nitrogen mustard which reacts with the N-7 position of guanine (Hemminki, 1985). Another compound, *cis*-diamminedichloroplatinum (II) (cisplatin), is a very effective component of chemotherapy of a variety of human cancers (Prestayko *et al.*, 1980). DNA interstrand cross-links are formed with cisplatin probably between two N-7 sites of guanine (Ploory *et al.*, 1985; Marcelis and Reedijk, 1983). How significant the various cross-links are in the dual antineoplastic and genotoxic action of cisplatin is not yet clearly understood.

Some agents exert their cytotoxicity by binding to chromatin and chromosomal proteins instead of, or in addition to, covalent binding to DNA. Histone H1 is a principal target molecule for the binding of several mutagens and/or carcinogens, such as aflatoxin B (Prince and Campbell, 1982), 1,2-dimethylhydrazine (Boffa *et al.*, 1982), ‡-7β, 8α-dihydroxy-9α,10α-epoxy-7,8,9,10-tetrahydrobenzo[*a*]pyrene (Sculley and Zytkovicz, 1983), and activated B[*a*]P (Bresnick *et al.*, 1977; Jenson *et al.*, 1982a). In addition, 9,10-dihydroxy-7,8-oxy-7,8,9,10-tetrahydrobenzo[*a*]pyrene associates virtually exclusively with nonhistone proteins comigrating with H1 (Selkirk *et al.*, 1982). Lysine residues of H1 are the principal target for covalent binding of activated B[*a*]P *in vitro* (Jenson *et al.*, 1982b).

The highly toxic acetylcholinesterase-inhibiting organophosphate, soman, also induces alterations in nuclear liver chromatin. Thirty minutes after an injection to rats of 0.9 LD$_{50}$ (120 μg/kg) soman, increased polyploidization, expansion of the nuclear envelope, and elevated deoxyribonucleoprotein (DNP) lability to acid hydrolysis were observed (Moore *et al.*, 1984). The enhanced susceptibility to acid hydrolysis may stem from increased accessibility of aldehyde groups as the DNP complex enters a more dispersed state. Such "chromatin activation" may be the recruitment of regulatory molecular events leading to an enhancement of detoxification by protein synthesis, since the induction of microsomal enzyme systems by a variety of xenobiotics involves accelerated protein synthesis (Perry and Swartz, 1967).

Another class of drugs, antitumor compounds such as adriamycin, actinomycin D, 4^1-(9-acridinylamino)methanesulfon-*m*-anisidide (m-AMSA), and 5-iminodaunorubicin, intercalate DNA and induce reversible protein-linked DNA breaks in cultured cells (Pommier *et al.*, 1985; Chen *et al.*, 1984; Ross *et al.*, 1978). DNA breakage induced by intercalative antitumor drugs is mediated by mammalian DNA topoisomerase II (Tewey *et al.*, 1984; Chen *et al.*, 1984; Ross *et al.*, 1984). Topoisomerase II is an ATP-dependent enzyme which enables one DNA helix to pass through another and may function in mediating the condensation and decondensation of eukaryotic chromatin (Sevall, 1983, for review). Many antitumor drugs block the rejoining reaction of mammalian topoisomerase II and cause protein-linked DNA single-stranded and double-stranded breaks (Tewey *et al.*, 1984; Chen *et al.*, 1984; Ross *et al.*, 1984; Nelson *et al.*, 1984). Pommier *et al.* (1985) showed that double-stranded DNA breaks (but not single-stranded breaks) induced by m-AMSA and 5-iminodaunorubicin at DNA topoisomerase II binding sites correlate closely with sister chromatid exchanges, mutations, and cell killing, and may be responsible for their production. These intercalative antitumor drugs inhibit the breakage–reunion reaction of DNA topoisomerase II by stabilizing a cleavable complex. Treatment of the cleavable complex with protein denaturants results in DNA breakage and covalent linking of one topoisomerase subunit to each 5′-phosphoryl end of the disrupted DNA strand (Nelson *et al.*, 1984; Tewey *et al.*, 1984). Double-stranded DNA breaks on SV40 viral DNA introduced into monkey cells have been mapped at multiple topoisomerase II cleavage sites (Yang *et al.*, 1985). A major cleavage site preferentially induced during late infection is localized on a region of SV40 chromatin that is hypersensitive to deoxyribonuclease I. Nuclease-hypersensitive regions are usually located at the 3′ and 5′ ends of transcribed genes (Elgin, 1981) and are probably under torsional stress (Larsen and Weintraub, 1982). The significance of torsional stress or negative DNA supercoiling to transcription and chromatin organization has been suggested (Ryoji and Worcel, 1984; Glikin *et al.*, 1984). The intercalating drug-induced stabilization of a cleavable complex between DNA and topoisomerase II may be the prerequisite of genotoxicity of antitumor drugs.

A. Nutritional Modulation of Chromatin Structure

Chromatin structure is a key determinant in gene expression and regulation. Eukaryotic interphase chromatin has multiple levels of organization: the nucleosome (Kornberg, 1974; McGhee and Felsenfeld, 1980, for review), the solenoid, which consists of 6–10 nucleosomes (Finch and Klug, 1976), and the supercoiled DNA loops or domains (Benyajati and Worcel, 1976; Paulson and Laemmli, 1977; Igo-Kemenes and Zachau, 1977). The higher order organization of chromatin characterized by successively coiled loops can be altered by nutrient intake. One method of determining the higher order configuration of chromatin is by the measurement of the amount of nuclease-sensitive chromatin. Micrococcal nuclease (EC 3.1.31.1) digests approximately 50% of nuclear DNA or chromatin into acid-soluble nucleotides. The remainder of the DNA is resistant to micrococcal nuclease because of associated nuclear proteins (Clark and Felsenfeld, 1974). Micrococcal nuclease digests nuclear DNA and purified chromatin into oligonucleosomes and subsequently into nucleosomes (Compton *et al.*, 1976).

When nuclear DNA from liver of rats fed a basal diet for 5 days is digested with micrococcal nuclease, 50.3% of the DNA is converted into acid-soluble oligonucleotides (Castro and Sevall, 1980). If nuclei are isolated from animals fed for 5 days with experimental diets which vary in the proportion of macronutrient components, the percentage of total DNA hydrolyzed by micrococcal nuclease varies as a function of diet ($p < .0001$) (Table I). After feeding a high-carbohydrate, fat-free (HCFF) diet, greater than 70% of nuclear chromatin is solubilized by micrococcal nuclease to acid-soluble oligonucleotides. In contrast, a protein-free, low-carbohydrate diet renders only 39% of nuclear chromatin as acid-soluble. These differential amounts of acid-soluble DNA at the limit digest suggest that the higher order organization of chromatin can be altered by dietary composition.

Nuclease sensitivity of chromatin is a structural modification that distinguishes transcriptionally active genes from inactive genes. Weintraub and Groudine

TABLE I

Effect of Dietary Composition on the Percentage of Total DNA Susceptible to Micrococcal Nuclease Hydrolysis[a]

Diet number	Dietary treatment	Acid-soluble DNA at limit digest	p[b]
1	High carbohydrate, fat-free	71.4	0.0022
2	Low carbohydrate, high fat	56.5	0.0002
3	Low carbohydrate, high protein	51.5	0.2655 (NS)[c]
4	High carbohydrate, low protein	60.1	0.0112
5	High carbohydrate, protein-free	45.7	0.0437
6	Low carbohydrate, protein-free	38.8	0.0001
7	Stock diet	50.3	—

[a]From Castro and Sevall (1980). © *J. Nutr.*, American Institute of Nutrition.

[b]Probability value at which slope differs from that of stock diet control by least-squares analysis of homogeneity of slopes.

[c]NS, Not significant.

(1976) demonstrated that chicken globin genes are preferentially digested by deoxyribonuclease I (DNase I) in erythrocyte nuclei, where they are actively transcribed, but not in fibroblast or brain nuclei, where they are not actively transcribed. In addition, nontranscribed ovalbumin sequences in erythrocytes or fibroblasts are not preferentially digested. Subsequently, Wood and Felsenfeld (1982), using a cloned fragment spanning 6.2 kilobase pairs (kbp) of the chicken globin gene, examined its chromatin structure by probing with three nucleases: DNase I, deoxyribonuclease II (DNase II), and micrococcal nuclease. The entire 6.2-kbp region in nuclei from chick embryo erythrocytes shows a 10- to 20-fold increase in sensitivity to DNase I, a sixfold increase in sensitivity to DNase II, and a threefold increase in sensitivity to micrococcal nuclease. These and other studies (Giri and Gorovsky, 1980; Levy-Wilon *et al.*, 1980; Storb *et al.*, 1981; Groudine *et al.*, 1981) reveal that actively transcribing genes are packaged differently than nontranscribed regions of the genome. A gene need not be actively transcribing to exhibit enhanced sensitivity to DNase I. Genes with a history of transcription (Mathis *et al.*, 1980) or a programmed future of transcription (Stalder *et al.*, 1980) exhibit sensitivity to DNase I. In contrast, enhanced sensitivity of genes to micrococcal nuclease depends on the expression of the gene (Bloom and Anderson, 1979; Smith and Yu, 1984).

The use of micrococcal nuclease as a probe for higher order chromatin structure has certain limitations. In addition to recognizing the tertiary structure of DNA, the enzyme also recognizes mucleotide composition and nucleotide sequences, with a particular preference for A-T rich regions (Hörz and Altenburger, 1981; Dingwall *et al.*, 1981). However, the enzyme shows a general preference for internucleosomal DNA rather than the DNA within the nucleosomal core particle. Therefore, the preference for A-T rich regions is most apparent in the generation of subnucleosomal particles (McGhee and Felsenfeld, 1983), rather than in the digestion of bulk chromatin (Castro and Sevall, 1980).

Not only does the total amount of nuclease-sensitive DNA vary as a function of dietary intake, the rate at which nuclear DNA is solubilized is also diet-dependent. After 30 min of incubation with micrococcal nuclease, 43.7% of liver nuclear chromatin from rats fed a protein-free, low-carbohydrate diet is present as undigested high molecular weight oligonucleosomes (> pentanucleosomes). After the same length of incubation time, 26.5 and 25.7% of nuclear chromatin is of the comparable size when the source of liver DNA was from rats fed stock diet or HCFF diet, respectively (Castro, 1983). The ultimate product of digestion, the mononucleosome, accounts for 20.6, 9.9, and 32.4% of the total-input DNA from rats fed stock, protein-free, or HCFF diets, respectively (Fig. 2).

Nutrient-mediated alteration in higher order chromatin structure has been demonstrated not only in rodents but also in the lower eukaryote, *Euglena gracilis* (Stankiewicz *et al.*, 1983). Zinc deficiency in *E. gracilis* is related to extensive repression of genomic activities, including a virtual disappearance of histone proteins (Mazus *et al.*, 1984) and repressed transcription (Falchuk *et al.*, 1975).

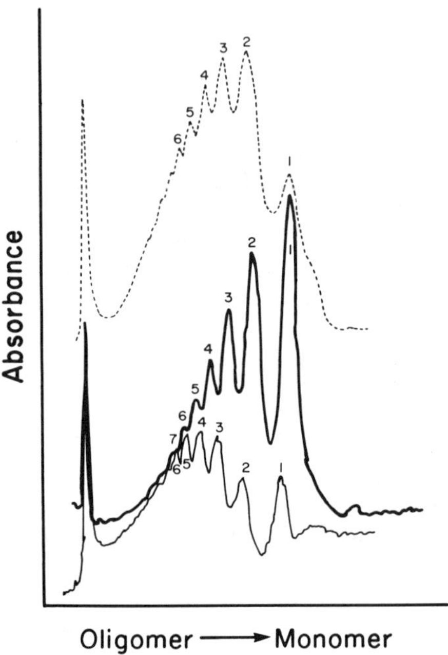

Fig. 2. Densitometric scan of DNA digestion products after 30 min of incubation with micrococcal nuclease at a ratio of 1 unit enzyme per A_{260} unit. The DNA was purified and separated on a 2% agarose gel in 40 mM Tris HCl (pH 8.0), 20 mM sodium acetate, 2 mM EDTA for 205 volt-hours. After the gel was stained with ethidium bromide and photographed, a negative was scanned at 500 nm. Stock diet (- - - -); carbohydrate-rich diet (—); protein-free diet (————). (From Castro *et al.*, 1986b. *Federation Proceedings*, Federation of American Societies for Experimental Biology.)

Nuclear DNA of *E. gracilis* grown in zinc-depleted ($-$Zn) or zinc-containing ($+$Zn) media with 0.1 μM and 10 μM Zn^{2+}, respectively, was digested with micrococcal nuclease. The accessibility of $-$Zn and $+$Zn chromatins to micrococcal nuclease differs substantially (Fig. 3). Micrococcal nuclease solubilizes $+$Zn chromatin at a rate 10- to 30-fold greater than that of $-$Zn chromatin. A 10-fold higher amount of nuclease digests the $+$Zn chromatin completely in 10 min, whereas only 20% of the $-$Zn chromatin is solubilized in the same time interval. The micrococcal nuclease digestion of $+$Zn chromatin is not affected by the addition of $-$Zn chromatin. A novel nuclear histone discussed below is responsible for the altered nuclease sensitivity of $-$Zn chromatin.

In a mammalian system, zinc deficiency alters the sensitivity of rat liver chromatin to micrococcal nuclease (Castro *et al.*, 1986b), although not to the same extent as in *E. gracilis*. If zinc deficiency is imposed on young male rats by feeding a diet containing 0.9 ppm, 34.6% of liver nuclear chromatin is solubilized by micrococcal nuclease. Nuclear chromatin of rats pair-fed or fed *ad libitum* a diet containing 40 ppm, the amount of nuclease-sensitive DNA is 53.5

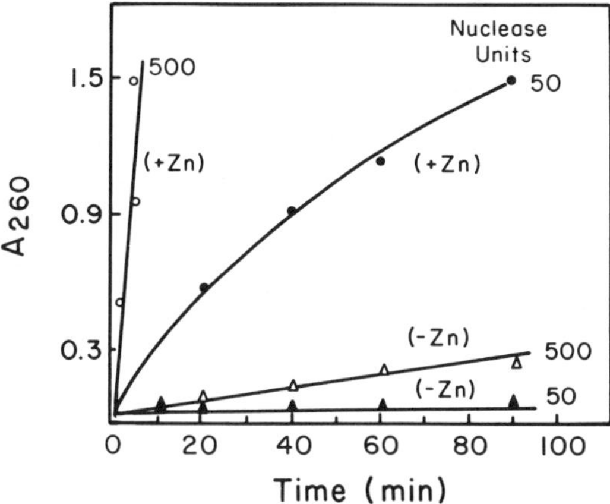

Fig. 3. Comparison of acid-soluble material resulting from micrococcal nuclease (50 or 500 units) digestion of ±Zn chromatins (400 µg of DNA). The digestion of +Zn chromatin with 500 units of nuclease was nearly complete within 10 min, and hence, the material is solubilized totally. A_{260} was measured in 5% perchloric acid-soluble supernatants of these digests. (Reprinted with permission from Stankiewicz *et al.*, 1983. *Biochemistry,* The American Chemical Society.)

and 45.1%, respectively (Fig. 4) (Castro *et al.*, 1986b). The amount of acid-soluble DNA in nuclei of zinc-deficient rats is similar to that from rats fed a protein-free, low-carbohydrate diet (Castro and Sevall, 1980). Similarly, magnesium deficiency decreases the amount of nuclease-sensitive chromatin in rat liver (C. E. Castro, M. E. Ramirez, and J. S. Sevall, unpublished observations). Deficiencies of protein, zinc, or magnesium all increase the resistance of bulk liver chromatin to micrococcal nuclease, suggesting a greater degree of chromatin condensation. Increased chromatin condensation may decrease the available binding sites for polymerases, effector molecules, or genotoxic agents which bind DNA.

B. Nutritional Modulation of the Fine Structure of Chromatin

The nucleosome is the fundamental packaging unit of eukaryotic chromatin. It consists of 146 base pairs (bp) of DNA wrapped around an octomer protein core of histones H2a, H2b, H3, and H4 plus 40–60 bp DNA (linker DNA) bound to histone H1 (Kornberg, 1974; Camerini-Otero *et al.*, 1976; Allan *et al.*, 1980; Thoma *et al.*, 1979). The nucleosome repeat length is the average of the combined lengths of the linker DNA (DNA which joins adjacent nucleosomes) and the invariant core DNA (the 146-bp DNA wrapped around the protein complex). An understanding of changes in overall nucleosome repeat length, particularly those mediated by nutritional intake, is important because such changes could

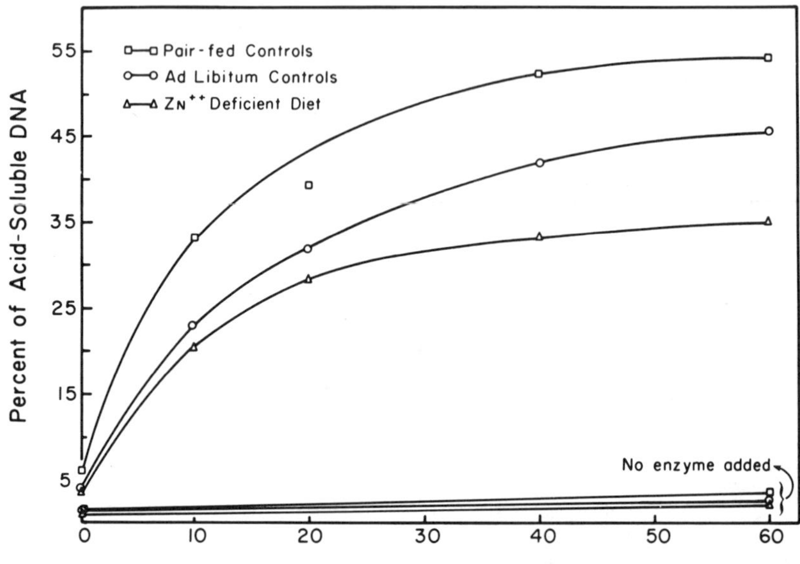

Fig. 4. Percentage of acid-soluble DNA generated by incubating liver nuclei with micrococcal nuclease. Nuclei from rats fed a Zn-deficient diet, pair-fed a Zn-supplemented diet, or fed the Zn-supplemented diet *ad libitum* were digested with 1 unit enzyme per 0.4 μg nuclear DNA. The digested DNA that is soluble in 1 *M* perchloric acid–1 *M* NaCl is expressed as a percentage of the total-input DNA. (From Castro *et al.,* 1986b. *Federation Proceedings,* Federation of American Societies for Experimental Biology.)

alter significantly the structure of the chromatin fiber, since even minute variations in repeat length would change the orientation of adjoining nucleosomes.

Nucleosome repeat length can be measured by briefly digesting nuclei with micrococcal nuclease and purifying the acid-soluble products by pronase incubation. The length of DNA products in base pair is calibrated by electrophoresis with fragments of known length. The nucleosome repeat length is quantitated either arithemtically or by linear regression (Castro, 1983). The repeat length has been quantitated for liver nuclear DNA from rats fed a commercial chow diet, a HCFF diet, or a low-carbohydrate, protein-free diet. A comparison among all three diets showed that the nucleosome repeat unit of liver nuclei from rats fed a HCFF diet is consistently 6–14% shorter than that of rats fed stock or protein-free diet. The nucleosome repeat length in nuclei from HCFF-fed rats is 28–13 bp shorter than that of chow-fed rats.

Associated with the HCFF diet are an increase in nuclease sensitivity of bulk chromatin and a decreased nucleosome repeat length. The increased susceptibility to micrococcal nuclease implies a greater degree of decondensation of chromatin after consuming a HCFF diet. Perhaps this is a compensatory response to some increased functional demand similar to that observed after challenge of rat liver with the organophosphate compound soman, which was postulated to mobilize regulatory molecular events leading to enhancement of detoxification (Moore *et al.*, 1984). After feeding a HCFF diet, there is an induction of protein synthesis and of mRNAs for a family of lipogenic enzymes (Morris *et al.*, 1982; Alberts *et al.*, 1975; Winberry and Holten, 1977; Morikawa *et al.*, 1984; Procsal *et al.*, 1976; Miksicek and Towle, 1983) required for the biosynthesis of fat.

Another aspect of nutritional modulation of the fine structure of chromatin involves the specific alkylation of DNA by dimethylnitrosamine. Alkylation of DNA bases by *N*-nitroso compounds in one or several positions weakens base-pairing accuracies and generates incorrect nucleotide insertion during replication and possibly during transcription (Klaude and von der Decken, 1985). DNA alkylation and the subsequent DNA repair mechanisms seem to be the most relevant determinants (Goth and Rajewsky, 1974; Montesano, 1981; Pegg, 1984a) in the initiation of carcinogenesis by nitrosamines (Bartsch and Montesano, 1984). Particularly critical to the process of carcinogenesis is the repair of alkylation damage at the oxygen atoms of purine and pyrimidine bases (Pegg, 1984b).

A decrease in dietary methionine and cysteine to 10% of control values markedly alters the methylation pattern of guanine after a single dose of dimethylnitrosamine (Klaude and von der Decken, 1985). Using column chromatography (Sephadex G10) to detect methylated bases, it was shown that the methionine- and cysteine-deficient diet increased the level of O^6-methylquanine in the liver of adult and subadult rats (Table II). The ratio of O^6-methylguanine to 7-methylguanine was likewise elevated. In lung, but not kidney or liver, there was an increase in 7-methylguanine after methionine–cysteine deficiency in both subadult and adult animals. Since the amino acid deficiency causes a general decrease in protein synthesis in liver (Omstedt and von der Decken, 1974), the increase in O^6-methylguanine may be due to quantitative or qualitative alterations in chromosomal proteins. Alternately, there may be modulation of repair of O^6-methylguanine induced by dimethylnitrosamine (Planche-Martel *et al.*, 1985).

C. Nutritional Modulation of Chromatin Composition

Chromatin consists of DNA, basic histone proteins, acidic nonhistone proteins, and nuclear RNA. The mass ratios of DNA : histone : nonhistone : RNA are modified by dietary composition (Castro and Sevall, 1982; Canfield and Chytil, 1978). Alterations in the chromosomal proteins are likely to be very subtle, since two-dimensional electrophoresis of nonhistone proteins from liver indicates virtually no qualitative differences in proteins isolated from rats fed a HCFF diet, a protein-free diet, or a stock diet.

One histone protein that could potentially account for diet-associated dif-

TABLE II

Diet- and Age-Dependent Methylation of DNA Purines from [^{14}C]Dimethylnitrosamine[a,b]

| Mice | Tissue | Experiment number | Methylation (μmol/mol of parent base) | | | | Ratio O^6-methylguanine/7-methylguanine | |
| | | | 7-methylguanine | | O^6-methylguanine | | | |
			Contr	Def	Contr	Def	Contr	Def
Subadult	Liver	1	116.1	93.8	5.6	5.0[c]	0.048	0.053[d]
		2	96.2	109.6	1.7	4.0[c]	0.018	0.037[d]
		3	123.0	129.8	5.5	8.8[c]	0.045	0.067[d]
	Kidney	1	23.6	17.4	1.3	2.1		
		2	27.2	30.3	UD	4.2		
		3	30.1	17.6	1.7	1.3		
	Lung	1	8.2	20.6[e]	5.1	UD		
		2	5.2	14.0[e]	2.0	1.9		
Adult	Liver	1	106.0	91.9	2.7	5.5[c]	0.025	0.060[d]
		2	121.4	133.8	1.7	5.4[c]	0.014	0.040[d]
	Kidney	1	15.6	33.4	0.9	2.2		
		2	18.0	25.7	1.5	0.7		
	Lung	1	1.7	15.0[e]	1.2	UD		
		2	4.8	15.9[e]	UD	UD		

[a]Reprinted with permission from Klaude and von der Decken (1985). *Biochem. Pharmacol.*, copyright © Pergamon Press, Ltd.

[b]Mice were injected with [^{14}C]dimethynitrosamine, 0.5 mg/kg body weight, and killed 45 min later. UD, under detection limit. Data were computed with the use of two ways analysis of variance. Contr, Controls; Def, fed diet deficient in cysteine and methionine; UD, under detection limit.

[c]Significantly different from controls, subadult and adult mice considered together, $p < .05$.

[d]Significantly different from controls, subadult and adult mice considered together, $p < .025$.

[e]Significantly different from controls, subadult and adult mice considered together, $p < .01$.

ferences in higher order chromatin structure is histone H1. Histone H1 exhibits an integral and dynamic role in maintaining the higher orders of chromatin organization (Allan *et al.*, 1980; Thoma *et al.*, 1979; Karnik, 1983), as well as the stability of the nucleosome (Thoma *et al.*, 1979; Simpson, 1978). H1 consists of at least five closely related subtypes or variants (Bustin and Cole, 1968), which differ in amino acid sequence, molecular size, and postsynthetic modifications (Langan, 1982; Lennox *et al.*, 1982). Various H1 subtype profiles are present during developmental growth (Larue *et al.*, 1983; Lennox and Cohen, 1983), liver regeneration (Ohba *et al.*, 1984), or partial pancreatectomy (Varricchio *et al.*, 1977). Normal and neoplastic human cells have different H1 compositions such that the ratio of two H1 variants (H1A : H1B) is correlated with tumorigenicity (Tan *et al.*, 1982). The covalent binding of B[*a*]P metabolites to H1 has already been discussed. Histone H1 subtypes may be significant in generating variegated chromatin structures important in differential gene expression and cell differentiation (Lennox, 1984).

TABLE III

Composition of Histone H1 from Liver Chromatin of Rats Fed Zinc-Deficient or Control Diets[a]

Source of nuclear chromatin	Percentage of total[b] H1 as		
	H1.1	H1.2	H1°
Zinc-deficient liver			
$(N = 3)$[c]	74.57 ± 3.67	21.62 ± 2.69	3.81 ± 1.42
Pair-fed control			
$(N = 3)$	72.62 ± 6.79	19.54 ± 4.91	7.84 ± 1.94
Ad libitum control			
$(N \pm 3)$	72.71 ± 1.57	21.67 ± 1.47	5.62 ± 0.17

[a]From Castro *et al.* (1986a). (© *Nutr. Rep. Int.*, Geron-X, Inc.).
[b]Total is taken as 100%.
[c]N is the number of individual isolations of histone H1.

The histone H1 profile in liver is modulated during zinc deficiency in rats (Castro *et al.*, 1986a) and in *E. gracilis* (Stankiewicz *et al.*, 1983). The major H1 subtypes in rat liver are H1.1, H1.2 and H1°. During zinc deficiency, there is as much as a 50% decrease in the H1° variant subtype ($p < .05$) (Table III; Fig. 5). H1° has an implied role in cellular differentiation (Gjerset *et al.*, 1982) and is decreased or extinguished during active proliferative growth of many developing tissues and increased in the corresponding nondividing mature system (Gjerset *et al.*, 1982; Lennox and Cohen, 1983). In some, although not all, neoplastic tissue the amount of H1° is inversely correlated with both the state of morphological differentiation and the proliferative rate of the cells (Marks *et al.*, 1975). In chromatin of $-$Zn *E. gracilis* the histone content, including H1, decreases markedly, concomitant with an increased resistance to micrococcal nuclease (Stan-

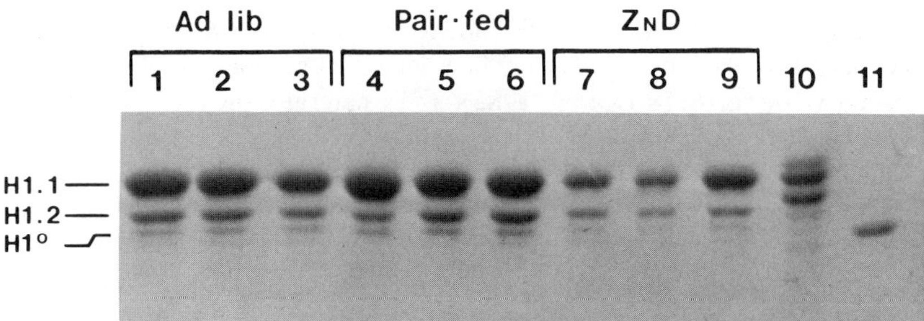

Fig. 5. Histone H1 isolated from liver of zinc-deficient or control rats. H1 subtypes from *ad libitum*-fed control (lanes 1–3), pair-fed (lanes 4–6), and zinc-deficient rats (ZnD) (lanes 7–9) were separated on a 10% polyacrylamide gel. Lanes 10 and 11 contain 3 μg of calf histone H1 and 15 ng of carbonic anhydrase, respectively. (From Castro *et al.*, 1986a. © *Nutr. Rep. Int.*, Geron-X, Inc.)

kiewicz *et al.*, 1983). The major protein constituent of this $-$Zn chromatin is a novel polypeptide of less than 3000 Da which differs electrophoretically from any known constituent of chromatin. This protein is required for the 10- to 30-fold decrease in the rate and extent of $-$Zn chromatin, which is reversed by the removal of the protein from $-$Zn chromatin. The addition of this protein to chromatin of zinc-supplemented ($+$Zn) *E. gracilis* or calf thymus DNA heightens the resistance of both to micrococcal nuclease. The observations demonstrate that the micronutrient zinc specifically affects the composition and the structure of chromatin.

III. NUTRITIONAL EFFECTS ON EXPRESSION OF GENES INVOLVED IN TOXIGEN METABOLISM

A. Metallothionein

Metallothioneins (MTs) are cysteine-rich, ubiquitous low molecular weight proteins that exhibit a selective capacity to bind heavy metals, such as zinc, copper, or cadmium (Karin, 1985, for review). Based on electrophoretic mobilities, there are two major subgroups of MTs, MT-I and MT-II. The MT-I group can be further resolved into distinct molecular isoforms known as MT-I$_A$ and MT-I$_B$ which exhibit slight differences in their affinity for metal ion ligands.

Rapid increases in MTs and their mRNAs occur if tissue culture cells are incubated with heavy-metal ions or glucocorticoid hormones (Karin and Herchman, 1979; Karin *et al.*, 1980), or if a single dose of parenteral zinc is administered *in vivo* to rats (Swerdel and Cousins, 1982). The accumulation of MTs and their mRNAs is due to transcriptional activation of the MT genes by heavy metal ions that bind to the proteins (Durnam and Palmiter, 1981). The mouse MT-I gene and the human MT-II$_A$ gene have been cloned (Durnam *et al.*, 1980; Karin and Richards, 1982), and the DNA sites that control the expression of these genes are under intense investigation (Karin *et al.*, 1984; Stuart *et al.*, 1984).

It is generally accepted that MTs function as protective mechanisms against heavy metal toxicity, although it may be argued that such a protective role is not the primary role of MTs (Karin, 1985). MTs naturally present in mammalian liver and kidney serve as major storage sites for the trace elements, zinc and copper. Dietary status of the animal greatly affects the level of these elements. In addition to the clearance of heavy metals, there may be a role for MTs in the intracellular and extracellular metabolism of zinc and copper.

B. Cytochrome *P*-450

The cytochrome *P*-450 enzyme system metabolizes numerous xenobiotics and endogenous compounds. Enzyme levels and concentrations of several members of the cytochrome *P*-450 family are altered by intake of proteins, carbohydrates, and lipids (Hathcock, 1982; Boyd and Campbell, 1983). In addition, deficiencies of nicotinic acid or riboflavin, because of their integral role in the *P*-450 system, are associated with decreased oxidase activity (Zannoni and Sato, 1976; Miltenberger and Oltersdorf, 1978). Whether the level of control of such interactions is transcriptional, posttranscriptional, or translational has not been determined.

A unique role in *P*-450 induction may be attributed to tryptophan and other naturally occurring indoles. These molecules increase the concentration of *P*-450 microsomal protein (Jorgensen and Majumdar, 1976). Tryptophan specifically induces activities of aniline hydroxylase and dimethylnitrosamine (Jorgensen and Majumdar, 1976; Everts and Mostafa, 1981).

Tryptophan has a specific function in supporting general hepatic protein synthesis (Sidransky *et al.*, 1968, 1981; Pronezuk *et al.*, 1968). With one exception, when a complex amino acid mixture devoid of a single amino acid is tube-fed to fasted animals, it stimulates a recovery shift toward heavier polysomes. The one exception is tryptophan. There is evidence that tryptophan exerts its effects on protein synthesis at multiple points of regulation (Sidransky, 1985). Tryptophan may stimulate protein synthesis by enhancement of mRNA synthesis (Vesley and Cihak, 1970; Henderson, 1970; Oravec and Korner, 1971), and/or posttranscriptionally by increasing nucleocytoplasmic translocation of mRNA (Murty *et al.*, 1982; Sidransky, 1985).

A cytochrome *P*-450 gene induced by 3-methylcholanthrene (*P*-450M) has been isolated and is the first gene coding for a member of the cytochrome *P*-450 family of enzymes for which chromatin structure as been examined (Einck *et al.*, 1985). The chromatin structure of a gene is central to its expression and will facilitate an understanding of its regulation. The *P*-450M gene, which is expressed constitutively at low levels in the uninduced liver is not organized into the typical 200-bp nucleosomal repeat. Four DNase I-hypersensitive sites occur at the 5′-terminal region of the gene (Einck *et al.*, 1985). DNase I-hypersensitive sites are features of transcriptionally active chromatin that have been identified at the 5′ or 3′ end of many genes (Wu *et al.*, 1979; Wu, 1980; Elgin, 1981). Since the induction of the *P*-450 gene by 3-methylcholanthrene does not alter detectably the DNase I-hypersensitive sites, the primary mechanism of regulation for this gene is probably developmentally determined (Einck *et al.*, 1985). However, an understanding of how this *P*-450M gene is organized will enhance the study of *P*-450 genes that are modulated by nutritional intake.

C. Albumin

Plasma albumin is the most common binding and transport system for many drugs (Hathcock, 1985), as well as for endogenous biomolecules such as fatty acids and bilirubin (Burckart *et al.*, 1982). Nutrient intake greatly influences the serum levels (Enwonwu and Sreebny, 1971; Anthony and Edozien, 1975; Lunn

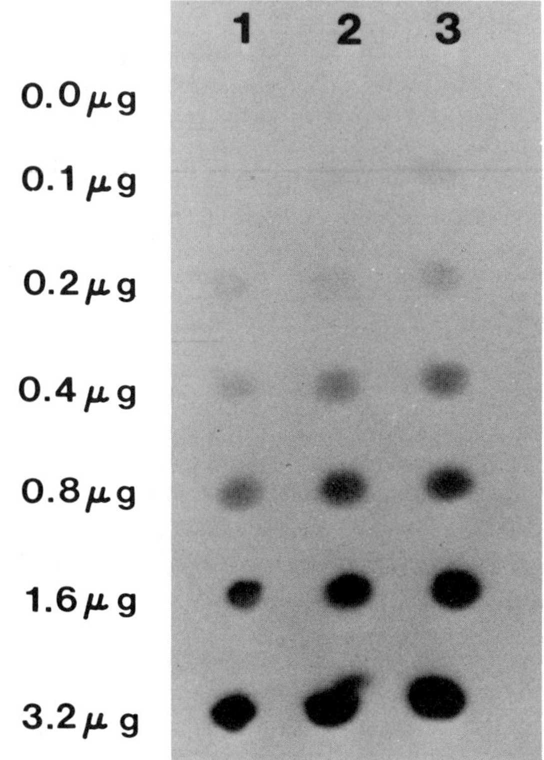

A
1   2   3
0.0 μg
0.1 μg
0.2 μg
0.4 μg
0.8 μg
1.6 μg
3.2 μg

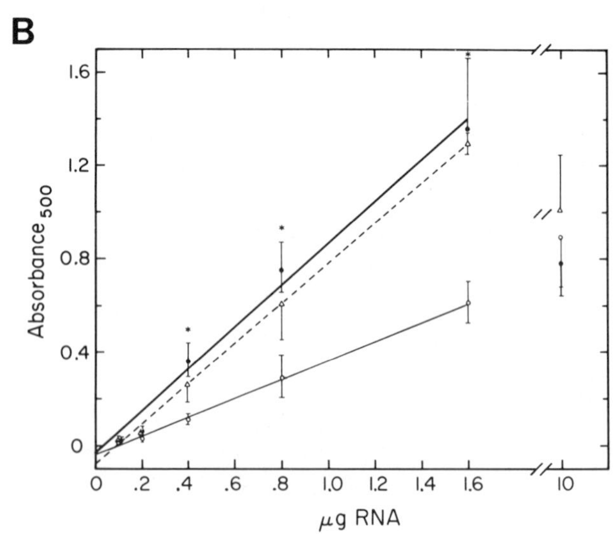

B
Absorbance 500
1.6
1.2
0.8
0.4
0
0   .2 .4 .6 .8 1.0 1.2 1.4 1.6   10
μg RNA

and Austin, 1983), the synthesis (Pain *et al.*, 1978; Kirsch *et al.*, 1968), and the mRNA levels (Castro and Sevall, 1985; Yap *et al.*, 1978) of albumin.

The rat serum albumin gene has been cloned and its fine structure examined in detail (Sargent *et al.*, 1979). Hybridizing a complementary DNA (cDNA) clone to isolated mRNA, it has been possible to measure the relative albumin mRNA in liver of rats fed a HCFF diet, a high-fat diet, or a basal diet containing 4% fat (Castro and Sevall, 1985). The level of albumin mRNA in rats fed the HCFF diet was 30–45% of the level in animals fed the basal 4% fat diet (Fig. 6). The concentration of another mRNA, that for α-fetoprotein, remained unchanged. It had been established by others that albumin mRNA levels and albumin synthesis are diminished in response to low levels of dietary protein (Pain *et al.*, 1978; Kirsch *et al.*, 1968). However, even when dietary protein is adequate (30% wt/wt), albumin mRNA level is decreased if all of the nonprotein calories are derived from carbohydrate.

Differential levels of albumin mRNA are related to rates of transcription of the gene, since many studies indicate that the production of albumin is regulated mainly at the transcriptional level (Nahon *et al.*, 1982; Tilghman and Belayew, 1982; Princen *et al.*, 1981). As for other structural genes, a study of the chromatin structure of the rat albumin gene is essential to understanding its expression. A provocative observation for the albumin gene has been the preferential *in vitro* binding of histone H1 to a 5′ site on the gene (Berent and Sevall, 1984). The potential significance of this H1-binding activity to the regulation of gene expression is under active investigation.

IV. ROLE OF THE NUCLEUS IN DETOXIFICATION

Nuclear metabolism of toxigens has been recognized for many years. The metabolites formed in nuclei are potentially immediately available to interact with DNA and chromatin. In contrast, metabolites generated by the microsomal fraction must diffuse from the point of production to the nucleus (Romano *et al.*, 1983, for review). Nuclear metabolism becomes more significant if (1) a metabolite has a short half-life, and (2) the nuclear metabolizing capacity generates ultimate mutagens or reactive compounds. Many microsomal enzymes that metabolize xenobiotics have nuclear counterparts (Table IV).

Fig. 6. Analysis by dot hybridization of relative concentrations of albumin mRNA. (A) Liver poly(A)$^+$ mRNA (0.1–3.2 µg) from rats fed a fat-free (1), high-fat (2), or basal (3) diet was applied to a nitrocellulose filter. An α-^{32}P-labeled *Pst*I fragment of a cDNA probe (pRSA 57) representing the 5′ end of the albumin mRNA was hybridized to filter-bound poly(A)$^+$ mRNA. (B) Relative optical density of hybridization between albumin cDNA and poly(A)$^+$ mRNA from rats fed fat-free (○), high-fat (△), or basal (●) diet. The asterisk denotes significant difference at $p < .05$. (From Castro and Sevall, 1985. © *J. Nutr.*, American Institute of Nutrition.)

TABLE IV

Nuclear Detoxifying Enzyme Activities

Enzyme	Reference
Cytochrome *P*-450	Romano *et al.* (1985)
	Hennig *et al.* (1983)
	Baker *et al.* (1983)
	Kennedy *et al.* (1982)
	Cheng *et al.* (1981)
	Holder *et al.* (1981)
	Gontovnick and Bellward (1981)
	Yoshizawa *et al.* (1981)
	Patton *et al.* (1980a)
Cytochrome *c* reductase	Romano *et al.* (1985)
Epoxide hydrolase	Romano *et al.* (1985)
	Pacifici *et al.* (1983)
	Gontovnick and Bellward (1981)
	Gazzotti *et al.* (1981)
Superoxide dismutase	Patton *et al.* (1980b)
UDP-Glucuronyltransferase	Zaleski *et al.* (1982)
	Elmamlouk *et al.* (1981)

Certain differences exist between microsomal and nuclear detoxifying enzymes, such as the developmental time of activation and the inducibility of the two subcellular counterparts. Romano *et al.* (1985) determined that nuclear cytochrome *P*-450, aryl hydrocarbon hydroxylase, and styrene epoxide hydrolase (EH) develop later than their microsomal counterparts in rabbit liver, whereas nuclear cytochrome *c* reductase develops earlier than the comparable microsomal enzyme. As for differences in inducibility between nuclear and microsomal enzyme, it is observed generally that responses to inducers are qualitatively similar but quantitatively distinct. Phenobarbital, 1α-acetylmethadol and *trans*-stibene oxide induce nuclear EH but to a level threefold lower than that of microsomal EH (Gontovnick and Bellward, 1981). Nuclear UDP-glucuronosyltransferase is stimulated about 1.5-fold by Lubrol WX, whereas under the same conditions the microsomal enzyme is activated up to 10-fold (Zaleski *et al.*, 1982).

Are the nuclear *P*-450-dependent enzymes responsive to nutrient intake as are their microsomal counterparts? Although a definitive answer cannot be given, there likely is qualitative similarity in the response of nuclear and microsomal enzymes to nutrient intake. Microsomal activation of B[*a*]P is greater in liver of rats fed a 10% corn oil diet rather than a fat-free diet. A similar increase in nuclear B[*a*]P hydroxylase occurs by feeding the corn oil diet (Baker *et al.*, 1983).

V. FUTURE DIRECTIONS

Nutrient–genome interaction is a fundamental relationship significant to toxicological processes. There are multiple levels of nutrient interaction with chromatin, from specific gene activation to alteration of the structure of chromatin. An area of investigation that will add to the understanding of gene regulation is the chromatin arrangement of specific gene sequences, such as the P-450M gene. Characterization of gene sequences coding for cytochrome P-450M and its isozymes will be important in understanding the mechanisms of coordinate regulation of gene expression involved in toxicogenesis. Another point of interest is whether nutrient intake affects the chromatin structure of specific gene sequences, such as by alteration of the degree of methylation, or by the formation or extinction of nuclease-hypersensitive sites. In addition, the mechanism(s) by which nutritional state alters higher order chromatin structure need to be elucidated. Are structural changes due to quantitative and/or qualitative differences in histone H1 subtypes? Is topoisomerase II involved in the nutrient-associated alteration of chromatin structure? The importance of topoisomerase II–DNA complexes to toxigen intercalation has been discussed. Information generated from answering these questions about nutrient–genome interaction will provide insight as to how nutrients influence the binding of toxigens to DNA.

REFERENCES

Alberts, A. W., Strauss, A. W., Hennessy, S., and Vagelos, P. R. (1975). Regulation of synthesis of hepatic fatty acid synthetase: Binding of fatty acid synthetase antibodies to polysomes. *Proc. Natl. Acad. Sci. U.S.A.* **72**, 3956–3960.

Allan, J., Hartman, P. G., Crane-Robinson. C., and Aviles, F. X. (1980). The structure of histone H1 and its location in chromatin. *Nature (London)* **288**, 675–679.

Anthony, L. E., and Edozien, J. C. (1975). Experimental protein and energy deficiencies in the rat. *J. Nutr.* **105**, 631–648.

Ariëns, E. J., and Simonis, A. M. (1982). General principles of nutritional toxicology. *In* "Nutritional Toxicology" (J. N. Hathcock, ed.), Vol. 1, pp. 17–80. Academic Press, New York.

Baker, M. T., Karr, S. W., and Wade, A. E. (1983). The effects of dietary corn oil on the metabolism and activation of benzo[*a*]pyrene by the benzo[*a*]pyrene metabolizing enzymes of the mouse. *Carcinogenesis (London)* **4**, 9–15.

Bartsch, H., and Montesano, R. (1984). Relevance of nitrosamines to human cancer. *Carcinogenesis (London)* **5**, 1381–1393.

Benyajati, C., and Worcel, A. (1976). Isolation, characterization, and structure of the folded interphase genome of *Drosophila melanogaster. Cell (Cambridge, Mass.)* **9**, 393–407.

Berent, S. L., and Sevall, J. S. (1984). Histone H1 binding at the 5′ end of the rat albumin gene. *Biochemistry* **23**, 2977–2983.

Bloom, K. S., and Anderson, J. N. (1979). Conformation of ovalbumin and globin genes in chromatin during differential gene expression. *J. Biol. Chem.* **254**, 10532–10539.

Boffa, L. C., Gruss, R. J., and Allfrey, V. G. (1982). Aberrant and nonrandom methylation of chromosomal DNA-binding proteins of colonic epithelial cells by 1,2-dimethylhydrazine. *Cancer Res.* **42**, 382–388.

Boyd, J. N., and Campbell, T. C. (1983). Impact of nutrition on detoxication. *In* "Biological Basis of Detoxication" C. J. Caldwell and W. B. Jakoby, eds.), pp. 287–306. Academic Press, New York.

Bresnick, E., Vaught, J. B., Chuang, A. H. L., Stoming, T. A., Bockman, D., and Mukhtar, H. (1977). Nuclear aryl hydrocarbon hydroxylase and interaction of polycyclic hydrocarbons with nuclear components. *Arch. Biochem. Biophys.* **181**, 257–269.

Brookes, P., and Lawley, P. D. (1964). Evidence for the binding of polynuclear aromatic hydrocarbons to the nucleic acids of mouse skin: Relation between carcinogenic power of hydrocarbons and their binding to deoxyribonucleic acid. *Nature (London)* **202**, 781–784.

Burckart, G. J., Whitington, P. F., and Helms, R. A. (1982). The effect of two intravenous fat emulsions and their components on bilirubin binding to albumin. *Am. J. Clin. Nutr.* **36**, 521–526.

Bustin, M., and Cole, R. D. (1968). The applicability of extraction by trichloroacetic acid to the preparation of very lysine-rich histones from the mammary gland. *Arch. Biochem. Biophys.* **127**, 457–462.

Camerini-Otero, R. D., Stollner-Webb, B., and Felsenfeld, G. (1976). The organization of histones and DNA in chromatin: Evidence for an arginine-rich histone kernel. *Cell (Cambridge, Mass.)* **8**, 333–347.

Canfield, L. M., and Chytil, F. (1978). Effect of low lysine diet on rat liver nuclear metabolism. *J. Nutr.* **108**, 1336–1342.

Castro, C. E. (1983). Nucleosomal repeat length in rat liver nuclei is decreased by a high carbohydrate, fat-free diet. *J. Nutr.* **113**, 557–565.

Castro, C. E., and Sevall, J. S. (1980). Alteration of higher order structure of rat liver chromatin by dietary composition. *J. Nutr.* **110**, 105–116.

Castro, C. E., and Sevall, J. S. (1982). Analysis of rat liver chromatin and nuclear proteins after nutritional variation. *J. Nutr.* **112**, 1203–1211.

Castro, C. E., and Sevall, J. S. (1983). Variations in chromatin structure and nucleosomal DNA repeat length with nutritional manipulation. *In* "Nutritional Factors in the Induction and Maintenance of Malignancy" (C. E. Butterworth, Jr. and M. L. Hutchinson, eds.), pp. 75–99. Academic Press, New York.

Castro, C. E., and Sevall, J. S. (1985). Hepatic level of rat albumin messenger RNA is influenced by factors other than dietary protein. *J. Nutr.* **115**, 491–495.

Castro, C. E., Alvares, O. F., and Sevall, J. S. (1986a). Zinc deficiency alters the proportion of histone H1 molecular subtypes in rat liver. *Nutr. Rep. Int.* **34**, 67–74.

Castro, C. E., Armstrong-Major, J., and Ramirez, M. E. (1986b). Diet-mediated alteration of chromatin structure. *Fed. Proc., Fed. Am. Soc. Exp. Biol.* **45**, 2394–2398.

Chen, G. L., Yang, L., Rowe, T. C., Halligan, B. D., Tewey, K. M., and Liu, L. F. (1984). Nonintercalative antitumor drugs interfere with the breakage–reunion reaction of mammalian DNA topoisomerase. II. *J. Biol. Chem.* **259**, 13560–13566.

Cheng, K.-C., Ragland, W. L., and Wade, A. E. (1981). Dietary fat and 3-MC induction of hepatic nuclear and microsomal cytochrome *P*-450. *Drug-Nutr. Interact.* **1**, 63–74.

Clark, R. J., and Felsenfeld, G. (1974). Chemical probles of chromatin structure. *Biochemistry* **13**, 3622–3628.

Compton, J. L., Bellard, M., and Chambon, P. (1976). Biochemical evidence of variability in the DNA repeat length in the chromatin of higher eucaryotes. *Proc. Natl. Acad. Sci. U.S.A.* **73**, 4382–4386.

Dingwall, C., Lomonossoff, G. P., and Laskey, R. A. (1981). High sequence specificity of micrococcal nuclease. *Nucleic Acids Res.* **9**, 2659–2673.

Durnam, D. M., and Palmiter, R. D. (1981). Transcriptional regulation of the mouse metallothionein-I gene by heavy metals. *J. Biol. Chem.* **256**, 5712–5716.

Durnam, D. M., Perrin, F., Gannon, F., and Palmiter, R. D. (1980). Isolation and characterization of the mouse metallothionein-I gene. *Proc. Natl. Acad. Sci. U.S.A.* **77**, 6511–6515.

Einck, L., Fagan, J., and Bustin, M. (1985). Chromatin structure of a 3-methylcholanthrene-induced cytochrome *P*-450 gene. *Biochemistry* **24**, 5269–5275.

Elgin, S. C. R. (1981). DNaseI—hypersensitive sites of chromatin. *Cell (Cambridge, Mass.)* **27**, 413–415.

Elmamlouk, T. H. H., Mukhtar, H., and Bend, J. R. (1981). The nuclear envelope as a site of glucuronyltransferase in rat liver: Properties of and effect of inducers on enzyme activity. *J. Pharmacol. Exp. Ther.* **219**, 27–34.

Enwonwu, C. O., and Sreebny, L. M. (1971). Studies of hepatic lesions of experimental protein–calorie malnutrition in rats and immediate effects of refeeding an adequate protein diet. *J. Nutr.* **101**, 501–514.

Everts, R. P., and Mostafa, M. H. (1981). Effects of indole and tryptophan on cytochrome *P*-450, dimethylnitrosamine demethylase, and arylhydrocarbon hydroxylase activities. *Biochem. Pharmacol.* **30**, 517–522.

Falchuk, K. H., Fawcett, D. W., and Vallee, B. L. (1975). Role of zinc in cell division of *Euglena gracilus*. *J. Cell Sci.* **17**, 57–78.

Finch, J. T., and Klug, A. (1976). Solenoidal model for superstructure in chromatin. *Proc. Natl. Acad. Sci. U.S.A.* **73**, 1897–1901.

Frederick, C. B., Mays, J. B., Ziegler, D. M., Guengerich, F. P., and Kadlubar, F. F. (1982). Cytochrome *P*-450- and flavin-containing monooxygenase-catalyzed formation of the carcinogen *N*-hydroxy-2-aminofluorene and its covalent binding to nuclear DNA. *Cancer Res.* **42**, 2671–2677.

Gazzotti, G., Garattini, E., and Salmona, M. (1981). Nuclear metabolism. II. Further studies on epoxide hydrolase activity. *Chem.-Biol. Interact.* **35**, 311–318.

Giri, C. P., and Gorovsky, M. A. (1980). DNase I sensitivity of ribosomal genes in isolated nucleosome core particles. *Nucleic Acids Res.* **8**, 197–214.

Gjerset, R., Gorka, C., Hasthorpe, S., Lawrence, J. J., and Eisen, H. (1982). Developmental and hormonal regulation of protein H1° in rodents. *Proc. Natl. Acad. Sci. U.S.A.* **79**, 2333–2337.

Glikin, G. C., Ruberti, I., and Worcel, A. (1984). Chromatin assembly in *Xenopus* oocytes: *In vitro* studies. *Cell (Cambridge, Mass.)* **37**, 33–41.

Gontovnick, L. S., and Bellward, G. D. (1981). A comparative study of benzo[*a*]pyrene hydroxylase and epoxide hydrolase derived from isolated rat hepatic nuclei and microsomes. *Drug Metab. Dispos.* **9**, 265–269.

Goth, R., and Rajewsky, M. F. (1974). Persistence of O^6-ethylguanine in rat-brain DNA: Correlation with nervous system-specific carcinogenesis by ethylnitrosourea. *Proc. Natl. Acad. Sci. U.S.A.* **71**, 639–643.

Groudine, M., Eisenman, R., and Weintraub, H. (1981). Chromatin structure of endogenous retroviral genes and activation by an inhibitor of DNA methylation. *Nature (London)* **292**, 311–317.

Gupta, R. C., Dighe, N. R., Randerath, K., and Smith, H. C. (1985). Distribution of initial and persistent 2-acetylaminofluorene-induced DNA adducts within DNA loops. *Proc. Natl. Acad. Sci. U.S.A.* **82**, 6605–6608.

Hathcock, J. N. (1982). Nutritional toxicology: Definition and scope. *In* ''Nutritional Toxicology'' (J. N. Hathcock, ed.), Vol. 1. pp. 1–15. Academic Press, New York.

Hathcock, J. N. (1985). Metabolic mechanisms of drug-nutrient interactions. *Fed. Proc., Fed. Am. Soc. Exp. Biol.* **44**, 124–129.

Hemminki, K. (1985). Binding of metabolites of cyclophosphamide to DNA in a rat liver microsomal system and *in vivo* in mice. *Cancer Res.* **45**, 4237–4243.

Henderson, A. R. (1970). The effect of feeding with a tryptophan-free amino acid mixture on rat liver magnesium ion-activated deoxyribonucleic acid-dependent ribonucleic acid-dependent polymerase. *Biochem. J.* **120**, 205–214.

Hennig, E. W., Demkowicz-Dobrzański, K. K., Sawicki, J. T., Mojska, H., and Kujawa, M. (1983). Effect of dietary butylated hydroxyanisole on the mouse hepatic monooxygenase system of nuclear and microsomal fractions. *Carcinogenesis (London)* **4**, 1243–1246.

Holder, G. M., Tierney, B., and Bresnick, E. (1981). Nuclear uptake and subsequent nuclear metabolism of benzo[*a*]pyrene complexed to cytosolic proteins. *Cancer Res.* **41**, 4408–4414.

Hörz, W., and Altenburger, W. (1981). Sequence specific cleavage of DNA by micrococcal nuclease. *Nucleic Acids Res.* **9**, 2643–2658.

Huberman, E., Sachs, L., Yang, S. K., and Gelboin, H. V. (1976). Identification of mutagenic metabolites of benzo[*a*]pyrene in mammalian cells. *Proc. Natl. Acad. Sci. U.S.A.* **73**, 607–611.

Igo-Kemenes, T., and Zachau, H. G. (1977). Domains in chromatin structure. *Cold Spring Harbor Symp. Quant. Biol.* **42**, 109–118.

Jeffrey, A. M., Weinstein, I. B., Jennette, K. W., Grezeskowiak, K., Nakanishi, K., Harvey, R. G., Autrup, H., and Harris, C. (1977). Structures of benzo[*a*]pyrene–nucleic acid adducts formed in human and bovine bronchial explants. *Nature (London)* **269**, 348–350.

Jenson, J. C., FitzGibbon, J., Brennan, L. A., and Litman, G. W. (1982a). Binding of benzo[*a*]pyrene to histones and altered affinity of modified histone 1 for deoxyribonucleic acid. *Biochemistry* **21**, 601–607.

Jenson, J. C., Gerber-Jenson, B., and Litman, G. W. (1982b). Lysines of histone 1 represent the principal target for covalent binding of microsomally activated benzo[*a*]pyrene *in vitro*. *Carcinogenesis (London)* **3**, 999–1003.

Jorgensen, A. J. F., and Majumdar, A. P. N. (1976). Influence of tryptophan on the level of hepatic microsomal cytochrome *P*-450 in well-fed normal, adrenalectomized, and phenobarbital-treated rats. *Biochim. Biophys. Acta* **444**, 453–460.

Karin, M. (1985). Metallothioneins: Proteins in search of function. *Cell (Cambridge, Mass.)* **41**, 9–10.

Karin, M., and Herchman, H. R. (1979). Dexamethasone stimulation of metallothionein synthesis in HeLa cell cultures. *Science* **204**, 176–177.

Karin, M., and Richards, R. I. (1982). Human metallothionein genes—primary structure of the metallothionein-II gene and a related processed gene. *Nature (London)* **299**, 797–802.

Karin, M., Andersen, R. D., Slater, E., Smith, K., and Herschman, H. R. (1980). Metallothionein mRNA induction in HeLa cells in response to zinc or dexamethasone is a primary induction response. *Nature (London)* **286**, 295–297.

Karin, M., Haslinger, A., Holtgreve, H., Cathala, G., Slater, E., and Baxter, J. D. (1984). Activation of a heterologous promoter in response to dexamethasone and cadmium by metallothionein gene 5′-flanking DNA. *Cell (Cambridge, Mass.)* **36**, 371–379.

Karnik, P. S. (1983). Correlation between phosphorylated H1 histone and condensed chromatin in *Planococcus citri*. *FEBS Lett.* **163**, 128–131.

Kennedy, K., Sligar, S. G., Polomski, L., and Sartorelli, A. C. (1982). Metabolic activation of mitomycin C by liver microsomes and nuclei. *Biochem. Pharmacol.* **31**, 2011–2016.

Kensler, T. W., Egner, P. A., Trush, M. A., Bueding, E., and Groopman, J. D. (1985). Modification of alfatoxin β_1, binding to DNA *in vivo* in rats fed phenolic antioxidants, ethoxyquin and a dithiothione. *Carcinogenesis (London)* **6**, 759–763.

Kirsch, R., Frith, L., Black, E., and Hoffenberg, R. (1968). Regulation of albumin synthesis and catabolism by alteration of dietary protein. *Nature (London)* **217**, 578–579.

Klaude, M., and von der Decken, A. (1985). Methionine-cysteine deficiency and alkylation of DNA in liver, kidney and lung of mice administered dimethylnitrosamine. *Biochem. Pharmacol.* **34,** 3627–3631.

Kornberg, R. D. (1974). Chromatin structure: A repeating unit of histones and DNA. *Science* **184,** 868–871.

Kriek, E., and Westra, J. G. (1979). Metabolic activation of aromatic amines and amides and interactions with nucleic acids. *In* ''Chemical Carcinogens and DNA'' (P. L. Grover, ed.), Vol. 2, pp. 1–28. CRC Press, Boca Raton, Florida.

Langan, T. A. (1982). Characterization of highly phosphorylated subcomponents of rat thymus H1 histone. *J. Biol. Chem.* **257,** 14835–14846.

Larsen, A., and Weintraub, H. (1982). An altered DNA conformation detected by S1 nuclease occurs at specific regions in active chick globin chromatin. *Cell (Cambridge, Mass.)* **29,** 609–622.

Larue, H., Bissonnette, E., and Bélanger, L. (1983). Histone H1° expression during developmental growth of rat liver. *Can. J. Biochem. Cell Biol.* **61,** 1197–1200.

Lennox, R. W. (1984). Differences in evolutionary stability among mammalian H1 subtypes. Implications for the roles of H1 subtypes in chromatin. *J. Biol. Chem.* **259,** 669–672.

Lennox, R. W., and Cohen, L. H. (1983). The histone H1 complements of dividing and nondividing cells of the mouse. *J. Biol. Chem.* **258,** 262–268.

Lennox, R. W., Oshima, R. G., and Cohen, L. H. (1982). The H1 histones and their interphase phosphorylated states in differentiated and undifferentiated cell lines derived from murine teratocarcinomas. *J. Biol. Chem.* **257,** 5183–5189.

Levy-Wilson, B., Kuehl, L., and Dixon, G. H. (1980). The release of high mobility group protein H6 and protamine gene sequences upon selective DNase I degradation of trout testis chromatin. *Nucleic Acids Res.* **8,** 2859–2869.

Lunn, P. G., and Austin, S. (1983). Dietary manipulation of plasma albumin concentration. *J. Nutr.* **113,** 1791–1802.

Lutz, W. K. (1979). *In vivo* covalent binding of organic chemicals to DNA as a quantitative indicator in the process of chemical carcinogenesis. *Mutat. Res.* **65,** 289–356.

McGhee, J. D., and Felsenfeld, G. (1983). Another potential artifact in the study of nucleosome phasing by chromatin digestion with micrococcal nuclease. *Cell (Cambridge, Mass.)* **32,** 1205–1215.

McGhee, J. D., and Felsenfeld, G. (1980). Nucleosome structure. *Annu. Rev. Biochem.* **49,** 1115–1156.

Marcelis, A. T. M., and Reedijk, J. (1983). Binding of platinum compounds to nucleic acids with respect to the antitumor activity of *cis*-diammine-dichloroplatinum (II) and derivatives. *Recl. Tran. Chim. Pays-Bas* **102,** 121–129.

Marks, D. B., Kanefsky, T., Keller, B. J., and Marks, A. D. (1975). The presence of histone H1° in human tissues. *Cancer Res.* **35,** 886–889.

Mathis, D., Oudet, P., and Chambon, P. (1980). Structure of transcribing chromatin. *Prog. Nucleic Acid Res. Mol. Biol.* **24,** 1–55.

Mazus, B., Falchuk, K. H., and Vallee, B. L. (1984). Histone formation, gene expression, and zinc deficiency in *Euglena gracilis*. *Biochemistry* **23,** 42–47.

Miksicek, R. J., and Towle, H. C. (1983). Use of a cloned cDNA sequence to measure changes in 6-phosphogluconate dehydrogenase mRNA levels caused by thyroid hormone and dietary carbohydrate. *J. Biol. Chem.* **258,** 9575–9579.

Miller, E. C., and Miller, J. A. (1981). Mechanisms of chemical carcinogenesis. *Cancer (Philadelphia)* **47,** 1055–1064.

Miller, E. C., Miller, J. A., and Enomoto, M. (1964). The comparative carcinogenicities of 2-acetylaminofluorene and its *N*-hydroxy metabolite in mice, hamsters, and guinea pigs. *Cancer Res.* **24,** 2018–2031.

Miltenberger, R., and Oltersdorf, U. (1978). The B-vitamin group and the activity of hepatic microsomal mixed-function oxidases of the growing Wistar rat. *Br. J. Nutr.* **39**, 127–137.

Mita, S., Ishii, K., Yamazoe, Y., Kamataki, T., Kato, R., and Sugimura, T. (1981). Evidence for the involvement of *N*-hydroxylation of 3-amino-1-methyl-5*H*-pyrido[4,3-6]indole by cytochrome *P*-450 in the covalent binding to DNA. *Cancer Res.* **41**, 3610–3614.

Mitchell, C. E. (1985). Effect of aryl hydrocarbon hydroxylase induction of the *in vivo* covalent binding of 1-nitropyrene, benzo[*a*]pyrene, 2-aminoanthracene, and phenanthridone to mouse lung deoxyribonucleic acid. *Biochem. Pharmacol.* **34**, 545–551.

Montesano, R. (1981). Alkylation of DNA and tissue specificity in nitrosamine carcinogenesis. *J. Supramol. Struct. Cell. Biochem.* **17**, 259–273.

Moore, R. A., Doebler, J. A., Shih, T.-M., and Anthony, A. (1984). Nuclear chromatin changes in hepatocytes of soman treated rats. *Toxicology* **31**, 99–108.

Morikawa, N., Nakayama, R., and Holten, D. (1984). Dietary induction of glucose-6-phosphate dehydrogenase synthesis. *Biochem. Biophys. Res. Commun.* **120**, 1022–1029.

Morris, S. M., Jr., Nilson, J. H., Jenik, R. A., Winberry, L. K., McDevitt, M. A., and Goodridge, A. G. (1982). Molecular cloning of gene sequences for avian fatty acid synthase and evidence for nutritional regulation of fatty acid synthase mRNA concentration. *J. Biol. Chem.* **257**, 3225–3229.

Murty, C. N., Verney, E., and Sidransky, H. (1982). Effect of tryptophan on nuclear envelope in rat liver: Evidence for increased nuclear RNA release. *In* "The Nuclear Envelope and the Nuclear Matrix" (G. G. Maul, ed.), pp. 111–127. Alan R. Liss, Inc., New York.

Nahon, J. L., Gal, A., Frain, M., Sell, S., and Sala-Trepat, J. M. (1982). No evidence for post-transcriptional control of albumin and α-fetoprotein gene expression in developing rat liver and neoplasia. *Nucleic Acids Res.* **10**, 1895–1911.

Nelson, E. M., Tewey, K. M., and Liu, L. F. (1984). Mechanism of antitumor drug action: Poisoning of mammalian DNA topoisomerase II on DNA by 4'-(9-acridinylamino)-methanesulfon-*m*-anisidide. *Proc. Natl. Acad. Sci. U.S.A.* **81**, 1361–1365.

Ohba, Y., Higurashi, M., and Hayashi, Y. (1984). Phosphorylation of H1 subtypes in regenerating rat liver. *J. Biol. Chem.* **259**, 2942–2948.

Omstedt, P. T., and von der Decken, A. (1974). Dietary amino acids. Effect of depletion and recovery on protein synthesis *in vitro* in rat skeletal muscle and liver. *Br. J. Nutr.* **31**, 67–76.

Oravec, M., and Korner, A. (1971). Stimulation of ribosomal and DNA-like RNA synthesis by tryptophan. *Biochim. Biophys. Acta* **247**, 404–407.

Pacifici, G. M., Lindberg, B., Glaumann, H., and Rane, A. (1983). Styrene oxide metabolism in Rhesus monkey liver: Enzyme activities in subcellular fractions and in isolated hepatocytes. *J. Pharmacol. Exp. Ther.* **226**, 869–875.

Pain, V. M., Clemens, M. J., and Garlick, P. J. (1978). The effect of dietary protein deficiency on albumin synthesis and on the concentration of active albumin messenger ribonucleic acid in rat liver. *Biochem. J.* **172**, 129–135.

Patton, S. E., Rosen, G. M., Rauckman, E. J., Graham, D. G., Small, B., and Ziegler, D. M. (1980a). Hamster hepatic nuclear mixed-function amine oxidase: Location and specific activity. *Mol. Pharmacol.* **18**, 151–156.

Patton, S. E., Rosen, G. M., and Rauckman, E. J. (1980b). Superoxide production by purified hamster hepatic nuclei. *Mol. Pharmacol.* **18**, 588–593.

Paulson, J. R., and Laemmli, U. K. (1977). The structure of histone-depleted metaphase chromosomes. *Cell (Cambridge, Mass.)* **12**, 817–828.

Pegg, A. E. (1984a). Repair of O^6-methylguanine in DNA by mammalian tissues. *Biochem. Basis Chem. Carcinog., Workshop Conf. Hoechst, 13th, 1982*, pp. 265–274.

Pegg, A. E. (1984b). Methylation of the O^6 position of guanine in DNA is the most likely initiating event in carcinogenesis by methylating agents. *Cancer Invest.* **2**, 223–231.

Perry, L. D., and Swartz, F. J. (1967). Evidence for a subpopulation of cells with an extended G_2 period in normal adult mouse liver. *Exp. Cell Res.* **48**, 155–157.

Planche-Martel, G., Likhachev, A., Wild, C. P., and Montesano, R. (1985). Modulation of repair of O^6-methylguanine in parenchymal and nonparenchymal liver cells of rats treated with dimethylnitrosamine. *Cancer Res.* **45,** 4768–4773.

Ploory, A. C. M., van Dijk, M., Berends, F., and Lohman. P. H. M. (1985). Formation and repair of DNA interstrand cross-links in relation to cytotoxicity and unscheduled DNA synthesis induced in control and mutant human cells treated with *cis*-diamminedichloroplatinum (II). *Cancer Res.* **45,** 4178–4184.

Pommier, Y., Zwelling, L. A., Kao-Shan, C.-S., Whang-Peng, J., and Bradley, M. O. (1985). Correlations between intercalator-induced DNA strand breaks and sister chromatid exchanges, mutations, and cytotoxicity in Chinese hamster cells. *Cancer Res.* **45,** 3143–3149.

Prestayko, A. W., Crooke, S. T., and Carter, S. K., eds. (1980). "Cisplatin: Current Status and New Developments." Academic Press, New York.

Prince, L. O., and Campbell, T. C. (1982). Effects of sex difference and dietary protein level on the binding of aflatoxin B_1, to rat liver chromatin *in vivo. Cancer Res.* **42,** 5053–5059.

Princen, J. M. G., Nieuwenhuizen, W., Mol-Backx, G. P. B. M., and Yap, S. H. (1981). Direct evidence of transcriptional control of fibrinogen and albumin synthesis in rat liver during the acute phase response. *Biochem. Biophys. Res. Commun.* **102,** 717–723.

Procsal, D., Winberry, L., and Holten, D. (1976). Dietary regulation of 6-phosphogluconate dehydrogenase synthesis. *J. Biol. Chem.* **251,** 3539–3544.

Pronezuk, A. W., Baliga, S., Triant, J. W., and Munro, H. N. (1968). Comparison of the effect of amino acid supply on hepatic polyribosome profiles in vivo and in vitro. *Biochim. Biophys. Acta* **157,** 204–206.

Radomski, J. L. (1979). The primary aromatic amines: Their biological properties and structure–activity relationships. *Annu. Rev. Pharmacol. Toxicol.* **19,** 129–157.

Romano, M., Facchinetti, T., and Salmona, M. (1983). Is there a role for nuclei in the metabolism of xenobiotics? A review. *Drug Metab. Rev.* **14,** 803–829.

Romano, M., Garattini, E., and Salmona, M. (1985). Perinatal development of cytochrome *P*-450, cytochrome *c* reductase, aryl hydrocarbon hydroxylase, styrene monooxygenase, and styrene epoxide hydrolase in rabbit liver microsomes and nuclei. *Dev. Pharmacol. Ther.* **8,** 232–242.

Ross, W. E., Glaubiger, Y. L., and Kohn, K. W. (1978). Protein-associated DNA breaks in cells treated with adriamycin or ellipticine. *Biochim. Biophys. Acta* **519,** 23–30.

Ross, W. E., Rowe, T., Glisson, B., Yalowich, J., and Liu, L. (1984). Role of topoisomerase II in mediating epipodophyllotoxin-induced DNA cleavage. *Cancer Res.* **44,** 5857–5860.

Ryoji, M., and Worcel, A. (1984). Chromatin assembly in *Xenopus* oocytes: *In vivo* studies. *Cell (Cambridge, Mass.)* **37,** 21–32.

Sargent, T. D., Wu, J.-R., Sala-Trepat, J. M., Wallace, R. B., Reyes, A. A., and Bonner, J. (1979). The rat serum albumin gene: Analysis of cloned sequences. *Proc. Natl. Acad. Sci. U.S.A.* **76,** 3256–3260.

Sculley, T. B., and Zytkovicz, T. H. (1983). Binding of benzo[*a*]pyrene and ($\pm$)-7β,8α-dihydroxy-9α,10α-epoxy-7.8,9,10-tetrahydrobenzo[*a*]pyrene to histones. *Cancer Res.* **43,** 1688–1695.

Selkirk, J. K., MacLeod, M. C., Kuroki, T., Drevon, C., Piccoli, C., and Montesano, R. (1982). Benzo[*a*]pyrene metabolites: Formation in rat liver cell-culture lines, binding to macromolecules, and mutagenesis in V79 hamster cells. *Carcinogenesis (London)* **3,** 635–639.

Sevall, J. S. (1983). DNA-binding nonhistone proteins. *In* "Chromosomal Nonhistone Proteins" (L. S. Hnilica, ed.), Vol. 1, pp. 25–46. CRC Press, Boca Raton, Florida.

Sidransky, H. (1985). Tryptophan. Unique action by an essential amino acid. *In* "Nutritional Pathology. Pathobiochemistry of Dietary Imbalances" (H. Sidransky, ed.), pp. 1–62. Dekker, New York.

Sidransky, H., Sarma, D. S. R., Bongiorno, M., and Verney, E. (1968). Effect of dietary tryptophan on hepatic polyribosomes and protein synthesis in fasted mice. *J. Biol. Chem.* **243,** 1123–1131.

Sidransky, H., Verney, E., and Murty, C. N. (1981). Effect of elevated dietary tryptophan on protein synthesis in rat liver. *J. Nutr.* **111,** 1942–1948.

Simpson, R. T. (1978). Structure of the chromatosome, a chromatin particle containing 160 base pairs of DNA and all the histones. *Biochemistry* **17,** 5524–5531.

Smith, R. D., and Yu, J. (1984). Alterations in globin gene chromatin conformation during murine erythroleukemia cell differentiation. *J. Biol. Chem.* **259,** 4609–4615.

Stalder, J., Groudine, M., Dodgson, J. B., Engel, J. D., and Weintraub, H. (1980). Hb switching in chickens. *Cell (Cambridge, Mass.)* **19,** 973–980.

Stankiewicz, A. J., Falchuk, K. H., and Vallee, B. L. (1983). Composition and structure of zinc-deficient *Euglena gracilis* chormatin. *Biochemistry* **22,** 5150–5156.

Storb, U., Wilson, R., Selsing, E., Walfield, A. (1981). Rearranged and germline immunoglobulin *k* genes: Different states of DNase I sensitivity of constant *k* genes in immunocompetent and nonimmune cells. *Biochemistry* **20,** 990–996.

Stuart, G. W., Searle, P. F., Chen, H. Y., Brinster, R. L., and Palmiter, R. D. (1984). A 12-base-pair DNA motif that is repeated several times in metallothionein gene promoters confers metal regulation to a heterologous gene. *Proc. Natl. Acad. Sci. U.S.A.* **81,** 7318–7322.

Swerdel, M. R., and Cousins, R. J. (1982). Induction of kidney metallothionein and metallothionein messenger RNA by zinc and cadmium. *J. Nutr.* **112,** 801–809.

Tan, K. B., Borun, T. W., Charpentier, R., Cristofalo, V. J., and Croce, C. M. (1982). Normal and neoplastic human cells have different histone H1 compositions. *J. Biol. Chem.* **257,** 5337–5338.

Tewey, K. M., Chen, G. L., Nelson, E. M., and Liu, L. F. (1984). Intercalative antitumor drugs interfere with the breakage–reunion reaction of mammalian DNA topoisomerase II. *J. Biol. Chem.* **259,** 9182–9187.

Thoma, F., Koller, T., and Klug, A. (1979). Involvement of histone H1 in the organization of the nucleosome and of the salt-dependent superstructures of chromatin. *J. Cell Biol.* **83,** 403–427.

Tilghman, S. M., and Belayew, A. (1982). Transcriptional control of the murine albumin/α-fetoprotein locus during development. *Proc. Natl. Acad. Sci. U.S.A.* **79,** 5254–5257.

Varricchio, F., Mabogunje, O., Kim, D., Fortner, J. G., and Fitzgerald, P. J. (1977). Pancreas acinar cell regeneration and histone (H1 and H1°) modifications after parital pancreatectomy or after a protein-free ethionine regimen. *Cancer Res.* **37,** 3964–3969.

Vesley, J., and Cihak, A. (1970). Enhanced DNA-dependent RNA polymerase and RNA synthesis in rat liver nuclei after administration of L-tryptophan. *Biochim. Biophys. Acta* **204,** 614–616.

Weintraub, H., and Groudine, M. (1976). Chromosomal subunits in active genes have an altered conformation. Globin genes are digested by deoxyribonuclease I in red blood cell nuclei but not in fibroblast nuclei. *Science* **193,** 848–856.

Winberry, L., and Holten, D. (1977). Rat liver glucose-6-P dehydrogenase. Dietary regulation of the rate of synthesis. *J. Biol. Chem.* **252,** 7796–7801.

Wood, W. I., and Felsenfeld, G. (1982). Chromatin structure of the chicken β-globin gene region. Sensitivity to DNase I, micrococcal nuclease, and DNase II. *J. Biol. Chem.* **257,** 7730–7736.

Wu, C. (1980). The 5′ ends of *Drosophila* heat shock genes in chromatin are hypersensitive to DNase I. *Nature (London)* **286,** 854–860.

Wu, C., Bingham, P. M., Livak, K. J., Holmgren, R., and Elgin, S. C. R. (1979). The chromatin structure of specific genes. 1. Evidence for higher order domains of defined DNA sequence. *Cell (Cambridge, Mass.)* **16,** 797–806.

Yang, L., Rowe, T. C., Nelson, E. M., and Liu, L. F. (1985). *In vivo* mapping of DNA topoisomerase II-specific cleavage sites on SV40 chromatin. *Cell (Cambridge, Mass.)* **41,** 127–132.

Yap, S. H., Strair, R. K., and Shafritz, D. A. (1978). Effect of a short-term fast on the distribution of cytoplasmic albumin messenger ribonucleic acid in rat liver. Evidence for formation of free albumin messenger ribonucleoprotein particles. *J. Biol. Chem.* **253,** 4944–4950.

Yoshizawa, H., Uchimaru, R., and Ueno, Y. (1981). Metabolism of aflatoxin B_1 in the isolated nuclei of rat liver. *J. Biochem. (Tokyo)* **89**, 443–452.

Zaleski, J., Bansal, S. K., and Gessner, T. (1982). Nuclear membrane-bound UDP-glucuronosyltransferase of rat liver. *Can. J. Biochem.* **60**, 972–979.

Zannoni, V. G., and Sato, P. H. (1976). The effect of certain vitamin deficiencies on hepatic drug metabolism. *Fed. Proc., Fed. Am. Soc. Exp. Biol.* **35**, 2464–2469.

6

Mutagens in Cooked Foods

Walter A. Hargraves

I. INTRODUCTION

Over the past decade the role of diet in causation of cancer has caused great concern and controversy. The speculation that dietary factors can be responsible for 30% of reported human cancers (1) or even as much as 60% for men and 40% for women (2) has been the basis for the concern. However, it has also been suggested that the role of diet in cancer causation has been exaggerated (3,4), and, in an attempt to resolve some of the speculation, several investigators have conducted surveys aimed at a more quantitative analysis of mutagenic components in foods (4–6). On the basis of the available data it could be concluded that many of the food classes tested have some detectable mutagenic activity, but this is orders of magnitude below that which occurs in cooked and heat-processed foods. The data of these surveys on cooked foods have been recently summarized (7). The National Academy of Sciences (1982) has also concluded that ''with the exceptions of mutagens produced by cooking it seems unlikely that large numbers of mutagens remain to be discovered in common foods.'' Because of this

157

Copyright © 1987 by Academic Press, Inc.
All rights of reproduction in any form reserved.

TABLE I

Chemical Structures of Mutagens

Carbolines:

α-

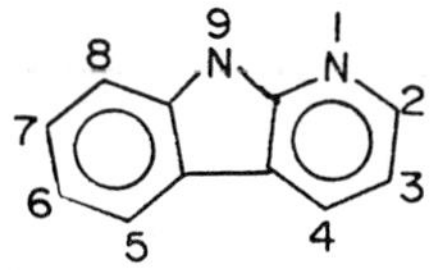

2-Amino-9*H*-pyrido{2,3-b}indole (2-amino-α-carboline, AαC)

2-Amino-3-methyl-9*H*-pyrido{2,3-b}indole (2-amino-3-methyl-α-carboline, MeAαC)

β-

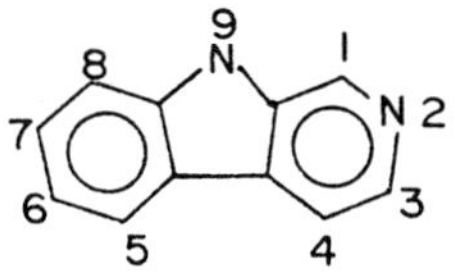

1-Amino-9*H*-pyrido{3,4-b}indole (1AN)

3-Amino-9*H*-pyrido{3,4-b}indole (3AN)

3-Amino-1-methyl-9*H*-pyrido{3,4-b}indole (3AH)

γ-

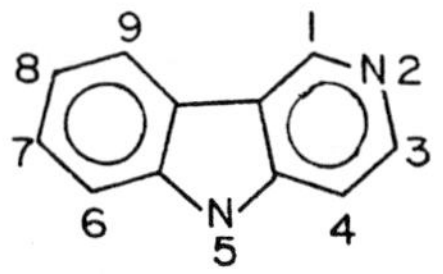

3-Amino-1-methyl-5*H*-pyrido{4,3-b}indole (Trp-P-2)

3-Amino-1,4-dimethyl-5*H*-pyrido{4,3-b}indole (Trp-P-1)

δ-

(amino-9*a*-aza-δ-carbolines)

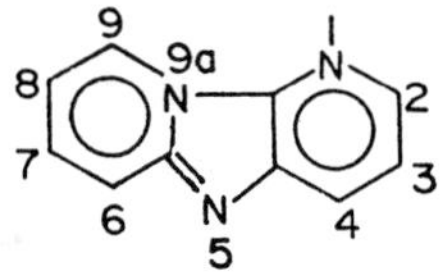

2-Aminodipyrido{1,2-*a*:3′,2′-*d*}imidazole (Glu-P-2)

2-Amino-6-methyl dipyrido{1,2-*a*:3′,2′-*d*}imidazole (Glu-P-1)

Quinolines:

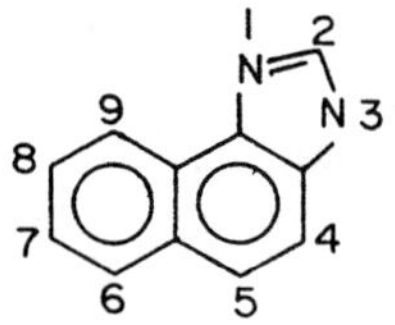

2-Amino-3-methylimidazo{4,5-*f*}₁quinoline (IQ)

2-Amino-3,4-dimethylimidazo{4,5-*f*}quinoline (MeIQ)

Quinoxalines:

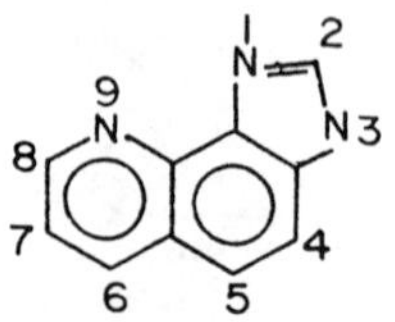

2-Amino-3,8-dimethylimidazo{4,5-*f*}quinoxaline (MeIQx)

2-Amino-3,4,8-trimethylimidazo{4,5-*f*}quinoxaline (4,8-DiMeIQx)

2-Amino-3,7,8-trimethylimidazo{4,5-*f*}quinoxaline (7,8-DiMeIQx)

conclusion and the available data, this review will be limited to the mutagenic activity found only in cooked foods.

It is now well established that mutagenic compounds are formed during the cooking or heat processing of foods, and those mutagens which have been structurally characterized are shown in Table I. The important question that remains to be answered is whether these compounds represent a health risk. Several of these mutagens have been synthesized and are undergoing carcinogenicity testing, but not much progress has been made in the chemical analysis for quantifying these compounds in foods. The data reported in this review are intended to describe the situation as presently known regarding the possible risk of ingesting these recently discovered mutagens.

II. OCCURRENCE AND EXPOSURE

Plumlee *et al.* (6) attempted to estimate the total mutagen content of an average American diet based on priority assessment of food consumption data from the USDA and the Health and Nutritional Examination study. After assaying the high-priority cooked foods, the authors estimated that the mutagenic activity equivalent of about 5600 revertants per day (Ames test) are consumed (8,9). However, based on the data in Ref. 1, the mutagenic activity from all reported values may be twice that estimated, and this does not take into account the cooking and, in particular, the extraction methods, which also have an effect on the estimate of the amount of mutagenic activity present. For example, Felton *et al.* (10) suggested that this estimate should be increased to 22,500 revertants per day to account for the fact that only 25% of the activity is extracted by the acetone method. These authors also noted that this level of activity is approximately equivalent to that in five cigarettes, but 200 times more than that contributed by aflatoxin B_1 in the diet. A consideration in such an evaluation is whether the mutagenic activity is as important as the actual amounts of mutagen consumed.

The specific mutagenic activity of the heterocyclic amine mutagens generated in food during cooking has been found to be considerably higher than B[*a*]P ($\sim 1000\times$), aflatoxin B_1 ($\sim 100\times$), and nitrosamines ($\sim 10^7\times$). Hence, although the mutagenic activity is high, the actual amounts of mutagens present in most foods is small. In fact, Dunn (11) calculated that in a charbroiled steak the activity would only comprise about 6 ng of the heterocyclic amine mutagens compared to about 1000 ng of B[*a*]P. Kawachi *et al.* (12) estimated that a 50-year-old person has eaten about 7.5 metric tons of food. If the heterocyclic amine mutagens are present at levels of about 1 part per billion (ppb), then the total 50-year exposure would only be about 7.5 mg. Moreover, by extrapolation of the estimated values of Felton *et al.* (10), the total exposure over 50 years would be only about 1 mg of heterocyclic amine mutagen. However, based on a chemical method of analysis, Takahashi *et al.* (13) and Sugimura (14) have estimated that the amount of heterocyclic amines consumed per capita per day could be as high as 100 μg. The complete answer to the question of activity versus concentration can only be determined when the carcinogenic potency of these mutagens is also known.

III. QUANTITATION

The most important step in answering the questions brought out in the previous section will be establishing a reliable method for quantifying the mutagenic compounds. The initial problems in separation and cleanup have already been addressed, but the best detection and quantifying techniques have not yet been determined. Once IQ, MeIQ, and MeIQx have been adequately separated from a food extract, the concentrations of these mutagens could be estimated utilizing the known specific activity of the synthetic compounds. This has been done with commercial beef extract (15–17). Although the method is not rigorous, it can, if done carefully, provide an initial estimate of the amounts of IQ, MeIQ, and MeIQx present in the food. The levels reported in commercial beef extract using this method have not been in close agreement: IQ $\simeq$ 18 ppb, MeIQx $\simeq$ 3 ppb, MeIQ $\simeq$ 34 ppb (15), as compared to IQ $\simeq$ 41–142 ppb, MeIQ, not found, MeIQ× $\simeq$ 142–527 ppb (16), and IQ $\simeq$ 20–40 ppb, MeIQx $\simeq$ 200–300 ppb, MeIQ not found (17).

A more analytical approach has been proposed for estimation of the amount of IQ in food extracts, utilizing HPLC for separation and UV absorption for detection and quantitation (18). This method is dependent on the purity of the chromatographic peak corresponding to the retention time of a standard IQ sample, and on the resolving power of the HPLC system. The results obtained with an extract of a cooked ground beef sample suggests that the IQ concentration is only about 0.53 ppb. Because the limit of detection of this method was reported to be about 0.1 ppb for an extract to which IQ had been purposely added (spiked extract), the general utility of this method is unclear. However, the concentration of IQ in fried ground beef is expected to be quite low, since some investigators have not been able to detect it at all in the majority of their samples (10, 15, 19, 20). A more recent combination of HPLC with electrochemical detection has lowered the detection limit to 0.5–1.5 pmol. No analyses of actual food products were carried out in this report (21), but Takahashi *et al.* (22, 23), with a similar method, have quantified IQ, MeIQx, and 4,8-DiMeIQx in commercial beef extract, and found 41.6, 58.7, and 10.0 ng/gm, respectively.

A potentially useful analytical method emplying a gas chromatograph for separation and a mass spectrometer for detection and quantitation has also been attempted (24–26). The chromatograph is fitted with a capillary column which has been coated with SE54. The underivatized mutagens are separated in the gas chromatograph by using a temperature gradient of 190°C for 3 min followed by raising the temperature to 235°C at 35°C/min. Only Glu-P-2 and Lys-P-1 could not be eluted from this column. The sensitivity and selectivity of this method can be enhanced by using the selected-ion mode of the mass spectrometer. By this technique it was found that fried beef contained 0.59 ppb of IQ and 2.4 ppb of MeIQx, while MeIQ was not detected. Data for other foods analyzed by this method have been reported elsewhere (27). The method has not yet been fully developed or extended to a systematic survey of cooked foods. Perhaps this is due to the extensive cleanup procedures and the influence of contaminants on the retention times and peak widths of the eluted mutagens (28). Gas chromatography using a fused-silica capillary column has also recently been employed for separation of the mutagenic components (29), but the sensitivity was still not as good as the electrochemical method.

IV. FORMATION

It has often been suggested in the literature that the mutagenic products formed during the cooking of food result from the reaction pathways originally described by Maillard. This seems to be a reasonable assumption, since foods contain proteins, carbohydrates, simple sugars, and free amino acids which possess the necessary functional groups for amine-carbonyl reactions. The Maillard reactions (30) which have been systematized by Hodge (31) have been the subject of several recent reviews (32–35) and will not be further discussed here. The model systems involve mainly simple sugars and a source of nitrogen such as NH_3, ammonium salts, amino acids, or various other amino compounds. It is perhaps not surprising that mutagenic activity has been observed in many of these reaction systems and that the activity is correlated with the extent of browning.

The simplest systems using sugar or sugar dehydration products and ammonia as reactants resulted in substantial mutagenic activity in the products after refluxing for several hours (36–40). The only mutagenic product isolated and identified from any of these systems was 1,5(or 7)-2,3,6,7-tetrahydro-1H,5H-biscyclopentapyrazine (40), which was obtained from a reaction between cyclotene and ammonia (39). Reactions between sugars and amino acids have also resulted in the formation of mutagenic (41–44), and clastogenic (45) products, as have reactions of cysteamine–glucose (46), creatine–glucose (47, 48), creatinine–fatty acids (49), starch–glycine at 290°C for 40 min (50), and triose reductone–nucleic acids (51).

In a model system consisting of creatinine, glucose, and glycine refluxed at 130°–190°C for 20 hr in diethylene glycol–H_2O (6 : 1) (52, 53), it was claimed that IQ was isolated in high yields, a noteworthy observation, since this is the same mutagen found in cooked beef and fish. Unfortunately, the experiments could not be successfully repeated, but subsequently Jagerstad *et al.* (54) and

Negishi *et al.* (55) did isolate and identify MeIQx (90% of the activity) and 7,8-DiMeIQx (10% of the activity) from a creatinine, glycine, and glucose mixture heated at 128°C for 2 hr. If alanine was used in place of glycine the products were MeIQx and 4,8-DiMeIQx, and if threonine was used the products were MeIQx and 7,8-DiMeIQx (1 : 3). IQ, MeIQx, and 4,8-DiMeIQx have also been isolated and identified from reaction systems consisting of creatinine, fructose, and amino acids (56). IQ has been isolated from a mixture of proline and creatinine heated to 180°C for 1 hr (57). In a complicated system more closely resembling beef extract, Taylor *et al.* (58) have found that, although IQ is initially present, the amount can be increased by boiling with added creatine phosphate. In fact, all these heterocyclic amine mutagens could be identified as products in this model system.

These data indicate that the mutagens found in cooked foods can definitely be formed by reaction pathways which at some step involve Maillard products as originally outlined by Jagerstad *et al.* (153).

V. GENOTOXIC AND CARCINOGENIC EFFECTS

The short-term *in vitro* and *in vivo* assays discussed in our previous review indicate that the heterocyclic amine mutagens in cooked foods are, or are likely to be, carcinogens. More recently Bird and Bruce (59) have shown that MeIQ is much more potent than IQ, Trp-P-2, Trp-P-1, or Glu-P-1 for inducing nuclear aberration in colon epithelial cells after oral administration to C57BL/67 mice. In other moderate-term assays, Barnes *et al.* (60) found that in the Sencar mouse skin assay IQ induced tumors at an incidence of only 7% compared to 70% for quinoline, while Pariza *et al.* (61) found that, although the incidence of hepatomas in fetal mouse liver induced by IQ was approximately 90% and for MeIQ about 50%, compared to N-OH-AAF the potency was orders of magitude lower.

The carcinogenic potential of some of these mutagens has been investigated in several longer term mouse-feeding studies. In an experiment with 7-week-old CDF$_1$ mice fed purified Trp-P-1 and Trp-P-2 (200 ppm) for 621 days, both compounds were found to induce hepatocellular carcinomas (62). In this study females were more susceptible than males and Trp-P-2 was slightly more potent. Implantation of pellets containing crude tryptophan pyrolyzate, purified Trp-P-1, or Trp-P-2 into the bladder of female ddy mice induced a high incidence of transitional cell carcinomas at 40 weeks (63). The percentage of mice with carcinomas which were histologically malignant was 47% for the crude extract and for Trp-P-1, but only 22% for Trp-P-2. Female mice fed a diet containing 0.05% Glu-P-1 or Glu-P-2, or 0.08% MeAαC also developed a higher incidence of hepatic tumors than males (64). This experiment was repeated using CDF$_1$ mice of both sexes and again it was found that the females were more susceptible than the males (65), a result which is in agreement with the Trp-P-1 and Trp-P-2 cited above. The IQ at 300 ppm fed continuously in the diet was also carcinogenic for CDF_1 mice of both sexes, but in this case males appeared to be slightly more susceptible (66). At 400 ppm MeIQ also induced carcinomas in CDF_1 mice (females greater than males), but the incidence seemed to be lower than any of the other heterocyclic amines tested (67).

In a 2-year experiment a crude tryptophan pyrolyzate was given orally to Wistar rats (68), and at the highest concentration(0.2%), two neoplastic nodules were found in males and five in females (25 rats in each group). This low incidence of lesions indicates the weak carcinogenic effect of the crude extract.

A purified component of the pyrolyzate, Trp-P-2, was further tested in an inbred strain of ACI rats by feeding at 0.01% for 870 days (67). Of 10 female rats, only one hemangioendothelial sarcoma was found, but 6 rats had neoplastic nodules in the liver. No liver tumors were found among the 10 male rats.

Takayama *et al.* (70) have reported that Glu-P-1 and Glu-P-2 at 500 ppm fed in the diet to F344 rats induced multipotent carcinomas, apparently more potent in this species than in the Wistar or ACI rats even though they were fed five times more carcinogen. This group has also reported that IQ is carcinogenic in F344 rats at 300 ppm in the diet, and it was concluded that IQ was more potent in this model than Glu-P-1 or Glu-P-2 (71). This was based on the dose and latency period; however, if only the liver tumor incidence is compared, IQ induced 40% whereas Glu-P-1 induced 83% in the male rats. It should also be noted that the male rats were much more susceptible than the females overall. This result is exactly the opposite of tumor incidence in mice, where the female was most susceptible and where Glu-P-2 was slightly more potent (65).

VI.   METABOLIC ACTIVATION AND DETOXIFICATION

Active metabolites of Trp-P-1 and Trp-P-2 could be isolated from the bile of cannulated but uninduced living rats, but no activity was found if isolated perfused livers were used for metabolism of these compounds (72). Nevertheless, isolated rat hepatocytes were shown to activate these molecules if the rat was previously induced with 3-MC (73). Primary monolayer cultures of hepatocytes from uninduced rats readily activated IQ for bacterial mutagenesis and 2-(2,4-dichloro-6-phenyl)phenoxyl ethylamine, an inhibitor of cytochrome P-448/-P-450, inhibited the activity by about 95% (74). We have reported elsewhere that covalent binding of activated IQ to hepatocyte macromolecules is particularly sensitive to intracellular glutathione levels (75).

Rat liver S-9 has most commonly been used to activate the heterocyclic amines, but it has also been shown that rat liver nuclei (76) and rat intestinal S-9 (77), if induced with 3-MC, will activate these molecules. The cytosolic fraction of the S-9 apparently does not participate in activation of the parent compounds to mutagens (78), but it does have an enhancing effect on the binding to DNA (79). The microsomal fraction of livers from various species exhibit both quantitative and qualitative differences in activating ability (80, 81). For uninduced microsomes the activity is in the order of hamster > mouse > rabbit > guinea pig > rat ~ human. On the other hand, PCB-induced rat microsomes display the highest activity among all other PCB-induced species tested (80).

Because the molecules being activated are amines and bear some structural resemblance to the known mutagenic/carcinogenic aromatic amines and amides, it is reasonable to assume that they may be activated at the amino nitrogen. In fact it has been demonstrated that cytochrome P_1-450 is involved in the activation of 2-acetylaminofluorene (AAF) as well as the heterocyclic aromatic amines from pyrolysis products (82). Isolation of the metabolites of Trp-P-2 from a microsomal incubation mixture after 30 min and subsequent separation by HPLC indicated that at least four metabolites are formed (77, 80, 83, 84). Assay of the HPLC fractions for direct-acting mutagenic activity revealed that 95% of the activity had been recovered and that about 80% of the activity was in a single fraction (83). The interpretation of these data assumed that the specific activity of the direct-acting metabolite was the same as that of the activated parent compound. The active metabolite was subsequently purified and identified as 3-hydroxyamino-1-methyl-5H-pyrido{4,3-b}indole (83, 84). The active metabolite of Trp-P-1 has not yet been identified, although it is presumed to be similar to that of Trp-P-2. The same procedures were used to determine the active metabolite of Glu-P-1 (85) and AαC (86). As might be expected, N-hydroxylated metabolites were identified as the direct-acting mutagens (85, 87).

The N-hydroxylated metabolite of IQ has also been isolated and identified (88), but in this case the metabolite was formed very early in the incubation (1 min), was not found in incubations stopped at 10 min, and was unstable at room temperature (half-life ≃ 1 min). More recently Yamazoe *et al.* (89) reported that NADPH may play a role in the stabilization of the hydroxylated metabolite of IQ.

Although it appears that in all cases metabolic activation involves N-hydroxylation, some differences in subsequent metabolism may exist. Evidence was recently reported suggesting that sulfate esters of the hydroxylamine metabolites of Glu-P-1, Glu-P-2, IQ, MeIQ, and MeIQx were generated within the bacteria by bacterial enzymes and represented the ultimate mutagenic species, but this was apparently not so for Trp-P-1, Trp-P-2, AαC, or MeAαC (90). In general, a more thorough elucidation of all the metabolites formed from these compounds is needed.

It was shown that the hydroxylamine metabolite of Trp-P-2 (OH-Trp-P-2) isolated from the incubation medium had a much higher rate of nonenzymatic binding to DNA at pH 7.4 than did the parent compound, Trp-P-2, as might be expected (91). However, it had been previously reported that the synthetic OH-

Trp-P-2 did not react appreciably with DNA under neutral conditions unless it had been O-acetylated (92). The possible requirement for further activation of the OH-Trp-P-2 metabolite is suggested by enhancement of its binding to DNA in the presence of seryl-tRNA synthetase (93), prolyl-tRNA synthetase (94), acetyl-CoA (95), and O-acetyltransferase (96). However, the acetylation is not necessarily required for mutagenicity. In contrast, acylation of N-hydroxy-Glu-P-2 seems to be important in binding to DNA and for mutagenicity (97). The OH-Trp-P-2 DNA complex has been hydrolyzed, and the specific metabolite–base adduct has been isolated and identified (92). The covalent bond of the Trp-P-2 guanine adduct which was formed is between the amino nitrogen of the metabolite and C-8 of the nucleotide and is similar to that of the 2-aminofluorene–base complex (98). This adduct is also formed with Glu-P-1 (99), and it has recently been shown that the N-acetoxyacetyl derivative of Glu-P-3 also binds to the C-8 of guanidine in DNA (100).

In summary, the activation of the heterocyclic amine mutagens from cooked foods proceeds through N-hydroxylation, which may then be followed by acylation leading to DNA binding, or esterification, which in some cases leads to enhanced mutagenicity. However, none of the acetyl or ester derivatives have been isolated or identified in any of the metabolizing model systems to date. Furthermore, strong noncovalent intercalation may be a prerequisite for subsequent covalent binding.

Relative rates of activation versus detoxification are important in assessing the potential toxicity of any compound, but only recently have the detoxification pathways of the heterocyclic amines in cooked foods been investigated. In the case of Trp-P-2 it was found that the enzymatic reaction of N-OH-Trp-P-2 with glutathione produced three adducts (101). Two of these adducts were not mutagenic (by definition detoxified), but the third adduct was even more mutagenic than the N-OH-Trp-P-2. In fact, the overall effect of the incubation mixture which contained all three adducts was still more mutagenic than N-OH-Trp-P-2. In a latter study this was again observed for Trp-P-2 but not for Trp-P-1 (102). However, in this study it was shown that the glucuronic acid conjugates always detoxified (measured by decreased mutagenicity) the heterocyclic amines. Lipids have also been shown to have a role in detoxification of these compounds. Fatty acids inhibit the formation of N-OH-Trp-P-2 by inhibiting the P-450 enzymes, while the microsomal lipids decreased the amount of active metabolite by direct action without inhibiting the formation of the metabolites of Trp-P-2 (103). It was postulated that lipid peroxides react with the N-OH-Trp-P-2 to form adducts of aryl hydroxyamines and the lipids. Another direct-acting compound which decreases the mutagenicity of Trp-P-2 is N-acetylcysteine (104). However, this compound might be considered to be a modifier of mutagenic activity, since at lower concentrations it can enhance the mutagenicity. Compounds of this type will be further discussed in the next section.

VII. MODIFIERS OF MUTAGENIC ACTIVITY

Aside from the mutagenic and carcinogenic compounds which are present in food, compounds which modify the mutagenic and/or carcinogenic activity have also been found. These substances can either enhance (105–107) or inhibit (106–109) mutagenic or carcinogenic activity. Probably the best-known mutagenesis enhancers are the comutagens harman and norharman (110–112), but recently it has been shown that certain chalcones can also enhance as well as inhibit the activity of polycyclic aromatic hydrocarbons (107).

In general, those compounds which inhibit mutagenic activity can be classified into the following groups: antioxidants (106), peroxidases (113), hydrocarbons (114), and inorganic metal salts (115). Many of these antimutagens have previously been reviewed (105, 109, 116–121), but in our view only those which are heat-stable are relevant to the health risk posed by the mutagens in cooked foods per se. We are currently investigating an antimutagen other than oleic acid which is present in cooked ground beef and appears to act by inhibiting or altering metabolic activation of promutagens in the Ames test (108, 122, 123). Heat-stable antimutagenic factors have also been found in ammonia-processed caramel (124) and in model browning reaction products (125), but none of the antimutagens from these systems has been structurally identified.

Many of the antimutagens isolated from vegetables (126, 127) and fruits (128) are proteins and therefore not heat-stable. Even though such substances may not persist during cooking, their presence in uncooked foods such as raw vegetables may contribute to the beneficial aspects of consuming a mixed diet.

VIII. CONCLUSIONS

Although the heterocyclic amines produced by cooking foods are indeed carcinogenic, their potency is only moderate and certainly magnitudes lower than that for aflatoxin. Because these compounds are highly mutagenic, it might have been predicted that they would also be highly carcinogenic. The correlation in this case is not good, and this is probably due to the lack of detoxifying components in the *in vitro* mutagenicity models. It seems readily apparent that more needs to be known about the detoxification pathways involved *in vivo*, because, in comparison with the mutagenic effects observed in the *in vitro* systems, these pathways contribute significantly to the less than expected carcinogenicity. The carcinogenic potency of these compounds in the presence of the antimutagens also known to coexist in the same food source has not been determined but is an important factor in the overall carcinogenicity of the diet.

In order to make a reasonable risk assessment, more data must be obtained about the carcinogenicity in species other than rats and mice. Just as important, a reliable method for quantifying the mutagens in various food sources must be developed. At present the methods which have been utilized suggest that the concentration of heterocyclic amines in cooked foods is quite low. Coupled with the moderate carcinogenicity and the presence of modifying factors in food, the potential risk of these compounds is still questionable.

ACKNOWLEDGMENTS

This work was supported in part by the College of Agricultural and Life Sciences, University of Wisconsin–Madison (CALS Research Division project number 2640), the University of Wisconsin–Madison Graduate School, the Wisconsin Agricultural Experiment Station, the United States Department of Agriculture, the University of Wisconsin–Madison Food Research Institute, and PHS research grant number R01-CA29618, awarded by the National Cancer Institute, DHHS.

REFERENCES

1. Doll, R., and Peto, R., *JNCI, J. Natl. Cancer Inst.* **66,** (U.S.) 1192 (1983).
2. Wynder, E. L., and Gori, G. B., *J. Natl. Cancer Inst. (U.S.)* **58,** 825–832 (1977).
3. Epstein, S. S., and Swartz, J. B., *Nature (London)* **289,** 127–130 (1981).
4. Stoltz, D. R., Stavric, B., Stapley, R., Klassen, R., Bendall, R., and Krewski, D., *Environ. Mutat.* **6,** 343–354 (1984).
5. Krone, C. A., and Iwaoka, W. T., *Mutat. Res.* **141,** 131–134 (1984).
6. Plumlee, C., Bjeldanes, L. F., and Hatch, F. T., *J. Am. Diet. Assoc.* **79,** 446 (1981).
7. Hargraves, W. A., and Pariza, M. W., *J. Environ. Sci. Health,* **C2**(1), 1–49 (1984).
8. Bjeldanes, L. F., Morris, M. M., Felton, J. S., Healy, S., Stuermer, D., Berry, P., Timourian, H., and Hatch, F. T., *Food Chem. Toxicol.* **20,** 357 (1982).
9. Bjeldanes, L. F., Morris, M. M., Felton, J. S., Healy, S., Stuermer, D., Berry, P., Timourian, H., and Hatch, F. T., *Food Chem. Toxicol.* **20,** 365 (1982).
10. Felton, J. S., Hatch, F. T., Knize, M. G., and Bjeldanes, L., *Curr. Top. Nutr. Dis.* **9,** 17 (1983).
11. Dunn, B. P., *in* "Carcinogens and Mutagens in the Environment" (H. F. Stich, ed.), Vol. 1, p. 175. CRC Press, Boca Raton. Florida, 1982.
12. Kawachi, T., Nagao, M., Yahgi, T., Takahashi, Y., Sugimura, T., Takayama, S., Kosuge, T., and Shudo, T., *Adv. Med. Oncol. Res. Educ., Proc. Int. Cancer Congr., 12th, 1978, Vol. 1,* p. 199 (1979).
13. Takahashi, M., Wakabayashi, K., Nago, M., Tomita, I., and Sugimura, T., *Mutat. Res.* (in press).
14. Sugimura, T., *Mutat. Res.* **150,** 33–41 (1985).
15. Hargraves, W. A., and Pariza, M. W., *Cancer Res.* **43,** 1467 (1983).
16. Turesky, T. J., Wishnok, J. S., Tannenbaum, S. R., Pfund, R. A., and Buchi, G. H. *Carcinogenesis (London)* **4,** 863 (1983).
17. Hikoya, H., Yukari, M., Ohara, Y., Oka, T., and Toshiko, H., *Gann* **74,** 472 (1983).
18. Barnes, W. S., Maher, J. C., and Weisburger, J. H., *J. Agric. Food Chem.* **31,** 883 (1983).
19. Hargraves, W. A., Dietrich, R., and Pariza, M. W., *in* "Carcinogens and Mutagens in the Environment" (H. F. Stich, ed.), Vol. 1, p. 223. CRC Press, Boca Raton, Florida, 1982.
20. Bjeldanes, L. F., Grose, K. R., Davis, P. H., Stuermer. D. H., Healy, S. K., and Felton, J. S., *Mutat. Res.* **105,** 43 (1982).

21. Grivas, S., and Nyhammer, T., *Mutat. Res.* **142,** 5–8 (1985).
22. Takahashi, M., Wakabayashi, K., Nagao, M., Yamamoto, M., Masui, T., Goto, T., Kinae, N., Tomita, I., and Sugimura, T., *Carcinogenesis (London)* **6**(8), 1195–1199 (1985).
23. Takahashi, M., Wakabayashi, K., Nagao, M., Yamaizumi, Z., Sato, S., Kinae, N., Tomita, I., and Sugimura, T., *Carcinogenesis (London)* **6**(10), 1537–1539 (1985).
24. Yokoyama, S., Miyazawa, T., Kasai, H., Nishimura, S., Sugimura, T., and Iitaka, Y., *FEBS Lett.* **122,** 251 (1980).
25. Sugimura, T., Nagao, M., and Wakabayashi, K., *IARC Sci. Publ.* **40,** 251 (1981).
26. Nishimura, S., and Yamaizumi, A., *Mass. Anal.* **29,** 151 (1981).
27. Sugimura, T., and Sato, S., *Cancer Res.* **43,** Suppl., 2415S (1983).
28. Yamaizumi, Z., Shiomi, T., Kasai, H., Nishimura, S., Takahashi, Y., Nagao, M., and Sugimura, T., *Cancer Lett.* **9,** 75 (1980).
29. Schunk, H., Hayashi, T., and Shibomoto, T., *HRC CC, J. High Resolut. Chromatogr. Chromatogr. Commun.* **7**(10), 563–565 (1984).
30. Maillard, L. C., *C. R. Hebd. Seances Acad. Sci.* **154,** 66 (1912).
31. Hodge, E., *J. Agric. Food Chem.* **1,** 928 (1953).
32. Nursten, H. E., *Food Chem.* **6,** 263 (1981).
33. Powrie, W. D., Wu, C. H., and Stich, H. F., *in* "Carcinogens and Mutagens in the Environment" (H. F. Stich, ed.), vol. 1, p. 121. CRC Press, Boca Raton, Florida, 1981.
34. Olsson, K., Apernamalm, P., and Theander, O., *Prog. Food Nutr. Sci.,* p. 47 (1981).
35. Kawamura, S., *ACS Symp. Ser.* **215,** 3 (1983).
36. Spingarn, N. E., and Garvie, C. T., *J. Agric. Food Chem.* **27,** 1319 (1979).
37. Yoshida, D., and Okamoto, H., *Agric. Biol. Chem.* **46,** 1067 (1982).
38. Shibumoto, T., Nishimura, O., and Mihara, S., *J. Agric. Food Chem.* **29,** 643 (1981).
39. Nishimura, O., Mihara, S., and Shibamoto, T., *J. Agric. Food Chem.* **28,** 39 (1980).
40. Shibamoto, T., *J. Agric. Food Chem.* **28,** 883 (1980).
41. Omura, H., Jahan, N., Shinohara, K., and Murakami, H., *ACS Symp. Ser.* **215,** 437 (1983).
42. Yoshida, D., and Okamoto, H., *Agric. Biol. Chem.* **44,** 2521 (1980).
43. Spingarn, N. E., Garvie-Gould, C. T., and Slocum, L. A., *J. Agric. Food Chem.* **31,** 301 (1983).
44. Shinohara, K., Wu, R. T., Jahan, N., Tanaka, M., Morinaga, N., Murakami, H., and Omura, H., *Agric. Biol. Chem.* **44,** 671 (1980).
45. Powrie, W. D., Wu, C. H., Rosin, M. P., and Stich, H. F., *J. Food Sci.* **46,** 1433 (1981).
46. Mihara, S., and Shibamoto, T., *J. Agric. Food Chem.* **28,** 62 (1980).
47. Yoshida, D., and Okamoto, H., *Biochem. Biophys. Res. Commun.* **96,** 844 (1980).
48. Yoshida, D., and Fukahara, Y., *Agric. Biol. Chem.* **46,** 1069 (1982).
49. Yoshida, D., and Okamoto, H., *Agric. Biol. Chem.* **44,** 3025 (1980).
50. Wu, C. I., Kitamura, K., and Shibamoto, T., *Food Cosmet. Toxicol.* **19,** 749 (1981).
51. Shinohara, K., Lee, J., Tanaka, M., Murakami, H., and Omura, H., *Agric. Biol. Chem.* **44,** 1737 (1980).
52. Jagerstad, M., Reutersward, A. L., Olsson, R., Grivas, S., Nyhammar, T., Olson, K., and Dahlquist, A., *Food Chem.* **12,** 255 (1983).
53. Jagerstad, M., Reutersward, A. L., Oste, R., and Dahlquist, A., *ACS Symp. Ser.* **215,** 507 (1983).
54. Jagerstad, M., Olsson, K., Grivas, S., Negishi, C., Wakabayashi, K., Tsuda, M., Sato, S., and Sugimura, T., *Mutat. Res.* **125,** 239–244 (1984).
55. Negishi, C., Wakabayashi, K., Tsuda, M., Sato, S., Sugimura, T., Sarto, H., Maeda, M., and Jagerstad, M., *Mutat. Res.* **140,** 55–59 (1984).
56. Grivas, S., Nyhammar, T., Olsson, K., and Jagerstad, M., to be published.
57. Yoshida, D., Saito, Y., and Mizusaki, S., *Agric. Biol. Chem.* **48**(1), 241–243 (1984).

58. Taylor, R. T., Fultz, E., and Knize, M., *J. Environ. Sci. Health Part A* **20**(2), 135–148 (1985).
59. Bird, R. P., and Bruce, W. R., *JNCI, J. Natl. Cancer Inst.* **73**(1), 237 (1984).
60. Barnes, W. S., Lovelette, C. A., Tong, C., Williams, G. M., and Weisburger, J. H., *Carcinogenesis (London)* **6**(3), 441–444 (1985).
61. Pariza, M. W., and Miller, J. M., in preparation.
62. Matsukura, N., Kawachi, T., Morino, K., Ohgaki, H., Sugimura, T., and Takayama, S., *Science* **213**, 346 (1981).
63. Hashida, C., Nagayama, K., and Takemura, N., *Cancer Lett.* **17**, 101 (1982).
64. Sugimura, T., *in* "Genetic Toxicology: An Agricultural Perspective" (A. Hollaender, ed.). Plenum, New York, 1982.
65. Ohgaki, H., Matsukura, N., Morino, K., Kawachi, T., Sugimura, T., and Takayama, S., *Carcinogenesis (London)* **5**(6), 815–819 (1984).
66. Ohgaki, H., Kusama, K., Matsukura, N., Morino, K., Hasegawa, H., Sato, S., Takayama, S., and Sugimura, T. *Carcinogenesis (London)* **5**(7), 921–924 (1984).
67. Ohgaki, H., Hasegawa, H., Kato, T., Suenaga, M., Ubukatu, M., Sato, S., Shozo, T., and Sugimura, T., *Proc. Jpn. Acad., Ser. B* **61**, 137–139 (1985).
68. Matsukura, N., Kawachi, T., Wakabayaski, K., Ohgaki, H., Morino, K., Sugimura, T., Nukaza, H., and Kosuge, T., *Cancer Lett.* **13**, 181 (1981).
69. Hosaka, S., Matsushima, T., Hirono, I., and Sugimura, T., *Cancer Lett.* **13**, 23 (1981).
70. Takayama, S., Masuda, M., Mogami, M., Ohagaki, H., Sato, S., and Sugimura, T., *Gann* **75**, 207–213 (1984).
71. Takayama, S., Nakatsuru, Y., Masuda, M., Ohgaki, H., Sato, S., and Sugimura, T., *Gann* **75**, 467–470 (1984).
72. Dolara, P., Caderni, G., and Benetti, D., *Nutr. Cancer* **3**, 168 (1982).
73. Mita, S., Yamazoe, Y., Kamataki, T., and Kato, R., *Biochem. Pharmacol.* **32**, 1179 (1983).
74. Gayda, D. P., and Pariza, M. W., *Mutat. Res.* **118**, 7 (1983).
75. Loretz, L. J., and Pariza, M. W., unpublished observations.
76. Mita, S., Yamazoe, Y., Kamataki, T., and Kato, R., *Cancer Lett.* **14**, 261 (1981).
77. de-Wazien, I., and Decloitre, F., *Mutat. Res.* **119**, 103 (1983).
78. Ishii, K., Yamazoe, Y., Kamataki, T., and Kato, R., *Cancer Res.* **40**, 2596 (1980).
79. Nemoto, N., Kusumi, S., Takayama, S., Nagao, M., and Sugimura, T., *Chem.-Biol. Interact.* **27**, 191 (1979).
80. Yamazoe, Y., Kamataki, T., and Kato, R., *Cancer Res.* **41**, 4518 (1981).
81. Kato, R., Yamazoe, Y., Ishii, K., Mita, S., Kamataki, T., and Sugimura, T., *Adv. Exp. Med. Biol.* **136B**, 997 (1982).
82. Nebert, D. W., Bigelow, S. W., Okey, A. B., Yahagi, T., Marie, Y., Nagao, M., and Sugimura, T., *Proc. Natl. Acad. Sci. U.S.A.* **76**, 5929 (1979).
83. Yamazoe, Y., Ishii, K., Kamataki, T., Kato, R., and Sugimura, T., *Chem.-Biol. Interact.* **30**, 125 (1980).
84. Yamazoe, Y., Ishii, K., Kamataki, T., and Kato, R., *Drug Metab. Dispos.* **9**, 292 (1981).
85. Ishii, K., Yamazoe, Y., Kamataki, T., and Kato, R., *Chem.-Biol. Interact.* **38**, 1 (1981).
86. Niwa, T., Yamazoe, Y., and Kato, R., *Mutat. Res.* **95**, 159 (1982).
87. Hashimoto, Y., Shudo, K., and Okamoto, T., *Biochem. Biophys. Res. Commun.* **92**, 971 (1980).
88. Okamoto, T., Shudo, K., Hasimoto, Y., Kosuge, T., Sugimura, T., and Nishimura, S., *Chem. Pharm. Bull.* **29**, 590 (1981).
89. Yamazoe, Y., Shimada, M., Karnatabu, T., and Kato, R., *Cancer Res.* **43**, 5768 (1983).
90. Nagao, M., Fujita, K., Wakabayashi, K., and Sugimura, T., *Biochem. Biophys. Res. Commun.* **114**, 626 (1983).

91. Mita, S., Ishii, K., Yamazoe, Y., Kamataki, T., Kato, R., and Sugimura, T., *Cancer Res.* **41**, 3610 (1981).

92. Hashimoto, Y., Shudo, K., and Okamoto, T., *Biochem. Biophys. Res. Commun.* **96**, 355 (1980).

93. Yamazoe, Y., Tada, M., Kamataki, T., and Kato, R., *Biochem. Biophys. Res. Commun.* **102**, 432 (1981).

94. Yamazoe, Y., Shimada, M., Kamataki, T., and Kato. R., *Biochem. Biophys. Res. Commun.* **107**, 165 (1982).

95. Saito, K., Yamazoe, Y., Kamataki, T., and Kato, R., *Biochem. Biophys. Res. Commun.* **116**, 141 (1983).

96. Saito, K., Shinohara, A., Kamataki, T., and Kato, R., *Arch. Biochem. Biophys.* **239**(1), 286–295 (1985).

97. Hasimoto, Y., Shudo, K., and Okamoto, T., *Biochem. Biophys. Res. Commun.* **92**, 971 (1980).

98. Beranek, D. T., White, G. L., Heflich, R. H., and Beland, F. A., *Proc. Natl. Acad. Sci. U.S.A.* **79**, 5175 (1982).

99. Hashimoti, Y., Shudo, K., and Okamoto, T., *J. Am. Chem. Soc.* **104**, 7636–7640 (1982).

100. Loukakau, B., Hebert, E., Saint-Ruf, G., and Leng, M., *Carcinogenesis (London)* **6**(3), 377–383 (1985).

101. Saito, K., Yamazoe, Y., Kamataki, T., and Kato, R., *Carcinogenesis (London)* **4**(12), 1551–1557 (1983).

102. deWaziers, I., and Decloitre, F., *Ultra. Res.* **139**, 15–19 (1984).

103. Saito, K., Yamazoe, Y., Kamataki, T., and Kato, R., *Chem.-Biol. Interact.* **45**, 295–304 (1983).

104. DeFlora, S., Bennicelli, C., Zanacchi, P., Camorano, A., Morelli, A., and DeFlora, A., *Carcinogenesis (London)* **5**(4), 505–510 (1984).

105. Ames, B. N., *Science* **221**, 1256 (1983).

106. Wattenburg, L. W., *Cancer Res.* **43**, Suppl., 2-48S, (1983).

107. Torigoe, T., Arisawa, M., Itoh, S., Fujui, M., and Maruyama, H. B., *Biochem. Biophys. Res. Commun.* **112**, 833 (1983).

108. Pariza, M. W., Loretz, L. J., Storkson, J. M., and Holland, N. C., *Cancer Res.* **43**, Suppl., 2444S (1983).

109. Wattenburg, L. W., Loub, W. D., Lam, L. K., and Spein, J. L., *Fed. Proc., Fed. Am. Soc. Exp. Biol.* **35**, 1327 (1976).

110. Pahlamn, R., Pelkmen, D., and Raumo, V., *Mutat. Res.* **97**, 210 (1982).

111. Nagao, M., Yahagi, T., Honda, M., Seino, Y., Matsushima, T., and Sugimura, T., *Proc. Jpn. Acad., Ser. B* **53**, 34 (1977).

112. Matsumoto, T., Yoshida, D., and Mizusaki, S., *Mutat. Res.* **56**, 85 (1977).

113. Morita, K., Yamada, H., Iwamoto, S., Sotomura, M., and Suzuki, A., *J. Food Saf.* **4**, 139 (1982).

114. Haugan, D. A., and Peak, M. J., *Mutat. Res.* **116**, 257 (1983).

115. Mochizuki, H., and Kada, T., *Mutat. Res.* **95**, 145 (1982).

116. Pariza, M. W., *Food Technol.* **36**, 53 (1982).

117. Barale, R., Zucconi, D., Bertani, R., and Lopriend, N., *Mutat. Res.* **120**, 145 (1983).

118. Stich, H. F., Wu, C., and Powrie, W., *in* "Environmental Mutagens and Carcinogens" (T. Sugimura, S. Knodo, and H. Takebe, eds.), p. 347. Alan R. Liss, Inc., New York, 1982.

119. Kada, T., *in* "Environmental Mutagens and Carcinogens" (T. Sugimura, S. Knodo, and H. Takabe, eds.), p. 355. Alan R. Liss, Inc., New York, 1982.

120. Fiala, E. S., Reddy, B. S., and Weisburger, J. H., *Annu. Rev. Nutr.* **5**, 295–321 (1985).

121. Kada, T., Kaneko, K., Matsuzaki, S., Matsuzaki, T., and Hara, Y., *Mutat. Res.* **150**, 127–132 (1985).

122. Krone, C. A., and Iwaoka, W. T., *J. Agric. Food Chem.* **31,** 428 (1983).
123. Pariza, M. W., and Hargraves, W. A., *Carcinogenesis (London)* **6,** 591–593 (1985).
124. Rosin, M. P., *in* ''Carcinogens and Mutagens in the Environment'' (H. F. Stich, ed.), Vol. 1, p. 260. CRC Press, Boca Raton, Florida, 1982.
125. Chan, R. I. M., Stich, H. F., Rosin, M. P., and Powrie, W. D., *Cancer Lett.* **15,** 27 (1982).
126. Kada, T., Morita, K., and Inone, T., *Mutat. Res.* **53,** 351 (1978).
127. Inoue, T., Morita, K., and Kada, T., *Agric. Biol. Chem.* **45,** 345 (1981).
128. Morita, K., Hara, M., and Kada, T., *Agric. Biol. Chem.* **42,** 1235 (1978).

7

Allergic and Sensitivity Reactions

to Food Components

Steve L. Taylor

I. INTRODUCTION AND CLASSIFICATION

One man's food may be another man's poison. Perhaps Lucretius was thinking of food sensitivities when he uttered those immortal words centuries ago. Food sensitivities are those food-related illnesses that afflict only a small proportion of the population. For many years, these individualistic adverse reactions to food were collectively referred to as "food allergies," a practice that is still common among some physicians and many consumers. However, in recent years, it has become widely recognized that many different diseases fall into this general category, and that true food allergies represent only one type of illness. Hence, food sensitivity has become the accepted term to describe the broad range of individualistic adverse reactions to foods.

The relationships between the major categories of food sensitivities are depicted in Fig. 1 (Institute of Food Technologist's Expert Panel on Food Safety and Nutrition, 1985). The two major subclassifications are the primary and secondary food sensitivities. The primary food sensitivities include the true food

173

Copyright © 1987 by Academic Press, Inc.
All rights of reproduction in any form reserved.

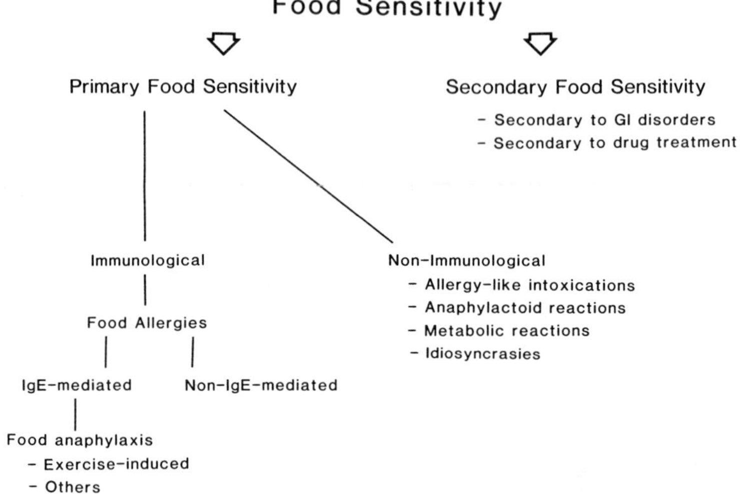

Fig. 1.   Relationships between the different types of food sensitivity.

allergies and a host of nonimmunological food sensitivities. The secondary food sensitivities, as suggested by the descriptor, are sensitivities that occur secondary to other events such as other illnesses or drug therapy. A variety of distinct disease processes is involved in each of the categories. As a consequence, a variety of procedures must be considered for the diagnosis, treatment, and management of these food sensitivities.

II. PRIMARY FOOD SENSITIVITIES

The primary food sensitivities are more common than secondary food sensitivities and do not require any predisposing conditions. Several different types of true food allergies and a variety of nonimmunological reactions including allergylike intoxications, anaphylactoid reactions, metabolic food disorders, and idiosyncratic illnesses fall within this category.

A. True Food Allergies

Food allergies are abnormal immunological reactions to a food or food component, usually a protein (Aas, 1983; Gallant, 1978: May, 1983; Taylor, 1980, 1985a). The involvement of the immune system distinguishes food allergies from other types of primary food sensitivities. Gell *et al.* (1975) classified true allergic reactions into four types, designated types I–IV, on the basis of the immunological mechanism of the reaction. Types I, III, and IV may occur with foods.

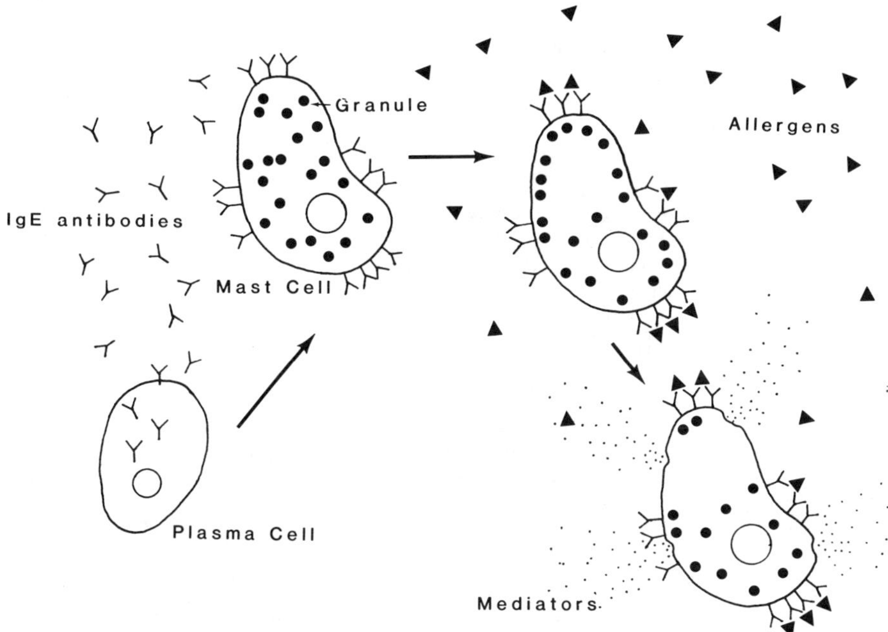

Fig. 2. Biochemical mechanism of a type I allergic reaction.

1. *Type I Reactions*

a. Mechanism and Symptomatology. The mechanism involved in type I reactions is depicted in Fig. 2. Type I reactions are often referred to as acute or immediate hypersensitivity reactions, because the onset time is very short. Type I reactions are characterized by this rapid onset of symptoms and are mediated by allergen-specific immunoglobulin E (IgE). With food allergies, the allergens initiating the allergic response are usually proteins. The initial event in type I reactions is the production of allergen-specific IgE in response to an exposure to an allergenic food protein. Allergen-specific IgE is produced by plasma cells and attaches itself to the outer membrane surfaces of tissue mast cells and/or circulating basophils. The mast cells and basophils are thus sensitized and become ready to respond to subsequent exposure to that particular food protein. This sensitization process distinguishes allergic individuals from nonallergic individuals in the population. Most people will not respond to exposure to a foreign food protein with production of allergen-specific IgE. Once the mast cells and basophils are sensitized, subsequent exposure to the allergen results in the release of allergic mediators from these sensitized cells. The allergen cross-links two IgE molecules on the surface of the mast cell or basophil, which causes the sensitized cells to degranulate. The granules of mast cells and basophils contain most of the impor-

TABLE I

Mast Cell Mediators of Type I Reactions

Preformed, rapidly secreted mediators
   Histamine
   Eosinophil chemotactic factor of anaphylaxis (ECF-A)
   ECF oligopeptides
   Neutrophil chemotactic factor
   T-Lymphocyte chemotactic factor
   B-Lymphocyte chemotactic factor
   Lymphocyte chemotactic factor
   Superoxide anions
   Exoglycosidases
   Arylsulfatase A

Generated mediators
   Leukotrienes or slow-reacting substances of anaphylaxis
   Monohydroxyeicosatetraenoic acids (HETEs)
   Hydroperoxyeicosatetraenoic acids (HPETEs)
   Thromboxanes
   Prostaglandins
   Platelet-activating factor (PAF)
   Prostaglandin-generating factor of anaphylaxis (PGF-A)

Preformed, granule-associated mediators
   Heparin
   Tryptase
   Myeloperoxidase
   Superoxide dismutase
   Arylsulfatase B
   Inflammatory factor of anaphylaxis (IFA)

tant mediators of the allergic reactions, although some mediators exist outside the granules (Table I) (Wasserman, 1983). Histamine is probably the most important mediator of the allergic reaction and is responsible for most of the immediate effects. The slow-reacting substances of anaphylaxis or leukotrienes may be responsible for many of the delayed effects observed occasionally in type I reactions. The mediators are secreted into the bloodstream and react with tissue receptors. The symptoms of an allergic reaction (Table II) are dependent on which tissue receptors are affected. A variety of symptoms can be associated with IgE-mediated reactions, but any single allergic individual is likely to suffer from only a few of them. Antihistamines are effective in blocking the allergic response by inhibiting the reaction between histamine and its tissue receptors (Beavan, 1978).

    b. Common Allergenic Foods and Allergens. The most common allergenic foods involved in type I reactions are listed in Table III. Cow's milk is, by far, the most common allergenic food among infants. Obviously, this is

TABLE II

Symptoms of Type I Allergic Reactions to Foods[a]

Gastrointestinal symptoms	Respiratory symptoms
Nausea	Rhinitis
Vomiting	Asthma
Diarrhea	
Cutaneous symptoms	Other symptoms
Urticaria	Laryngeal edema
Eczema or atopic dermatitis	Anaphylactic shock
Angioedema	Hypotension
	Headache

[a]Reprinted with permission from Institute of Food Technologists' Expert Panel on Food Safety and Nutrition (1985). Copyright © by Institute of Food Technologists.

related partially to the frequency of consumption of cow's milk in early infancy. Among adults, peanuts and crustacea are probably the most common allergenic foods, although accurate incidence data are not available. The allergens in most foods have not been specifically isolated and identified. Casein and β-lactoglobulin are the major allergens in cow's milk (Bleumink and Young, 1968; Goldman *et al.*, 1963b). Ovomucoid and ovalbumin are the major allergens in eggs (Hoffman, 1983; Langeland, 1982). Norwegian investigators have isolated the major allergen in codfish and identified it as a parvalbumin (Elsayed and Bennich, 1975). Partial purification of other allergenic food proteins has been achieved (Metcalfe, 1985). In many cases, multiple allergenic proteins occur in a single food. For example, more than a half-dozen allergenic proteins have been identified in peanuts (Barnett *et al.*, 1983). This multiplicity complicates the task of purification and characterization.

c.   Prevalence and Persistence.   In all likelihood, the incidence of type I reactions in the overall population is less than 1% (Golbert, 1972; Taylor,

TABLE III

**Common Allergenic Foods Involved in
Type I Reactions**[a]

Cows' milk	Crustacea (shrimp, crab, lobsters)
Eggs	Molluscs (clams, oysters, scallops)
Peanuts	Fish
Soybeans	Wheat
Other legumes	Tree nuts

[a]Reprinted with permission from Institute of Food Technologists' Expert Panel on Food Safety and Nutrition (1985). Copyright © by Institute of Food Technologists.

1985a). The perceived incidence of food allergy is much higher, but many of these illnesses are not true IgE-mediated reactions. Harris (1982) conducted a survey of the perceived incidence of allergic reactions to cows' milk in Britain by questioning 8749 people about their avoidance of cows' milk and their reasons for such avoidance. Within this group, 1.47% limited their consumption of milk for reasons that were related to allergies or other types of food sensitivities. Most likely, lactose intolerance was a more frequent problem than true cows' milk allergy. Accurate estimation of the prevalence of allergic reactions to foods is difficult due to diagnostic difficulties. Frequently, the occurrence of the adverse reaction to a specific food is not corroborated with double-blind food challenges. Even if a confirmed adverse reaction is identified, the physician may not seek evidence of any immunological involvement. Hence, it is impossible to ascertain whether an allergic mechanism is involved.

Certainly, infants and children are more likely to have food allergies than adults. Bock and Martin (1983) determined that 4% of a group of 500 non-selected infants developed allergies to cows' milk as defined by double-blind challenge tests (DBCTs) and positive immunological tests within the first 3 years of life. Most of these cases of cows' milk allergy were rather transitory; in some cases, sensitivity was lost within a matter of weeks (Bock, 1985). Children born to allergic parents are much more likely to devleop food allergies than children born to nonallergic parents. Infants with food allergies are likely to develop their initial symptoms very early in life, often before their first birthday (Minford *et al.*, 1982). Subsequent challenges of children with confirmed cases of IgE-mediated food allergy indicate that many infants outgrow these conditions (Bock, 1982; Dannaeus and Inganas, 1981; Ford and Taylor, 1982). Allergies to certain foods are more easily outgrown than others; milk and egg allergies are more often outgrown than peanut and fish allergies (Bock, 1982; Ford and Taylor, 1982). Presumably, this loss of sensitivity is due to enhanced protein processing in the gastrointestinal tract, increased maturity of the gastrointestinal barrier, and development of other types of antibody responses that might block the reaction with IgE (Dannaeus and Inganas, 1981).

d.   Diagnosis. Self-diagnosis and parental diagnosis of food allergies is a common practice. However, such evaluations are more often erroneous than correct (Bock *et al.*, 1978). Careful medical evaluation is needed to confirm a diagnosis of IgE-mediated food allergy. The first step is to determine that an adverse reaction actually occurs upon consumption of the suspected food. Once that has been established, the involvement of IgE must be determined.

Many physicians rely heavily on patients' historical accounts of their experiences with various foods for a diagnosis of food allergy. Since patients' impressions are often incorrect, such reliance on their accounts can be risky. Challenge tests are often needed to establish with certainty the role of specific foods in the reactions. The DBCT is the most reliable type of challenge procedure (Bernstein *et al.*, 1982; May and Bock, 1978; Simpson *et al.*, 1980). DBCTs have been particularly useful in assessing the role of foods in particular manifestations of the allergic response such as their role in atopic dermatitis (Sampson, 1983). DBCTs are contraindicated in some situations, especially in patients with severe reactions to foods (Taylor, 1985a). Single-blind challenge procedures can also be employed but are not as reliable as the DBCT. Another popular alternative to DBCTs is the elimination–challenge test, where patients are placed on an elimination diet until symptoms subside and then challenged openly with individual foods (Goldman *et al.*, 1963a; Johnstone, 1978). The use of open challenges can be less definitive, but this method is frequently employed because in some cases the patient can be challenged at home.

The diagnosis of IgE mediation of a confirmed adverse reaction to food can be made with either the skin prick test or the radioallergosorbent test (RAST). The simplest procedure is the skin prick test, where a small amount of a food extract is applied to the skin of the patient and the site is pricked to allow entry of the antigen. A wheal-and-flare response at the skin prick site demonstrates that IgE in the skin has reacted with some protein in the food extract. An alternative procedure is the RAST, an *in vitro* test utilizing a small sample of the patient's blood (Adolphson *et al.*, 1980). The binding of serum IgE to a food protein bound to some solid matrix is assessed with radiolabeled anti-IgE. The RAST is a considerably more expensive procedure, but is equally reliable and preferred for patients with extreme sensitivities (Metcalfe, 1984a). The leukocyte histamine release assay (Siraganian, 1976) is also a reliable method for detecting a type I reaction. This assay involves monitoring the release of histamine from the patient's leukocytes upon exposure to a food extract. This method is used infrequently because it requires specialized equipment.

e.   Treatment.   *i. Specific-Avoidance Diets.* The major means of treatment of true food allergies including the type I reactions is the specific-avoidance diet. The patients must carefully avoid the food(s) that provoke their reaction. With type I reactions, the degree of tolerance for the offending allergen is extremely low in some cases. Some examples of the exquisite sensitivity are provided in Table IV. Obviously, the amount of allergen exposure occurring in some of these circumstances is extremely small. The severity of the allergic reaction is dependent to some extent on the degree of exposure. Therefore, the reactions observed in these cases of exquisite sensitivity are often mild. However, adherence to such strict avoidance diets is difficult, and many inadvertent exposures to the offending food are likely. Patients must have considerable knowledge of food composition. They must carefully scrutinize food labels. However, undeclared uses of the food can occur, especially through restaurant meals but also through use of foods and food ingredients as processing aids and the occasional presence of allergenic residues.

Individuals with type I reactions often have many questions relating to the

TABLE IV

Exquisite Sensitivity of Some Individuals with Type I Food Allergies[a]

---

1. Traces of offending food contaminating other foods
   From inadequate cleaning of processing equipment
   From attempts to remove offending food from mixture by allergic individual or others
   From direct or indirect contact between two foods, such as using the same serving utensil for several different entrees
2. Touching utensils, bottles, other materials contaminated with the offending food
3. Kissing lips of person who is eating the offending food
4. Opening packages containing offending food
5. Inhalation of vapors from cooking of offending food
6. Transfer of food allergens from mother to infant via breast milk

---

[a]Reprinted with permission from Institute of Food Technologists' Expert Panel on Food Safety and Nutrition (1985). Copyright © by Institute of Food Technologists.

necessary degree of selectivity to institute in their diets. Should they avoid the offending food in all forms (e.g., soybean oil, soy sauce, and soya lecithin for soybean-allergic individuals)? The allergens in foods are usually proteins, and some foods such as oils contain no detectable proteins (Tattrie and Yaguchi, 1973) and other foods contain completely hydrolyzed forms of the protein. In most cases, the allergenicity of specific foods has not been determined. Exceptions are the known lack of allergenicity of peanut oil for peanut-sensitive individuals (Taylor *et al.*, 1981) and soybean oil for soybean-sensitive individuals (Bush *et al.*, 1985), and the demonstrated allergenicity of other peanut products as determined by the RAST inhibition test (Nordlee *et al.*, 1981).

Cross-reactivity is another serious concern for individuals with type I reactions. The peanut- or soybean-allergic individual must be aware of the possibility of reactions to other legumes. Cross-reactions do not always occur but must be considered during the construction of avoidance diets. Cross-reactions can occur within many classes of genetically related foods such as peanuts and soybeans, shrimp and crab, or cows' milk and goats' milk.

Very few specialized foods are available for consumers with food allergies. Infants with cows' milk allergies can select from a variety of alternative hypoallergenic formulas based on soybeans, hydrolyzed casein, and other foods. Substitute foods are not specifically available for other types of food allergies. With infants in particular, care must be taken in the selection of substitute formulas because allergies can develop to the substitute ingredients, especially soybeans and goats' milk (Bahna and Gandhi, 1983).

ii. Breast-Feeding. Breast-feeding has been advocated by some physicians as a prophylactic treatment to prevent the development of food allergies in early infancy. However, numerous studies on the effectiveness of breast feeding have been performed and the results are conflicting (Burr, 1983). The length of any recommended breast-feeding period is also subject to considerable debate. If breast milk is an effective prophylactic treatment, the presence of secretory IgA antibodies in breast milk likely plays a significant role (Hamburger *et al.*, 1983).

Food allergies can develop in children who have been exclusively breast-fed. These allergies can be manifested while the infant is still in the strict breast-feeding period, or they can occur on the first exposure to a specific food (Gerrard and Shenassa, 1983: Van Asperen *et al.*, 1983; Warner, 1980). Apparently the sensitization is caused by transmission of proteinaceous food allergens through the breast milk (Gibney, 1983).

iii.   Elimination Diets.   Overall elimination diets involve the simultaneous removal of a variety of possible allergenic foods (Dockhorn and Smith, 1981; Gallant *et al.*, 1977). Such diets are usually employed in clinical settings in an attempt to resolve chronic or mysterious symptoms. This approach might also be tried when multiple food allergies are suspected. If these diets are successful in leading to remission of symptoms, a series of food challenges would be conducted to identify any offending foods. While these diets are useful for clinical purposes, they are not sufficiently palatable for long-term use.

iv.   Pharmacological Treatment.   The symptoms of allergic reactions can be treated pharmacologically with drugs such as the antihistamines (Anderson and Lessof, 1983). Patients with histories of life-threatening reactions to foods are often advised to carry antihistamines and/or an epinephrine-filled syringe at all times (Atkins, 1983).

Prophylactic treatments of a pharmacological nature remain in the experimental stage of development. Prophylactic treatment with oral disodium cromoglycate (Businco *et al.*, 1983) or antihistamines (Bahna and Gandhi, 1983) has been successful on some occasions but has not been universally beneficial. Immunotherapy for food allergies is extremely controversial, and no definitive evidence of the value of this therapy exists (Atkins, 1983; Soothill, 1983).

2.   *Type III Reactions*

Type III reactions are also known as immune complex reactions and result from an inflammatory process initiated by antigen–antibody complexes. Type III reactions have typical onset times of 4–6 hr. IgG and IgM antibodies can participate in type III reactions. Complement also plays an essential role in immune complex reactions, since some of the complement activation products, such as C3a and C5a, which are produced during the activation of the complement system by the immune complexes, are potent inflammatory agents and leukocyte chemoattractants. The polymorphonuclear leukocytes, which are attracted to the immune complex site by the C3a and C5a components of complement, are responsible for much of the inflammatory tissue damage. The leukocytes release hydrolytic enzymes in an attempt to destroy the immune complexes, but these enzymes also initiate extensive tissue damage.

Type III reactions are likely to occur with food antigens (Stern and Walker,

1985), but no estimates of the prevalence of these reactions have been made. Circulating immune complexes containing specific food antigens have been demonstrated in patients with IgA deficiency (Cunningham-Rundles *et al.*, 1979) and in patients with cows' milk allergy (Paganelli *et al.*, 1979). Local deposits of cows' milk antigen (Bock *et al.*, 1983) and complement, IgG, and IgM (Shiner *et al.*, 1975) have been demonstrated. Immune complex reactions seem to be linked to the pathogenesis of delayed enteropathy, although the precise mechanism of tissue damage remains to be determined (Stern and Walker, 1985).

The diagnosis of type III reactions is difficult. The demonstration of circulating immune complexes is only partially definitive. The demonstration of tissue-bound immune complexes requires biopsy of inflamed tissues. Consequently, much more evaluation will be necessary to determine the role of immune complexes in food allergies.

The treatment of type III reactions would include specific avoidance diets primarily. Specific pharmacological approaches are not available.

3. Type IV Reactions

Type IV reactions are often called delayed-hypersensitivity reactions or cellular hypersensitivty. The symptoms of these reactions usually appear 6–24 hr after consumption of the offending food. These reactions develop slowly, reaching a peak at approximately 48 hr and subsiding after 72–96 hr. Type IV reactions involve interaction between specific antigens and sensitized T lymphocytes. In contrast to other mechanisms, these reactions occur without the involvement of complement or antibodies. The first step in type IV reactions is the binding of an antigen to a small number of sensitized T lymphocytes. This interaction results in lymphokine synthesis, lymphocyte proliferation, and the generation of cytotoxic T cells. Lymphokine production occurs first within a few hours of the interaction between the antigen and the sensitized lymphocytes. Lymphokines are soluble proteins and glycoproteins which exert potent effects on macrophages, polymorphonuclear leukocytes, lymphocytes, and other cells. A list of some of the known lymphokine activities is provided in Table V. The collective activities of these lymphokines and the inflammatory cells which they attract are principally responsible for the pathological events observed in type IV reactions. Lymphocyte proliferation, also known as transformation or blastogenesis, is the second event in type IV reactions. This proliferative process increases the number of antigen-responsive cells and amplifies the developing immune response. A third event occurring in type IV reactions is the generation of cytotoxic T cells. These killer cells can destroy cells which bear antigens identical to those that triggered the reaction.

T Lymphocytes are a major component of the gut-associated lymphoid tissue (Stern and Walker, 1985). Evidence for the involvement of type IV reactions in food allergies is sparse but reasonably compelling. Increased numbers of intestinal intraepithelial lymphocytes have been observed in cows' milk allergy (Phil-

TABLE V

Some of the Known Lymphokine Activities

Macrophage migration-inhibitory factor (MIF)
Macrophage-activating factor (MAF)
Lymphocyte-derived chemotactic factor for monocytes (LDCF)
Leukocyte-inhibitory factor (LIF)
Chemotactic factors for polymorphonuclear leukocytes, basophils, and
  eosinophils
Histamine-relasing factor
Lymphocyte mitogenic factor (LMF)
Transfer factor (TF)
Helper factors for antibody production
Suppressor factors for antibody production
Lymphotoxin (LT)
Interferon

lips *et al.*, 1979; Stern *et al.*, 1982). Peripheral lymphocytes in cows' milk allergy can be stimulated by cows' milk antigens with the production of lymphokines such as leukocyte migration-inhibitory factor (Ashkenazi *et al.*, 1980; Minor *et al.*, 1980). Impaired lymphoblastogenesis has also been observed in cows' milk allergy indicating altered T-cell reactivity (Fallstrom *et al.*, 1983). Again, these reactions may be involved in the development of enteropathy in some cows' milk-allergic individuals, but further evidence is needed. No estimates of the prevalence of type IV food allergies have been made.

The diagnosis of type IV reactions involves monitoring the production of lymphokines by lymphocytes or lymphoblastogenesis. Usually, these assays involve peripheral lymphocytes, although it would be desirable to have tests of the responsiveness of intestinal lymphocytes. The collection of intestinal lymphocytes for such tests would be difficult. The treatment of type IV reactions also involves specific avoidance diets.

B. Nonimmunological Food Sensitivities

Basically, any food-related illness that falls outside the limits of the true food allergies discussed above would be included in this category. A wide variety of disease mechanisms is possible.

1. Allergylike Intoxications

The sole example of an allergylike intoxication is histamine poisoning, also known as scombroid fish poisoning, an illness associated with the consumption of foods containing high levels of histamine. Histamine poisoning does not actually belong in a chapter on food sensitivities, since it is not an individualistic reaction. Presumably, everyone is susceptible to histamine poisoning. It is a classical type of intoxication rather than a form of food sensitivity. Histamine poisoning is included in this discussion because it is frequently confused with and misdiagnosed as true food allergy.

Histamine poisoning occurs rather sporadically. Few countries compile statistics on the prevalence of histamine poisoning episodes. The most frequent reports come from the United States, Japan, Britain, and several other European countries (Taylor, 1985b). In all likelihood, many histamine poisoning episodes are not reported in these countries because the illness is relatively mild and has a short duration. Histamine poisoning undoubtedly occurs in many other countries also. The true prevalence of histamine poisoning is difficult to estimate.

Histamine was discussed earlier as a primary mediator of allergic reactions. In the case of true food allergy, histamine is released from tissue mast cells following exposure to an allergen. In the case of histamine poisoning, the exogenous histamine from foods in the diet is the culprit rather than endogenously secreted histamine. Humans are relatively resistant to dietary histamine because of the presence of two histamine-metabolizing enzymes, histamine-N-methyltransferase (HMT) and diamine oxidase (DAO), in the small intestinal mucosa (Maslinski, 1975). These enzymes are sufficiently active to metabolize the levels of histamine normally present in the diet. The major products of these reactions do not possess the profound physiological properties of histamine. The mechanism of action of histamine poisoning apparently involves the coincident ingestion of histamine and some substances that potentiate its toxicity by inhibiting these hitamine-metabolizing enzymes (Hui and Taylor, 1985: Lyons *et al.*, 1983). Cadaverine and putrescine have been identified as potentiators of histamine toxicity (Bjeldanes *et al.*, 1978; Parrot and Nicot, 1966) and substances that can inhibit the intestinal metabolism of histamine (Hui and Taylor, 1985; Lyons *et al.*, 1983; Taylor and Lieber, 1979). The inhibition of the intestinal histamine-metabolizing enzymes allows enhanced transport of unmetabolized histamine across the mucosal barrier (Lyons *et al.*, 1983). Once this histamine reaches the portal blood, it can circulate and generate its well-known physiological effects. Extraintestinal metabolism of histamine is also inhibited by the presence of potentiators, such as cadaverine (Hui and Taylor, 1985). In foods where histamine is present at extremely high levels, such potentiation may not be necessary; the high levels of histamine could conceivably overwhelm the metabolic enzymes (Taylor *et al.*, 1984).

Histamine is formed in foods primarily as the result of bacterial action. Consequently, high levels of histamine are encountered most frequently in fermented foods or spoiled foods. Certain types of fish, including the scombroid fish (tuna, mackerel, bonito) and a few species of nonscombroid fish (mahi-mahi, sardines, bluefish), are most commonly implicated in outbreaks of histamine poisoning (Taylor, 1985b; Taylor *et al.*, 1984). The presence of high levels of the precursor amino acid, histidine, in the muscle tissues of these fish makes them especially susceptible to histamine formation during spoilage. In these fish, histamine can

TABLE VI

Symptoms of Histamine Poisoning

Cutaneous	Gastrointestinal
Rash	Nausea
Urticaria	Vomiting
Edema	Diarrhea
Localized inflammation	
	Neurological
Hemodynamic	Headache
Hypotension	Palpitations
	Tingling
	Burning
	Itching

form very rapidly, so that the fish displays no overt signs of spoilage even though it contains hazardous levels of histamine. The only other food implicated with any frequency in episodes of histamine poisoning is cheese, especially Swiss cheese (Taylor *et al.*, 1982).

Several species of bacteria are able to decarboxylate histidine to generate histamine, although it is not a common property of bacteria (Taylor *et al.*, 1978). In fish, *Morganella morganii*, *Klebsiella pneumoniae*, and *Hafnia alvei* have been implicated as the histamine-producing species in actual incidents of scombroid fish poisoning (Taylor, 1985b). In cheese, *Lactobacillus buchneri* is the only histamine-producing species implicated in an actual episode of histamine poisoning (Sumner *et al.*, 1985). Other bacterial species, including *Enterobacter aerogenes* and *Lactobacillus delbreuckii*, have been identified as prolific histamine producers, although their roles in actual episodes of histamine poisoning have not been established (Taylor, 1985b; Taylor *et al.*, 1978).

A variety of symptoms can occur during incidents of histamine poisoning (Table VI). The most prevalent symptoms are a bright red rash, an oral burning sensation, flushing and sweating, nausea, and abdominal cramps (Taylor, 1985b). Most individuals suffering from histamine poisoning experience only a few of the symptoms listed in Table VI. The onset time for histamine poisoning is relatively short, ranging from a few minutes to a few hours. The symptoms are often rather mild and subside rapidly within a few hours in most cases. The symptoms of histamine poisoning are similar to the symptoms observed with true food allergies.

Histamine poisoning is frequently misdiagnosed as food allergy because of the similar symptomatology. Antihistamine therapy is equally effective in treating the symptoms of both histamine poisoning and food allergies, which often reinforces the incorrect diagnosis. A possible diagnosis of histamine poisoning can be confirmed only by analysis of the incriminated food for histamine. However, several clues can often allow the clinician to distinguish between histamine poisoning and true food allergies: (1) the lack of a previous history of allergic reactions to the incriminated food, (2) the suspected food's being one of the few foods commonly implicated in episodes of histamine poisoning, and (3) a high attack rate in group outbreaks.

The primary treatment for histamine poisoning is the administration of antihistamines. The risk of histamine poisoning can be diminished by limiting consumption of certain types of raw fish such as tuna. Raw fish are particularly susceptible to histamine formation if stored at improper temperatures.

2. *Anaphylactoid Reactions*

Anaphylactoid reactions are caused by substances that induce the spontaneous release of histamine and other mediators from tissue mast cells without the intervention of IgE. The lack of involvement of IgE or other immunological factors distinguishes anaphylactoid reactions from true food allergies. Histamine poisoning is sometimes classified as an anaphylactoid reaction (Taylor, 1985a), although it clearly belongs in a unique category because of the involvement of exogenous histamine.

The evidence for the existence of anaphylactoid reactions is largely circumstantial. None of the histamine-releasing substances has ever been identified. Therefore, their very existence is somewhat speculative. However, several types of primary food sensitivities may fall into this category, because evidence of immunological involvement is lacking. The best example is "strawberry allergy." Evidence for strawberry-specific IgE has never been acquired, yet some individuals displayed documented sensitivities to strawberries, and the symptoms such as urticaria are reminiscent of those associated with true food allergies. Consequently, histamine and other mast cell mediators are likely to be involved. The diagnosis of anaphylactoid reactions is difficult, since the nature of the offending chemicals and the mechanism of the reaction are unknown. Treatment for such reactions involves avoidance of the offending food.

3. *Metabolic Food Disorders*

These adverse reactions result from defects in the ability to metabolize some component of the food. The defect is often genetically acquired. Examples include lactose intolerance, favism, and perhaps celiac disease.

a. Lactose Intolerance. Lactose intolerance results from a deficiency of the enzyme lactase or β-galactosidase in the intestinal mucosa (Sandine and Daly, 1979). As a result, lactose, the principal sugar in milk, cannot be metabolized into its constituent monosaccharides, galactose and glucose. Galactose and glucose are normally absorbed into the portal circulation and utilized metabolically. Lactose cannot be absorbed unless it is first hydrolyzed to galactose and glucose. As a result, the undigested lactose passes from the small intestine into the colon. Colonic bacteria metabolize the lactose into CO_2 and H_2O. The result is abdominal cramping, flatulence, and frothy diarrhea, the primary symptoms of lactose intolerance.

The prevalence of lactose intolerance increases with increasing age. Many individuals can tolerate normal levels of lactose at a young age, but, as they age, the activity of intestinal lactase decreases and they gradually develop an intolerance to lactose. The prevalence of lactose intolerance varies with different races and ethnic origins. The prevalence in the United States among Caucasians is about 6–12% (Sandine and Daly, 1979). However, it can occur in 60–90% of some ethnic groups, including Greeks, Arabs, Jews, black Americans, Japanese, and other Orientals (Sandine and Daly, 1979).

The most common method for the diagnosis of lactose intolerance is the lactose tolerance test (LTT). In the LTT, a fasting individual is challenged orally with 50 gm of lactose. Blood glucose concentration is monitored and an increase of 25 mg/dl or more is considered normal. Symptoms are also noted. Breath hydrogen levels can also be monitored as an alternative to measurement of serum glucose.

The results of the LTT are frequently overinterpreted. Fifty grams of lactose is equivalent to the amount of lactose in a liter or more of milk. Certainly, it would be unusual to consume a quart of milk in a single meal, especially on an empty stomach. Some individuals with a clinical diagnosis of lactose intolerance based on the 50-gm challenge can consume 8 oz of milk with no adverse effects (Lisker and Aguilas, 1978; Reddy and Pershad, 1972; Welsh, 1978). Consequently, a clinical diagnosis of lactose intolerance based on the 50-gm challenge does not mean that avoidance of all dairy products is a necessity. A more reasonable diagnostic approach would involve sequential oral challenges with increasing doses of lactose to obtain a better impression of individual tolerance for lactose in the diet.

The usual treatment for lactose intolerance involves the avoidance of dairy products containing lactose, even though that is probably sound advice for only a few of the individuals with lactose intolerance. Alternatives to the total avoidance of dairy products include a restriction on dairy product intake, consumption of smaller, divided doses of milk, consumption of lactose-hydrolyzed milk, and eating of fermented dairy products. Lactose-intolerant individuals seem to tolerate fermented dairy products such as yogurt and acidophilus milk even when they cannot tolerate milk (Gallagher *et al.*, 1977). Unnecessary exclusion of dairy products from the diet may present other problems. Birge *et al.* (1967) suggested that osteoporosis may result from the inadequate calcium intakes that often accompany diets devoid of dairy products. The most reasonable approach would be to characterize an individual's degree of tolerance to lactose and allow consumption of dairy products up to that level of lactose intake. Since lactose intolerance may worsen with age, this approach would require careful medical follow-up. However, it would allow the lactose-intolerant consumer the maximum benefit and enjoyment from dairy products.

b.   Favism. The acute hemolytic anemia experienced by some individuals following the ingestion of broad beans (fava beans) or the inhalation of pollen from the *Vicia faba* plant is known as favism (Mager *et al.*, 1980). The major manifestations of favism are typical of the symptoms inherent in a hemolytic event: pallor, fatigue, dyspnea, nausea, abdominal and/or back pain, fever, and chills. On rare occasions, more severe symptoms including hemoglobinuria, jaundice, and renal failure are encountered. The onset time can be quite rapid, but usually ranges between 5 and 24 hr. The disease is usually self-limited with a prompt and spontaneous recovery. Favism is most prevalent when the *Vicia faba* plant is blooming and the pollen is in the air and when the edible broad beans are available in the market.

Favism affects individuals with a deficiency of erythrocyte glucose-6-phosphate dehydrogenase (G6PDH). The red blood cells of individuals with G6PDH deficiency are susceptible to oxidative damage because G6PDH is critical for the maintenance of the reduced forms of glutathione and nicotinamide adenine dinucleotide phosphate, which prevent oxidation. Fava beans contain several oxidants, including vicine and convicine, which are able to damage the erythrocytes of sensitive individuals. G6PDH deficiency is genetically determined but may be the most common enzymatic defect in human populations worldwide, affecting about 100 million people. The highest incidence of G6PDH deficiency occurs among Oriental Jewish communities in Israel, Sardinians, Cypriot Greeks, American blacks, and certain African populations. The trait is virtually absent in northern European nations, North American Indians, and Eskimos. However, favism occurs primarily in the Mediterranean area, the Middle East, China, and Bulgaria where the genetic trait is fairly prevalent and where broad beans are frequently consumed.

G6PDH deficiency can be diagnosed with a simple assay for enzymatic activity on isolated red blood cells. A deficiency of G6PDH is not a particularly serious condition. However, to avoid favism, these individuals should avoid the consumption of fava beans.

c.   Celiac Disease. Celiac disease, also known as celiac sprue or gluten-sensitive enteropathy, is characterized by malabsorption of nutrients from the intestine as a consequence of damage to the absorptive epithelial cells of the small intestine. This intestinal damage occurs in susceptible individuals after they consume the protein fractions of wheat, rye, barley, or oats (Hartsook, 1984; Karsarda, 1978). The gliadin fraction of wheat protein and the equivalent prolamin fractions of barley, rye, and oats are responsible for the damage (Baker and Read, 1976; Van de Kamer *et al.*, 1953). The mechanism for producing this damage is not understood, although several hypotheses have been promulgated: (1) that sensitive individuals lack some enzyme necessary for the digestion of gliadin, (2) that gliadin acts like a lectin and binds to abnormal glycoprotein receptors on the surfaces of the epithelial cells of sensitive individuals and this interaction results in a cytotoxic effect, and (3) that the sensitive individuals mount an abnormal immunological response to the gliadin protein (Kasarda, 1978, 1981). The missing-enzyme theory would fit nicely into the metabolic disorders category. However, if celiac disease results from an abnormal immunological response, then it should properly be grouped with the true food allergies. The classification used for the purposes of this chapter is strictly arbitrary.

The symptoms of celiac disease are typical of a malabsorption syndrome. They include diarrhea, bloating, weight loss, anemia, bone pain, chronic fatigue, weakness, muscle cramps, and, in children, failure to grow. The symptoms of celiac disease may begin at any age. No evidence has been found of spontaneous recovery from this illness.

Celiac disease is an inherited trait, but its inheritance is complex and poorly understood. The prevalence of celiac disease in the United States is about 1 in every 3000 individuals (Hartsook, 1984; Kasarda, 1978). In County Galway, Ireland, the disease is much more prevalent, affecting 1 in every 300 persons (Kasarda, 1978). Genetic inheritance probably involves multiple genes. Environmental factors, such as viral illness, may contribute to the onset of the illness in some cases (Kasarda, 1978). The disease has appeared in only one of a set of identical twins (Kasarda, 1978).

The diagnosis of celiac disease usually involves an intestinal biopsy. The biopsy material is examined histologically for evidence of the flattened intestinal villi that are characteristic of celiac disease. Improvement on a diet free of wheat, rye, barley, and oats with a subsequent normal biopsy can confirm the diagnosis.

The treatment of celiac disease involves the complete avoidance of wheat, rye, barley, and oats and any products made from these grains. Adherence to such avoidance diets can be very difficult. However, exposure to small amounts of gliadin can theoretically damage the intestinal epithelial cells. Some celiac patients seem to be able to tolerate small amounts of gliadin, but this is not true for all patients (Hartsook, 1984). Since the tissue damage is initiated by the protein fractions, the advice to avoid all products made from wheat, rye, barley, and oats may be unnecessary provided some of these products are protein-free. Hydrolyzed vegetable protein should contain only amino acids and no intact protein. However, any traces of protein in these products could be damaging. Ciclitira *et al.* (1985) have recently developed a radioimmunoassay for wheat gliadin and used it to demonstrate that traces of the protein were present in some types of wheat starch. Another approach to the treatment of celiac disease may be the eventual development of grain varieties that do not contain the toxic protein (Kasarda, 1981).

4. *Idiosyncratic Reactions*

Idiosyncratic reactions are those individualistic adverse reactions to foods with unexplained mechanisms. A variety of different mechanisms is possible, al-

TABLE VII

Partial List of Food-Related Idiosyncratic Reactions

Reaction	Implicated food or ingredient
Migraine headache	Chocolate
Asthma	FD&C Yellow number 5 (tartrazine)
Asthma	Sulfites
Hyperkinesis	Food-coloring agents
Aggressive behavior	Sugar
Chinese restaurant syndrome	Monosodium glutamate

though considerable research efforts will be required to define these mechanisms. A list of some possible idiosyncratic reactions associated with foods is provided in Table VII. The role of foods or food ingredients in some of these reactions, such as tartrazine and sulfites in asthma, has been well documented, although the mechanisms involved remain unknown. With other reactions, the role of foods or food ingredients has not been firmly established. An example would be the role of sugar in aggressive, antisocial behavior (Gray and Gray, 1983; Harper and Gans, 1985). These relationships remain very speculative, and double-blind challenges are needed to determine if a relationship exists. In other cases, the role of foods or food ingredients is widely believed despite evidence suggesting that the reactions are not associated with foods or are only rarely associated with foods. An example would be the role of food colorants in hyperkinesis (Harley *et al.*, 1978a,b; Stare *et al.*, 1980). Obviously, celiac disease could also fit into the idiosyncratic category, since the mechanism of that illness is not understood.

The prevalence of these reactions is unknown and difficult to estimate, since the role of foods in some of these conditions remains ill-defined. The symptoms are also quite diverse, since a variety of foods and mechanisms are involved. The major diagnostic procedure for these idiosyncratic reactions involves the DBCT. This procedure serves to demonstrate the role of foods or food ingredients in the reaction. A negative DBCT may indicate that foods are not involved in the response or that the wrong food was incriminated as the causative agent. The only treatment available for food idiosyncrasies is a specific-avoidance diet. Obviously, it would be impossible to discuss the myriad of food idiosyncrasies in detail. Sulfite sensitivity will be discussed as an example.

Sulfites are widely used in the food and food service industries to control enzymatic and nonenzymatic browning, to prevent undesirable bacterial growth, to condition doughs, to provide antioxidant protection, and to bleach cherries in the processing of maraschino cherries. Several years ago, the association was made between ingestion of sulfites by certain sensitive individuals and the triggering of an asthmatic reaction (Baker *et al.*, 1981; Stevenson and Simon, 1981). These reactions occur within a few minutes and can be quite severe on occasion. The U.S. Food and Drug Administration has received reports of over 20 deaths alleged to be due to ingestion of sulfited foods since 1982. The most prominent response associated with sulfites has been asthma. Reports of other manifestations have appeared, but these reports are largely anecdotal and unconfirmed (Bush *et al.*, 1986). The mechanism of sulfite sensitivity is not understood, although the inhalation of SO_2 vapors during the ingestion of acidic foods and beverages may be important (Delohery *et al.*, 1984), and preliminary evidence of a deficiency of sulfite oxidase, the primary enzyme responsible for sulfite metabolism, in some sulfite-sensitive asthmatics exists (Jacobsen *et al.*, 1984).

The prevalence of sulfite sensitivity has been the subject of several reports. Early reports suggested that perhaps 5–10% of all asthmatics might be sulfite-sensitive, which would equate to 500,000–1 million individuals nationwide (Simon *et al.*, 1982; Buckley *et al.*, 1985). Bush *et al.* (1986) have concluded from challenges of over 200 asthmatics that sulfite sensitivity affects perhaps only 100,000–200,000 individuals in the United States. Sulfite-induced asthma affects about 5–10% of the severe or steroid-dependent asthmatics, who represent only about 20% of the asthmatic population (Bush *et al.*, 1986).

The diagnosis of sulfite sensitivity is based on a sulfite challenge test. These tests should be, but are not always, performed in a double-blind manner. Challenges have been conducted with capsules, acidic beverages (citric acid solutions, lemonade, apple juice), or some combination of capsules and acidic beverages. Asthmatics may be more sensitive to sulfites in acidic beverages than to sulfites in capsules, due to the release of SO_2 vapor from acidic beverages (Bush *et al.*, 1986; Delohery *et al.*, 1984). A standardized challenge procedure is needed and is being developed currently. It will probably involve some combination of capsule and acidic beverage challenges.

The treatment of sulfite sensitivity involves the avoidance of sulfited foods and beverages. However, many foods and beverages are sulfited, and many contain only low residual concentrations of sulfite. Table VIII provides a partial list of sulfited foods and beverages according to their residual sulfite content. A major question is whether sulfite-sensitive asthmatics really need to avoid foods with low residual sulfite levels. Sulfites are very reactive in food systems, and very little free sulfite remains in most products. Sulfites can volatilize from acidic foods and beverages and be lost as SO_2. Sulfites can be oxidized to sulfate, an innocuous anion that is easily excreted. Sulfites can also bind to a variety of food components including reducing sugars, starch, proteins, aldehydes, ketones, and vitamins. The reactivity of sulfite-sensitive asthmatics to these bound forms of sulfite is unknown. The bound forms of sulfites predominate in most foods, and the values in Table VIII represent largely bound forms of sulfite. This lack of information on the sensitivity of sulfite-sensitive asthmatics to the forms of sulfite that predominate in foods adds more uncertainty to the general advice to

TABLE VIII

Estimated Total SO_2 Level as Consumed for Some Sulfited Foods[a,b]

Foods containing SO_2	Total SO_2 (ppm)
≥ 100 ppm	
Dried fruit (excluding dark raisins and prunes)	1200
Lemon juice (nonfrozen)	800
Salad bar lettuce	400–950
Lime juice (nonfrozen)	160
Wine	150
Molasses	125
Sauerkraut juice	100
50–99.9 ppm	
Dried potatoes	35–90
Grape juice (white, white sparkling, pink sparkling, red sparkling)	85
Wine vinegar	75
Gravies, sauces	75
Fruit topping	60
Maraschino cherries	50
10.1–49.9 ppm	
Pectin	≤ 10–50
Shrimp (fresh)	≤ 10–40
Corn syrup	30
Sauerkraut	30
Pickled peppers	30
Pickled cocktail onions	30
Pickles/relishes	30
Cornstarch	20
Hominy	20
Frozen potatoes	20
Maple syrup	20
Imported jams and jellies	14
Fresh mushrooms	13
≤ 10 ppm	
Malt vinegar	10
Dried cod	10
Canned potatoes	10
Beer	10
Dry soup mix	≤ 10
Soft drinks	≤ 10
Instant tea	≤ 10
Pizza dough (frozen)	≤ 10
Pie dough	≤ 10
Sugar (esp. beet sugar)	7
Gelatin	6.6
Coconut	5

TABLE VIII (*Continued*)

Foods containing SO_2	Total SO_2 (ppm)
Fresh fruit salad	5
Domestic jams and jellies	5
Crackers	5
Cookies	5
Grapes	1–5
High-fructose corn syrup	3

[a]From Life Science Research Office, (1985).

[b]Total SO_2 levels based on titratable acidity in Monier–Williams assay.

avoid sulfited foods. Controlled challenges with various sulfited foods will be needed to provide better advice on avoidance diets to sulfite-sensitive asthmatics. Only one controlled-challenge study has been reported with sulfited foods, and that study documented the reactivity of sulfite-sensitive asthmatics to sulfited lettuce (Howland and Simon, 1985). However, lettuce contains 400 ppm or more of total SO_2 and is an unusual food in that most of the sulfite remains in the product as free sulfite (Martin *et al.,* 1985).

III. SECONDARY FOOD SENSITIVITIES

Secondary food sensitivities develop after some predisposing condition such as a preexisting illness or drug therapy. A variety of gastrointestinal conditions can enhance the chances of developing food allergies, lactose intolerance, or celiac disease. These illnesses include Crohn's disease, ulcerative colitis, cystic fibrosis, or bacterial or viral gastroenteritis (Metcalfe, 1984b). These secondary conditions are usually temporary, although permanent sensitization can occur via this route. The topic of drug-induced food sensitivity has been thoroughly reviewed (Smith and Bidlack, 1982). Several examples include an increased sensitivity to tyramine and other monamines among patients on monoamine oxidase-inhibiting drugs (Blackwell and Marley, 1969) and the enhanced sensitivity to histamine among tuberculosis patients on isoniazid therapy (Senanayake and Vyravanathan, 1981).

REFERENCES

Aas, K. (1983). The critical approach to food allergy. *Ann. Allergy* **51,** 256–259.

Adolphson, C. R., Yunginger, J. W., and Gleich, G. J. (1980). Standardization of allergens. *In* "Manual of Clinical Immunology" (N. R. Rose and H. Friedman, eds.), 2nd ed., pp. 778–788. Am. Soc. Microbiol., Washington, D.C.

Anderson, J. B., and Lessof, M. H. (1983). Diagnosis and treatment of food allergies. *Proc. Nutr. Soc.* **42,** 257–262.

Ashkenazi, A., Levin, S., Idar, D., Or, A., Rosenberg, I., and Handzel, Z. T. (1980). *In vitro* cell-mediated immunologic assay for cow's milk allergy. *Pediatrics* **65,** 399–402.

Atkins, F. M. (1983). The basis of immediate hypersensitivity reactions to foods. *Nutr. Rev.* **41,** 229–234.

Bahna, S. L., and Gandhi, M. D. (1983). Milk hypersensitivity. II. Practical aspects of diagnosis, treatment, and prevention. *Ann. Allergy* **50,** 295–301.

Baker, G. J., Collett, P., and Allen, D. H. (1981). Bronchospasm induced by metabisulfite-containing foods and drugs. *Med. J. Aust.* **2,** 614–616.

Baker, P. G., and Read, A. E. (1976). Oats and barley toxicity in coeliac patients. *Postgrad. Med. J.* **52,** 264–268.

Barnett, D., Baldo, B. A., and Howden, M. E. (1983). Multiplicity of allergens in peanuts. *J. Allergy Clin. Immunol.* **72,** 61–68.

Beavan, M. A. (1978). Histamine: Its role in physiological and pathological processes. *Monogr. Allergy* **13,** 1–113.

Bernstein, M., Day, J. H., and Welsh, A. (1982). Double-blind food challenge in the diagnosis of food sensitivity in the adult. *J. Allergy Clin. Immunol.* **70,** 205–210.

Birge, S. T., Kentmann, H. T., Cuatrecasas, P., and Whedon, G. D. (1967). Osteoporosis, intestinal lactase deficiency and low dietary calcium intake. *N. Engl. J. Med.* **276,** 445–448.

Bjeldanes, L. F., Schultz, D. E., and Morris, M. M. (1978). On the aetiology of scombroid poisoning: Cadaverine potentiation of histamine toxicity in the guinea pig. *Food Cosmet. Toxicol.* **16,** 157–159.

Blackwell, B., and Marley, E. (1969). Monoamine oxidase inhibition and intolerance to foodstuffs. *Bibl. Nutr. Diet.* **11,** 96–110.

Bleumink, E., and Young, E. (1968). Identification of the atopic allergen in cow's milk. *Int. Arch. Allergy Appl. Immunol.* **34,** 521–543.

Bock, S. A. (1982). The natural history of food sensitivity. *J. Allergy Clin. Immunol.* **69,** 173–177.

Bock, S. A. (1985). Adverse reactions to foods during the first three years of life. *J. Allergy Clin. Immunol.* **75,** 178.

Bock, S. A., and Martin, M. (1983). The incidence of adverse reactions to foods—a continuing study. *J. Allergy Clin. Immunol.* **71,** 98.

Bock, S. A., Lee, W. Y., Remigio, L., and May, C. D. (1978). Studies of hypersensitivity reactions to foods in infants and children. *J. Allergy Clin. Immunol.* **62,** 327–334.

Bock, S. A., Remigio, L. K., and Gordon, B. (1983). Immunochemical localization of proteins in the intestinal mucosa of children with diarrhea. *J. Allergy Clin. Immunol.* **72,** 262–268.

Buckley, C. E., III, Saltzman, H. A., and Sieker, H. O. (1985). The prevalence and degree of sensitivity to ingested sulfites. *J. Allergy Clin. Immunol.* **75,** 144.

Burr, M. L. (1983). Does infant feeding affect the risk of allergy? *Arch. Dis. Child.* **58,** 561–565.

Bush, R. K., Taylor, S. L., Nordlee, J. A., and Busse, W. W. (1985). Soybean oil is not allergenic to soybean-sensitive individuals. *J. Allergy Clin. Immunol.* **76,** 242–245.

Bush, R. K., Taylor, S. L., and Busse, W. W. (1986). A critical evaluation of clinical trials in reactions to sulfites. *J. Allergy Clin. Immunol.* **78,** 191–202.

Businco, L., Cantani, A., Benincori, N., Perlini, R., Infussi, R., De Angelis, M., and Businco, E. (1983). Effectiveness of oral sodium cromoglycate (SCG) in preventing food allergy in children. *Ann. Allergy* **51,** 47–49.

Ciclitira, P. J., Ellis, H. J., Evans, D. J., and Lennox, E. S. (1985). A radioimmunoassay for wheat gliadin to assess the suitability of gluten free foods for patients with coeliac disease. *Clin. Exp. Immunol.* **59,** 703–708.

Cunningham-Rundles, C., Brandeis, W. E., and Good, R. H. (1979). Bovine antigens and the formation of circulating immune complexes in selective immunoglobulin A deficiency. *J. Clin. Invest.* **64,** 272–279.

Dannaeus, A., and Inganas, M. (1981). A follow-up study of children with food allergy. Clinical course in relation to serum IgE- and IgG-antibody levels to milk, fish, and eggs. *Clin. Allergy* **11,** 533–539.

Delohery, J., Simmul, R., Castle, W. D., and Allen, D. (1984). The relationship of inhaled sulfur dioxide reactivity to ingested metabisulfite sensitivity in patients with asthma. *Am. Rev. Respir. Dis.* **130,** 1027–1032.

Dockhorn, R. J., and Smith, T. C. (1981). Use of a chemically defined hypoallergenic diet (Vivonex) in the management of patients with suspected food allergy/intolerance. *Ann. Allergy* **47,** 264–266.

Elsayed, S., and Bennich, H. (1975). The primary structure of allergen M from cod. *Scand. J. Immunol.* **4,** 203–208.

Fallstrom, S. P., Lindholm, L., and Ahlstedt, S. (1983). Cow's milk protein intolerance in children is connected with impaired lymphoblastic responses to mitogens. *Int. Arch. Allergy Appl. Immunol.* **70,** 205–206.

Ford, R. P. K., and Taylor, B. (1982). Natural history of egg hypersensitivity. *Arch. Dis. Child.* **57,** 649–652.

Gallagher, C. R., Molleson, A. L., and Caldwell, J. H. (1977). Lactose intolerance and fermented dairy products. *Cult. Dairy Prod. J.* **10**(1), 22, 24.

Gallant, S. P. (1978). Food sensitivity in infants. *Comp. Ther.* **4,** 57–60.

Gallant, S. P., Franz, M. L., Walker, P., Wells, I. D., and Lundak, R. L. (1977). A potential diagnostic method for food allergy: Clinical application and immunogenicity evaluation of an elemental diet. *Am. J. Clin. Nutr.* **30,** 512–516.

Gell, P. G. H., Coombs, R. R. A., and Lachmann, D. J. (1975). "Clinical Aspects of Immunology," 3rd ed., Lippincott, Philadelphia, Pennsylvania.

Gerrard, J. W., and Shenassa, M. (1983). Sensitization to substances in breast milk: Recognition, management, and significance. *Ann. Allergy* **61,** 300–302.

Gibney, M. J. (1983). Food allergy—fact of fiction? *Proc. Nutr. Soc.* **42,** 213–218.

Golbert, T. M. (1972). Food allergy and immunologic diseases of the gastrointestinal tract. *In* "Allergic Diseases: Diagnosis and Management" (R. Patterson, ed.), pp. 355–379. Lippincott, Philadelphia, Pennsylvania.

Goldman, A. S., Anderson, D. W., Sellars, W. A., Saperstein, S., Kniker, W. T., and Halpern, S. R. (1963a). Milk allergy. I. Oral challenge with milk and isolated milk proteins in allergic children. *Pediatrics* **32,** 425–443.

Goldman, A. S., Sellars, W. A., Halpern, S. R., Anderson, D. W., Furlow, T. E., and Johnson, C. H. (1963b). Milk allergy. II. Skin testing of allergic and normal children with purified milk proteins. *Pediatrics* **32,** 572–579.

Gray, G. E., and Gray, L. K. (1983). Diet and juvenile delinquency. *Nutr. Today* **18**(3), 14–22.

Hamburger, R. N., Heller, S., Mellon, M. H., O'Connor, R. D., and Zeiger, R. S. (1983). Current status of the clinical and immunological consequences of a prototype allergic disease prevention program. *Ann. Allergy* **51,** 281–290.

Harley, J. P., Ray, R. S., Tomasi, L., Eichman, P. L., Matthews, C. G., Chun, R., Cleeland, C. S., and Traisman, E. (1978a). Hyperkinesis and food additives: Testing the Feingold hypothesis. *Pediatrics* **61,** 818–828.

Harley, J. P., Matthews, C. G., and Eichman, P. (1978b). Synthetic food colors and hyperactivity in children: A double-blind challenge experiment. *Pediatrics* **62,** 975–983.

Harper, A. E., and Gans, D. A. (1986). Diet and behavior—an assessment of reports of aggressive, antisocial behavior from consumption of sugar. *Food Technol.* **40**(I), 142–149.

Harris, P. G. (1982). Perceived incidence of milk allergy and/or lactose intolerance in Great Britain. *J. Soc. Dairy Technol.* **35,** 104–108.

Hartsook, E. I. (1984). Celiac sprue: Sensitivity to gliadin. *Cereal Foods World* **29,** 157–158.

Hoffman, D. R. (1983). Immunochemical identification of the allergens in egg white. *J. Allergy Clin. Immunol.* **71,** 481–486.

Howland, W. C., and Simon, R. A. (1985). Restaurant-provoked asthma: Sulfite sensitivity. *J. Allergy Clin. Immunol.* **75,** 143.

Hui, J. Y., and Taylor, S. L. (1985). Inhibition of *in vivo* histamine metabolism in rats by foodborne and pharmacologic inhibitors of diamine oxidase, histamine *N*-methyltransferase, and monoamine oxidase. *Toxicol. Appl. Pharmacol.* **81,** 241–249.

Institute of Food Technologists' Expert Panel on Food Safety and Nutrition (1985). Food allergies and sensitivities. *Food Technol.* **39**(9), 65–71.

Jacobsen, D. W., Simon, R. A., and Singh, M. (1984). Sulfite oxidase deficiency and cobalamin protection in sulfite-sensitive asthmatics (SSA). *J. Allergy Clin. Immunol.* **73,** 135.

Johnstone, D. E. (1978). Diagnostic methods in food allergy in children. *Ann. Allergy* **40,** 110–113.

Kasarda, D. D. (1978). The relationship of wheat protein to celiac disease. *Cereal Foods World* **23,** 240–244, 262.

Kasarda, D. D. (1981). Toxic proteins and peptides in celiac disease: Relations to cereal genetics. *In* "Food, Nutrition, and Evolution: Food as an Environmental Factor in the Genesis of Human Variability" (D. Walcher and N. Kretchmer, eds.), pp. 201–216. Masson Publ., New York.

Langeland, T. (1982). A clinical and immunological study of allergy to hen's egg white. III. Allergens in hen's egg white studied by crossed radio-immunoelectrophoresis (CRIE). *Allergy* **37,** 521–530.

Life Sciences Research Office (1985). "The Re-examination of the GRAS Status of Sulfiting Agents." Fed. Am. Soc. Exp. Biol., Bethesda, Maryland.

Lisker, R., and Aguilas, L. (1978). Double blind study of milk lactose intolerance. *Gastroenterology* **74,** 1283–1285.

Lyons, D. E., Beery, J. T., Lyons, S. A., and Taylor, S. L. (1983). Cadaverine and aminoguanidine potentiate the uptake of histamine *in vitro* in perfused intestinal segments of rats. *Toxicol. Appl. Pharmacol.* **70,** 445–458.

Mager, J., Chevion, M., and Glaser, G. (1980). Favism. *In* "Toxic Constituents of Plant Foodstuffs" (I. E. Liener, ed.), 2nd ed., pp. 265–294. Academic Press, New York.

Martin, L. B., Nordlee, J. A., and Taylor, S. L. (1986). Sulfite residues in restaurant salads. *J. Food Prot.* **49,** 126–129.

Maslinski, C. (1975). Histamine and its metabolism in mammals. Part II. Catabolism of histamine and histamine liberation. *Agents Actions* **5,** 183–225.

May, C. D. (1983). Immunologic versus toxic adverse reactions to foodstuffs. *Ann. Allergy* **51,** 267–268.

May, C. D., and Bock, S. A. (1978). A modern clinical approach to food hypersensitivity. *Allergy* **33,** 166–188.

Metcalfe, D. D. (1984a). Diagnostic procedures for immunologically-mediated food sensitivity. *Nutr. Rev.* **42,** 92–97.

Metcalfe, D. D. (1984b). Food hypersensitivity. *J. Allergy Clin. Immunol.* **63,** 749–762.

Metcalfe, D. D. (1985). Food allergens. *Clin. Rev. Allergy* **3,** 331–349.

Minford, A. M. B., MacDonald, A., and Littlewood, J. M. (1982). Food intolerance and food allergy in children: A review of 68 cases. *Arch. Dis. Child.* **57,** 742–747.

Minor, J. D., Tolber, S. G., and Frick, O. L. (1980). Leukocyte inhibition factor in delayed-onset food allergy. *J. Allergy Clin. Immunol.* **66,** 314–321.

Nordlee, J. A., Taylor, S. L., Jones, R. T., and Yunginger, J. W. (1981). Allergenicity of various peanut products as determined by RAST inhibition. *J. Allergy Clin. Immunol.* **68,** 376–382.

Paganelli, R., Levinsky, R. J., Brostoff, J., and Wraith, D. G. (1979). Immune complexes containing food proteins in normal and atopic subjects after oral challenge and effect of sodium cromoglycate on antigen absorption. *Lancet* **1,** 1270–1272.

Parrot, J.-L., and Nicot, G. (1966). Pharmacology of histamine. Absorption de l'histamine par l'appareil digestif. *Handb. Exp. Pharmakol.* [N. S.] **18,** Part 1, 148–161.

Phillips, A. D., Rice, S. J., France, N. E., and Walker-Smith, J. A. (1979). Small intestinal intraepithelial lymphocyte levels in cow's milk protein intolerance. *Gut* **20,** 509–512.

Reddy, V., and Pershad, J. (1972). Lactose deficiency in Indians. *Am. J. Clin. Nutr.* **25,** 114–119.

Sampson, H. A. (1983). Role of immediate food hypersensitivity in the pathogenesis of atopic dermatitis. *J. Allergy Clin. Immunol.* **71,** 473–480.

Sandine, W. E., and Daly, M. (1979). Milk intolerance. *J. Food Prot.* **42,** 435–437.

Senanayake, N., and Vyranvanathan, S. (1981). Histamine reactions due to ingestion of tuna fish (*Thunnus argentivittatus*) in patients on anti-tuberculosis therapy. *Toxicon* **19,** 184–185.

Shiner, M., Ballard, J., and Smith, M. E. (1975). The small intestinal mucosa in cow's milk allergy. *Lancet* **1,** 136–140.

Simon, R. A., Green, L., and Stevenson, D. D. (1982). The incidence of ingested metabisulfite sensitivity in an asthmatic population. *J. Allergy Clin. Immunol.* **69,** 118.

Simpson, S. I., Somerfield, S. D., Wilson, J. D., and Hillas, J. L. (1980). A double-blind study for the diagnosis of cow's milk allergy. *N. Z. Med. J.* **92,** 457–459.

Siraganian, R. P. (1976). Histamine release and assay methods for the study of human allergy. *In* "Manual of Clinical Immunology" (N. R. Rose and H. Friedman, eds.), pp. 603–615. Am. Soc. Microbiol., Washington, D.C.

Smith, C. H., and Bidlack, W. R. (1982). Food and drug interactions. *Food Technol.* **36**(10), 99–103.

Soothill, J. F. (1983). Prevention of atopic allergic disease. *Ann. Allergy* **51,** 229–232.

Stare, F. J., Whelan, E. M., and Sheridan, M. (1980). Diet and hyperactivity: Is there a relationship? *Pediatrics* **66,** 521–525.

Stern, M., and Walker, W. A. (1985). Food allergy and intolerance. *Pediatr. Clin. North Am.* **32,** 471–492.

Stern, M., Dietrich, R., and Muller, J. (1982). Small intestinal mucosa in coeliac disease and cow's milk protein intolerance: Morphometric and immunofluorescent studies. *Eur. J. Pediatr.* **139,** 101–105.

Stevenson, D. D., and Simon, R. A. (1981). Sensitivity to ingested metabisulfites in asthmatic subjects. *J. Allergy Clin. Immunol.* **68,** 26–32.

Sumner, S. S., Speckhard, M. W., Somers, E. B., and Taylor, S. L. (1985). Isolation of histamine-producing *Lactobacillus buchneri* from Swiss cheese implicated in a food poisoning outbreak. *Appl. Environ. Microbiol.* **50,** 1094–1096.

Tattrie, N. H., and Yaguchi, M. (1973). Protein content of various processed edible oils. *Can. Inst. Food Sci. Technol. J.* **6,** 289–290.

Taylor, S. L. (1980). Food allergy—the enigma and some potential solutions. *J. Food Prot.* **43,** 300–306.

Taylor, S. L. (1985a). Food allergies. *Food Technol.* **39**(2), 98–105.

Taylor, S. L. (1985b). "Histamine Poisoning Associated with Fish, Cheese, and Other Foods," Monograph. World Health Organ., Geneva, Switzerland.

Taylor, S. L., and Lieber, E. R. (1979). *In vitro* inhibition of rat intestinal histamine-metabolizing enzymes. *Food Cosmet. Toxicol.* **17,** 237–240.

Taylor, S. L., Guthertz, L. S., Leatherwood, M., Tillman, F., and Lieber, E. R. (1978). Histamine production by food-borne bacterial species. *J. Food Saf.* **1,** 173–187.

Taylor, S. L., Busse, W. W., Sachs, M. I., Parker, J. L., and Yuninger, J. W. (1981). Peanut oil is not allergenic to peanut-sensitive individuals. *J. Allergy Clin. Immunol.* **68,** 372–375.

Taylor, S. L., Keefe, T. J., Windham, E. S., and Howell, J. F. (1982). Outbreak of histamine poisoning associated with consumption of Swiss cheese. *J. Food Prot.* **45,** 455–457.

Taylor, S. L., Hui, J. Y., and Lyons, D. E. (1984). Toxicology of scombroid poisoning. *In* "Seafood Toxins" (E. P. Ragelis, ed.), pp. 417–430. Am. Chem. Soc., Washington, D.C.

Van Asperen, P. P., Kemp, A. S., and Mellis, C. M. (1983). Immediate food hypersensitivity reactions on the first known exposure to the food. *Arch. Dis. Child.* **58,** 253–256.

Van de Kamer, J. H., Weijers, H. A., and Dicke, W. K. (1953). Coeliac disease. IV. An investigation into the injurious constituents of wheat in connection with their action on patients with coeliac disease. *Acta Paediatr.* **42,** 223–231.

Warner, J. O. (1980). Food allergy in fully breast-fed infants. *Clin. Allergy* **10,** 133–136.

Wasserman, S. I. (1983). Mediators of immediate hypersensitivity. *J. Allergy Clin. Immunol.* **72,** 101–115.

Welsh, J. D. (1978). Diet therapy in adult lactose malabsorption: Present practices. *Am. J. Clin. Nutr.* **31,** 592–596.

8

Dietary Caffeine and Its Toxicity

Jack Bergman and P. B. Dews

I. INTRODUCTION

Caffeine is part of the diet of most people. It is generally accepted that caffeine helps people work and enjoy their days a little better, but that has not been established by rigorous, objective, and quantitative studies. There is much more substantial evidence that dietary consumption is harmless in normal people. There has continued to be a perhaps never-ending series of suggestions of adverse effects which, so far, on further investigation have been shown to be ill-founded. Use of the term toxicity for the effects reported or suggested for

199

NUTRITIONAL TOXICOLOGY, VOL. II

Copyright © 1987 by Academic Press, Inc.
All rights of reproduction in any form reserved.

caffeine as a component of the diet, the main concern of this review, may therefore be misleading. What is toxic and what is not, what is sought after and what is unwanted side effect, depends on circumstances. A reduction in sleepiness (with consequent improved performance and efficiency) with caffeine may be a desired effect by a worker in the middle of the day, but a "toxic" effect to an agitated imsomniac in the middle of the night. Frank toxicity can arise with therapeutic, recreational, or abusive use of caffeine as a drug taken as a pill or a solution of caffeine. Such intakes are not a matter of "nutrition," and so their effects will be discussed only insofar as they provide useful information and perspective on the safety margins of dietary caffeine. Further, the recent fascinating studies relating antagonism of effects of endogenous adenosine to actions of caffeine have so far not revealed previously unrecognized toxic effects of caffeine, and they will not be reviewed.

Caffeine has been used as a tool in studies on mutagenesis and on DNA repair mechanisms, because in millimolar concentrations it produces interesting effects on those processes (Roberts, 1984). Extremely large doses of caffeine weakly induce increased levels of mixed-function oxidase (Mitoma *et al.*, 1969). Such studies will not be discussed here because the levels of caffeine from dietary consumption by people are some two orders of magnitude less than those necessary to cause the effects. The distribution of plasma caffeine levels of 300 men and 300 women coming from the street into a hospital outpatient department is shown in Fig. 1 (Smith *et al.*, 1982). Only one subject had a level as high as 10

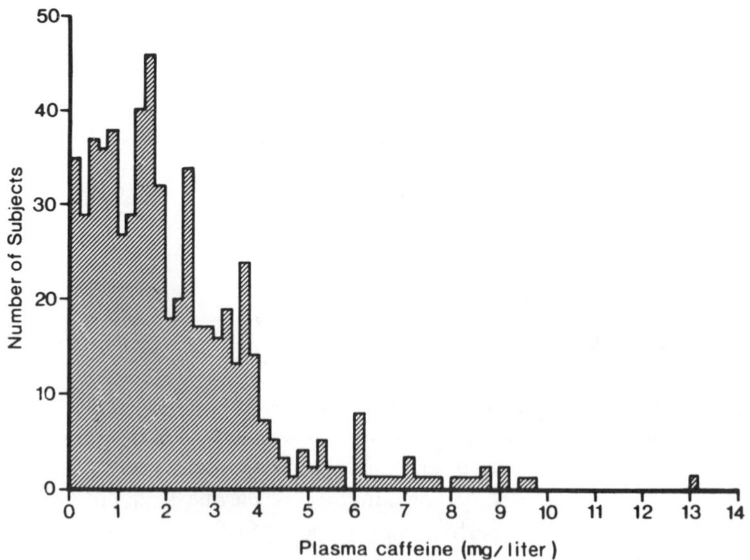

Fig. 1. Plasma caffeine concentrations.

mg/liter and 97% had levels below 6.5 mg/liter. Levels above 10 mg/liter may therefore be regarded as outside the range for normal consumption.

II. ACUTE TOXICITY

It appears that nobody has ever died, or even had life endangered, by the direct toxicity of caffeine ingested in dietary form. Less than a dozen human deaths have been reported as attributable to caffeine, all following intake of caffeine in drug rather than food form. Most of the victims were found dead, and the mechanism of death was not elucidated (Turner and Cravey, 1977). It is noteworthy that the reports describe no external evidence of convulsions such as bruises and contusions. One young woman was found alive and described as semicomatose (McGee, 1980). She died subsequently in a hospital with ventricular fibrillation that resisted repeated attempts at reversion. Her blood caffeine level after death was 181 mg/liter. A 42-year-old suicide victim had a blood caffeine level of 114 mg/liter (Bryant, 1981). She had died with ''no evidence of a struggle.'' The blood caffeine levels, when they were measured, of most of the people who succumbed were in excess of 100 mg/liter and at least one was over 1000 mg/liter. A 2-year-old boy survived a concentration of 190 mg/liter (Banner and Czajka, 1980). Premature newborns treated with caffeine for episodic apnea have had plasma caffeine levels of up to 80 mg/liter with few or no symptoms attributable to the caffeine and no recognizable deleterious aftermath (Aranda *et al.*, 1979). While opisthotonus is mentioned, full convulsions were not seen in human subjects.

The lack of convulsions may be surprising in view of the universal description of caffeine as a ''stimulant,'' indeed often as a ''potent stimulant'' of the central nervous system (CNS) (Goodman and Gilman, 1975). Yet convulsions are by no means a universal finding in all species and strains of laboratory animals at high and even with lethal doses of caffeine. ''True caffeine convulsions'' were described in anesthetized cats by Sollman and Pilcher (1911), but they seem to have been capricious and the authors raise the possibility they were secondary to some other effect. Convulsions in albino mice were described by Scott and Chen (1944), with CD_{50} of 84 mg/kg and by Vellucci and Webster (1984) in C3H mice. In that study 200 mg/kg produced no convulsions, 250 mg/kg produced 75% convulsions, and 300 mg/kg produced 100% convulsions; such dose levels produce substantial mortality. Similar results in C3H mice are reported by Marangos *et al.* (1981). Salant and Rieger (1909–1910) described ''symptoms'' in dogs, cats, and guinea pigs but convulsions only in rabbits. Although there appear to be strain differences, most workers have been impressed by the immobility of rodents given large doses of caffeine. Depending on strain, caffeine may cause increases in locomotor activity in mice at doses up to the range of 30 mg/kg. Above about that level, there is a progressive reduction of locomotor activity with increasing dose; activity was down to 20% of normal at 125 mg/kg in four of seven strains studied by Seale *et al.* (1984). Only two of the strains showed any convulsions at doses below 200 mg/kg. Mice are, of course, much more prone to convulsions then humans. Thus, over much the greatest part of the dose–effect curve, the effects of caffeine cannot be described as "stimulant." Boyd (1959) describes "schizophrenic withdrawal" and "little inclination to walk"; Maloney (1935) writes that "caffeine in lethal doses (in rats) does not cause death by convulsion but depression"; Campbell and Richter (1967) confess that they could not diagnose caffeinelike activity in their mouse screen because it caused no particular signs. Charles River CD1 mice do not convulse with caffeine, and only an occasional mouse shows evidence of tonic extension (personal observation). Marangos *et al.* (1981) noted that 50 mg/kg caffeine increased the proportion of mice convulsing after 80 mg/kg pentylenetertrazol from about 15% to 85%. It is clear that caffeine differs radically from metrazol, local anesthetics, antihistamines (such as in the over-the-counter sleeping pills), and even amphetamines that alone produce convulsions much more consistently. Caffeine certainly can produce modest increases in motor activity and in sleeplessness (Dews, 1982), but these are not effects that the term *potent CNS stimulant* leads one to expect. In fact, to be told that an agent is a CNS stimulant enables one to predict almost nothing of what to expect, so the term is useless. It appears that death from caffeine in humans is more likely to be due to cardiovascular than to CNS effects.

The lethal doses for mouse, rat, guinea pig, rabbit, cat, and dog are tabulated by Barnes and Eltherington (1973). The LD_{50}s range from about 100 mg/kg iv in mouse and rabbit to between 200 and 300 mg/kg by other routes in the species reported. Three points are noteworthy. First, there is unusually little influence of route of administration on toxicity, the LD_{50}s for oral administration being similar to those for sc, im, and ip dosing. The reason undoubtedly is the great ease of diffusion of caffeine from the gastrointestinal tract and then throughout body water which results from the solubility of caffeine in both water and lipids. Second, as caffeine diffuses freely throughout body water without selective concentration in any organ, and as body water is a more or less fixed fraction of body weight from species to species, the dose of caffeine for a given concentration in body water will be proportional to body weight. Hence, in contrast to the two-thirds power of body weight relation that is a better predictor of interspecies equivalence for most drugs than simply milligrams per kilogram (Dews, 1972), dosage for similar effects of caffeine tends to be similar in milligrams per kilogram even across species that differ as greatly in weight as mice and humans. Third, the mechanism of lethality seems to be similar in commonly studied species and, as in humans, is probably cardiovascular. As with amphetamines, the lethality of caffeine in mice can depend on conditions of housing. The LD_{50} in grouped mice has been reported to be half of that in solitary mice (Greenblatt and Osterberg, 1961).

III. CHRONIC TOXICITY

Effects of chronic intake of caffeine are unremarkable; that is, there are no selective toxic effects on specific organs. In the rodent, the kinetics of caffeine ($t_{1/2}$ ~3 hr) ensure that caffeine taken in food or drink does not accumulate and, indeed, that body burden falls to very low levels by the beginning of the feeding and drinking part of the diurnal cycle. Dosages of up to 100 mg/kg/day in the drinking water of rats for 2 years had no discernible effect on cumulative mortality, and even a reduction of weight gain required some 50 mg/kg/day (Mohr *et al.*, 1984). An intake of 50 mg/kg/day required a concentration in drinking water of 0.43 mg/ml, which is as high as in strong coffee and may be unpalatable to rodents.

Plasma levels of caffeine in CD1 mice at the end of 2 weeks of administration of 125 mg/kg/day in the drinking water are reported by Aeschbacher *et al.* (1978). Surprisingly, most showed less than 0.1 mg/liter most of the day, and the mean concentration at the time of day of highest levels was less than 2 mg/ml. Such low levels have serious implications for the interpretation of chronic toxicity studies of caffeine in rodents. Intakes even as high as 100 mg/kg/day cannot be assumed to produce substantial body levels of caffeine, not even as high as levels to which people are routinely exposed. The interpretation of chronic studies in which tissue levels were not measured must therefore be reappraised.

IV. ANATOMICAL EFFECTS

A. Teratogenesis

Administration of amounts of 100 mg–kg/day or more of caffeine to pregnant mice or rats results in an increase in the frequency of malformations in the offspring. Several independent investigators have obtained similar findings, putting them beyond dispute (Wilson and Scott, 1984). The commonest malformations are cleft palate and missing digits, which can result from nonspecific causes in rodents, such as weight loss in pregnant dams following interference with general nutrition. With doses below about 50 mg/kg/day, increase in malformations is no longer detectable. In seeking to interpret the findings for implications for human health, several factors must be considered. First, with certain salient exceptions (such as thalidomide) of which caffeine is certainly not one, rodents are generally much more suscpetible to teratogenic influences than are primates (Wilson and Scott, 1984). The great majority of agents that have been shown to be teratogenic in rodents are not found to have such effects in humans. Second, 50 mg/kg represents 3.5 gm in a 70-kg person, far more than can be achieved by sane dietary intake. Third, teratogenic effects at dosages below about 100 mg/

POLYTECHNIC OF NORTH LONDON
LIBRARY & INFORMATION SERVICE

kg/day are seen only when the total dose is given by injection or gavage (Collins *et al.*, 1981; Wilson and Scott, 1984), greatly accentuating peak concentrations. Properly conducted studies in humans have shown that sane caffeine consumption does not increase malformations (Heinonen *et al.*, 1977; van den Berg, 1977).

B. Delay of Ossification

At much lower intakes of caffeine by pregnant rodents, doses as low as 12.5 mg/kg/day [but not as low as 10 mg/kg every other day (Batirbaygil *et al.*, 1985)], there is a phenomenon in the fetuses that is called delayed ossification. Typically, pregnant rats are treated with caffeine and then are killed about day 21 of pregnancy. The fetuses are examined after soft tissue clearing and staining with alizarin. Some degree of slowing of bone maturation, particularly of sternebrae, relative to controls is seen in some pups of caffeine-treated dams in most of the studies (Wilson and Scott, 1984). The significance of the implications for human health has been questioned on the following grounds. First, around day 21, at the very end of pregnancy, changes in ossification are taking place rapidly, so that a slowing of bone maturation *in utero* of only a few hours could produce detectable effects. Second, any delay in maturation appears to disappear rapidly postnatally if the pups are allowed to live. Third, attempts to detect consequences of caffeine consumption on human pregnancy outcome have found no effects, even in very large series (Ernster, 1984). The conclusion seems to be that the delayed ossification in rodents should not be taken to have implications for human health requiring, for example, that attempts be made to persuade pregnant women to reduce their caffeine consumption below prevailing normal levels. But the phenomenon remains interesting scientifically, both for understanding implications of findings in rodents to humans and for learning more about ossification, so the mechanisms of the delayed ossification in rodents deserve to be studied. Is the delayed ossification a manifestation of a general slight slowing of maturation that happens to be easily observed in the skeleton? Or do toxic levels of caffeine have a selective effect on calcium metabolism? If the latter, further study conceivably could yield clues to mechanisms of decalcification, for example, in old people. An extensive literature does exist regarding the effects of high concentrations of caffeine on calcium of tissues *in vitro*. For example, caffeine is known to liberate calcium from the isolated endoplasmic reticulum (Weber and Herz, 1968) and from cardiac muscle (Konishi *et al.*, 1984). Interesting as these phenomena are for understanding fundamental physiology, however, the fact that they require millimolar concentrations makes their relevance to the subject of dietary intakes of caffeine questionable.

C. Fibrocystic Disease of the Breast (FDB)

An entirely different sort of anatomical effect that has been reported to be related to caffeine consumption is fibrocystic disease of the breast. FDB is a very common disorder. The pathological changes underlying the disorder were found in 58.5% of 725 women dying by misadventure (Davis *et al.*, 1964). Only a small proportion of women complain of symptoms. In women with symptoms the severity typically fluctuates greatly with time (Heyden and Muhlbaier, 1984). Assessment of treatment efficacy in disorders with statistically significant variations in time in the absence of deliberate therapeutic intervention is notoriously difficult. With disorders with fluctuating severity of symptoms, patients are more likely to seek help in the phase when the symptoms are more severe than less severe. There is therefore a biased intake into studies by self-selection and a good likelihood that there may be statistically significant regression of symptoms from their severity at intake even in the absence of intervention. Nonetheless, abstention from methylxanthines has been reported to ameliorate the symptoms of FDB (Minton *et al.*, 1979a,b). Criteria were subjective and poorly specified, subjects and "controls" (the patients who failed to comply with instructions) were self-selected, numbers were few, time was too short for the natural history of the disorder to compensate for nonrandom intake, and the effects of abstention were almost too dramatic to be credible. The conclusions, therefore, were not justified. That a study is scientifically unacceptable does not mean, however, that the conclusions are necessarily wrong, but merely that they should not be accepted until confirmed. Subsequent studies reviewed by Ernster (1984) have not confirmed the dramatic effect of abstention from ingestion of methylxanthines on FDB, although a slight effect has not been excluded (Ernster *et al.*, 1982). However, a recently published paper on risk factors for FDB does not rate caffeine worthy even of mention (Berkowitz *et al.*, 1985). Furthermore, even had benefit been derived from methylxanthine abstention in FDB, an etiological role for methylxanthines in FDB would not have been established. It appears that the report of substantial effects of caffeine on FDB is another example of an alleged bad effect of caffeine that more careful examination did not confirm.

D. Heart Size

Daily administration of 10 mg/kg/day caffeine to lactating rat dams and, subsequently, through day 88 in the food to their pups has been reported to increase heart weight of the pups (Temples *et al.*, 1985). There were concomitant decreases in stroke volume, cardiac output, and myocardial work measured at various atrial pressures in the isolated hearts of the pups. The authors speculated that the increased heart weight might be attributable to volume and/or pressure-overload hypertrophy, increased release of catecholamines, increased renin activity, or increased growth hormone levels. In contrast, Palm *et al.* (1984) found no difference from control values in the heart weights of rats exposed for as long as 2 years to concentrations of up to 100% coffee as drinking water. The daily caffeine intake was as high as approximately 100 mg/kg/day in female offspring after weaning. The finding of hypertrophy with doses almost an order of magnitude less by Temples *et al.* (1985) remains to be confirmed.

V. CARDIOVASCULAR EFFECTS

As mentioned, millimolar concentrations of caffeine have profound effects on cardiac muscle *in vitro* (Konishi *et al.*, 1984). Lethal doses of caffeine probably kill by cardiac effects in most strains of most species. The cardiovascular effects of levels of caffeine in the diet, however, are slight.

A. Conduction

In people, Prineas *et al.* (1980) found a positive correlation between levels of coffee or tea drinking and the incidence of ventricular extrasystole in a sample of over 700 middle-aged men. In subjects with history of cardiac arrhythmia, premature beats occurred twice as often when more than nine cups of coffee per day were consumed as when consumption averaged two cups or less per day. Attempts to substantiate these findings in other epidemiological and experimental investigations have resulted in mixed findings. In a well-conceived clinical study by Sutherland *et al.* (1985), periodic administration of 1 mg/kg caffeine was used to achieve steady-state levels of 2–3 mg/liter caffeine in plasma over a 24-hr period in subjects who were clinically normal and in subjects with frequent ventricular ectopy but, generally, without cardiac disease. An increased frequency of arrhythmia was found in subjects with preexisting ectopy but not in the clinically normal subjects. No effects were detected on prevailing cardiac rhythm, on rate, or on the rate of ventricular repolarization. Although clinical significance of the ventricular arrhythmias produced by caffeine in subjects with underlying cardiovascular disease is uncertain at this time, the association of these effects of caffeine with pathophysiological findings has been noted elsewhere. Dobmeyer *et al.* (1983) found that four of five patients who presented a history of dysrhythmia associated with caffeine consumption also suffered mitral valve-prolapse syndrome. These authors found, additionally, that iv administration of 200 mg caffeine was associated with supraventricular, but not ventricular, tachycardia in both patients and controls. Dobmeyer *et al.* (1983) speculate that the relationship between caffeine consumption and the production of dysrhythmia may be mediated by increased levels of catecholamines or, perhaps, by increased levels of intracellular cAMP consequent to stimulation of adenyl cyclase or to phosphodiesterase inhibition. Earlier studies by Gould *et al.* (1973) and DeBacker *et al.* (1979) on subjects with ventricular dysrhythmia did not find a decrease in incidence when caffeine consumption was decreased.

In sufficient concentrations, caffeine has interesting effects on both myocardial and junctional tissues. It is a positively inotropic agent. Isolated cardiac papillae show clear effect at 2–10 m*M* caffeine (Blinks *et al.*, 1972). The effects of caffeine in canine cardiac Purkinje fibers *in vitro* (Paspa and Vassale, 1984) or in dog hearts subjected to myocardial ischemia (Paulus *et al.*, 1982) suggest that increases in intracellular free calcium or in the sensitivity of myofilaments to calcium following caffeine administration also may result in conduction disturbances (Clusin, 1985). Such concentrations are, of course, far beyond those that result from dietary intakes of caffeine by human subjects.

In conclusion, the potential production of ventricular arrhythmias by caffeine in subjects with cardiovascular disease seems established although the clinical significance is uncertain. No hazard from caffeine consumption in persons with arrhythmias has been established, and it has not been shown that reduction in caffeine consumption leads to reductions in arrhythmias. Nevertheless, in view of the demonstrated effects of high concentrations of caffeine, it seems reasonable at present to recommend to those particularly at risk for arrhythmias that they limit their caffeine consumption.

B. Coronary Heart Disease

A connection has been made in epidemiological studies between caffeine consumption, by way of coffee intake, and coronary heart disease (CHD) through the intermediary link of increased levels of cholesterol. Initial longitudinal studies of CHD and caffeine found that coffee consumption correlated positively with the incidence of ischemic heart disease (Paul *et al.*, 1963; Jick *et al.*, 1973). It is now recognized that smoking was the likely causative agent in those studies; the positive association with coffee arose because smokers drink more coffee. Similarly, in almost every subsequent study that originally reported a correlation between coffee and CHD, the effect has been attributed to smoking (Heyden *et al.*, 1978; Curatolo and Robertson, 1983). Any study on associations of CHD and caffeine consumption, therefore, must take into account the effects of smoking to be of any value. In a 4.5-year *prospective* mortality study, no effects of caffeine consumption measured by coffee-drinking habits on CHD (or on total) mortality were detected by Heyden *et al.* (1978). More recently, however, an investigation in Norway, known as the Tromso heart study, has revealed a correlation between coffee intake and levels of serum cholesterol which did not disappear when smoking and other known risk factors were taken into account (Thelle *et al.*, 1983). Subsequent studies (Klatsky *et al.*, 1985; Forde *et al.*, 1985; Williams *et al.*, 1985) have confirmed the relationship. It should be noted that the effect in the Tromso study was small; the total cholesterol was 5.56 or 6.23 mM and the HDL fraction was 1.39 or 1.44 mM in drinkers of less than one cup or in drinkers of more than nine cups, respectively. Further, the correlation between the consumption of coffee and serum lipid levels generally has not been reported to extend to the consumption of tea (Thelle *et al.*, 1983; Klatsky *et al.*, 1985), nor has the degree of change in serum lipids been found to relate to the dose of caffeine consumed (Shirlow and Mathers, 1984). Observations such as these suggest that caffeine itself may not be causally related to increased levels of serum lipids in the populations studied. Finally, although undoubtedly there is a statistical association between serum lipids and CHD, it is now known to be a complicated matter. A causal relation between total lipids and CHD has not been established and the effects of interventions causing lowering of total lipids are still controversial. Any link between caffeine and CHD is, at most, very weak.

Some studies in other species also have found high levels of caffeine consumption to increase serum levels of cholesterol. Wurzner *et al.* (1977) measured serum cholesterol levels in rats ingesting diets containing 6% coffee solids in food for 2 years, representing intakes of up to about 200 mg/kg of caffeine per day. At 12 months the total cholesterol was 5.9 m*M* for controls and 10.3 m*M* for the highest caffeine intake group for males and 3.3 and 5.1 m*M* for females (our calculation). However, rabbits on an atherogenic diet given daily injections of 12–16 mg/kg caffeine for nearly 3 months showed no increase in plasma cholesterol above the already very high levels (almost 40 m*M*; Heyden *et al.*, 1969). There also was no increase in atherosclerosis in the rabbits given caffeine. In 15 monkeys eating an atherogenic diet for 6 months, 50% coffee as drinking water which yielded about 15 mg/kg caffeine per day, led to no convincing increase in plasma cholesterol above the level of some 12 m*M* produced by the atherogenic diet alone (Callahan *et al.*, 1979). There also was no increase in aortic atheroma. Robertson *et al.* (1985) studied the effects of approximately 12 mg/kg/day caffeine for 2 weeks on serum lipids in miniature swine that were genetically selected for their brisk response to high-fat diets and concluded that neither serum cholesterol nor HDL levels were altered from control values.

In conclusion, substantial increase in plasma cholesterol has been seen only with doses of caffeine far larger than dietary intakes, and increase in atherosclerosis attributable to caffeine has not been found in any species, no matter what the dosage.

C. Hemodynamics

The administration of a bolus dose of 250 mg caffeine in solution to non-tolerant individuals who have fasted overnight triggered increases in renin activity and in blood levels of epinephrine and of norepinephrine, and produced modest increases in blood pressure, heart rate, and cardiac output (Robertson *et al.*, 1978). Plasma levels of caffeine varied from 4.2 to 26 mg/liter from individual to individual, considerably higher than levels commonly encountered with dietary intakes of caffeine. When 250 mg was given three times per day tolerance developed rapidly, so that by the third day all the above effects were no longer seen (Robertson *et al.*, 1981; Smith *et al.*, 1985). Interestingly, when administration of the 750 mg/day was discontinued after the fifth day, no withdrawal symptoms were reported. The hemodynamic effects of dietary caffeine in regular users thus would be expected to be vanishingly slight.

In intact unanesthetized monkeys even concentrations as high as 30 mg/liter maintained by constant infusion, had relatively slight cardiovascular effects

(Dews, 1984a), confirming a great deal of earlier work on anesthetized dogs, cats, and other species already well reviewed (Eichler, 1976).

VI. BEHAVIORAL EFFECTS

A. Effects on Performance and Self Ratings

Behavioral effects of dietary caffeine as ordinarily taken are slight and unobtrusive, though unequivocally measurable under appropriate conditions. Most of the effects, such as reduction in sleepiness or slight enhancement of performance and efficiency, are sought and are not adverse. Goldstein, *et al.* (1965) found that administration in the morning of 150 or 300 mg caffeine produced reports of "nervousness" in nonusers but alleviated similar reports after placebo in individuals who normally consumed caffeine. Alleviation of the modest withdrawal effects were the most noteworthy consequences of caffeine administration among habitual users in that study. The point to be emphasized here is that the effects of caffeine on performance and on ratings depend largely on the condition of the subject being studied: a dose of caffeine that slightly disrupts behavior in the abstainer may be restorative in the habitual user. Furthermore, it should not be surprising that when abstention from caffeine leads to decrements in performance, simple recovery of normal levels of performance may be viewed as an enhancement.

In addition to the condition of the subject, the nature of the task being performed may influence the direction of the effects of caffeine on the performance. Battig *et al.* (1984) reported that 300 mg caffeine decreased variability of performance by human subjects in successive 20-sec periods of a letter cancellation task during the 30-min duration of the test, but did not improve performance on the task itself or in tasks that required the subject to determine what succession of key presses on a response panel had been programmed as correct. Also, Broverman and Casagrande (1982) found that approximately 110 mg caffeine could retard completion of an embedded-figures task by male undergraduates when it was first presented (by some 25%) but facilitated performance when the task had been learned previously (by some 30%). These are surprisingly large changes and illustrate how effects of caffeine may be influenced by test condition. The findings may not be replicable under a variety of conditions, however, and their generality remains to be established.

Another line of investigation has examined the relationship between caffeine and work-related performances, for example, among college students. Unfortunately, these studies most often employ questionnaires which require self-report and which are difficult to evaluate with respect to causal relationships. The association between caffeine intake and psychological well-being and academic performance has been assessed by Gilliland and Andress (1981) in 159 college students consuming up to the equivalent of eight cups of coffee (or ~600 mg caffeine) daily. Students consuming the highest levels of caffeine generally reported the lowest scores in psychological and somatic well-being and received the worst course grades. As high or low consumption of caffeine is self-selected and may be related to many other features of life-style, an association, as the authors recognize, in no way indicates a causal relationship between caffeine consumption and measures of academic performance and of well-being. One would not suggest that aspirin causes headache because there is an association of aspirin use with headache.

Overconsumption of caffeine is commonly thought to cause tremulousness. Objective recording of tremor, however, showed that finger tremor was significantly increased by fasting but not by 450 mg/day caffeine, which produced plasma levels of 4.9–16.7 mg/liter in subjects on a normal diet (Wharrad *et al.*, 1985).

The foregoing is by no means an exhaustive account of reports of deleterious effects of caffeine on performance. The great majority of studies, however, are single-dose studies, offering no information on dose–effect relations, and very few have been replicated, even in bare essentials. For studies to contribute to our understanding of the effects of caffeine, basic requirements for pharmacology, such as exploration of dose–effect relations, must be met.

With regard to physical or athletic performance, a review of evidence for the ergogenic potential of caffeine by Powers and Dodd (1985) led them to conclude that while results on the effects of caffeine on incremental, graded exercise or high-intensity, short-term work are equivocal, moderate doses of caffeine enhance rather than impair performance in submaximal long-term exercise such as cross-country skiing or marathon running (Berglund and Hemmingsson, 1982). This effect of caffeine may be due to an increase in free fatty acids and, hence, reduced rates of glycolysis after caffeine. It is noteworthy that, based probably on the attention paid in the lay press to possible ergogenic effects of caffeine, the International Olympic Committee has stipulated that athletes must not have blood levels of more than 15 mg/liter of caffeine. As Powers and Dodd (1985) point out, the level of plasma caffeine that is considered unacceptable exceeds levels that are obtained by dietary consumption.

Previously suspected deleterious effects of caffeine on thermoregulation in exercise were not found in careful study (Gordon *et al.*, 1982). Deleterious effects of caffeine on physical performance have been reported only following consumption of excessive amounts, usually under extreme conditions. For example, a case is reported by Stillner *et al.* (1978) of a 28-year-old male who experienced symptoms of delirium shortly after consuming in excess of 1000 mg of caffeine within a 3-hr period and following 48 hr of continuous mushing in the 1977 Iditarod Trail International Sled Dog Race. Noteworthy is that the driver continued mushing despite symptoms of tinnitus, vertigo, tremor, hallucinations, and paranoia. After approximately 6 hr the delirium abated without sequelae.

B. Effects on Sleep

The effects of moderate doses (1–3 mg/kg) of caffeine in delaying and modifying sleep in humans may vary depending on patterns of individual usage but are generally evident both in electroencephalographic–electrooculographic assessments and in subjective estimates of sleep characteristics. Karacan *et al.* (1976) found that the administration of 2.3 or 4.6 mg/kg caffeine 30 min prior to bedtime in young adults postponed onset of sleep by 10–20 min and decreased total sleep time by about the same amount. REM sleep and stages III, IV sleep changed in opposite directions: the former increased and the latter decreased in early sleep and vice versa later in the night.

The effects of moderate doses of the amphetamine-like agents pemoline, prolintane, and methylphenidate were compared to the effects of 100, 200, and 300 mg caffeine on the sleep of young adults by Nicholson and Stone (1980); they concluded that wakefulness following amphetamine intake was associated with marked disturbances of REM sleep, whereas wakefulness following xanthines is likely to be associated with reduced slow-wave sleep.

Increased wakefulness is not of itself a toxic effect, because often caffeine is consumed deliberately to delay the onset of sleep. However, inappropriate timing of dietary consumption of caffeine may lead to unwelcome effects in people who suffer from insomnia. Early studies suggested that effects on sleep were greater in older than young people (Gresham *et al.*, 1963), but more recent research in middle-aged subjects (Brezinova, 1974) and in young adults (Karacan *et al.*, 1976; Nicholson and Stone, 1977) suggests that the dose-related effects of caffeine, particularly on REM and slow-wave sleep stages, are relatively uniform in all ages, at least from 20 to 65. Much younger people are no more (and maybe less) sensitive to behavioral effects of caffeine than are adults, and there are no grounds for supposing that the same may not apply to effects on sleep (Elkins *et al.*, 1981). Insofar as insomnia may be a greater problem in older people than in young people, the sleep-postponing effects of caffeine may pose a relatively greater hazard to the sleep of older adults than to the sleep of young adults; nonetheless, the direct effects do not change with age.

The behavioral effects of caffeine in laboratory animals have been reviewed recently (Dews, 1984b) and do not bear repetition in the present context except to underscore that the effects of acute administration of amounts of caffeine comparable to amounts in human dietary intakes are slight in all species studied and do not in themselves represent toxicity. The effects depend greatly on the baseline conditions and often require sensitive methods to detect them.

Even chronic administration of high levels of caffeine may be without observable effects. Up to 100 mg/kg or more of caffeine through the drinking water was given daily to rodents during gestation and lactation and produced no overt behavioral effects in the dams and no consistent or convincing alterations in the performance of the postweanling adolescent subjects in a variety of tests including assessments of exploratory activity and schedule-controlled performance in rats (Sobotka *et al.*, 1979; Butcher *et al.*, 1984) or mice (Dews and Wenger, 1979).

The daily administration to rats of doses of caffeine over 100 mg/kg leads to mutilation of paws by self-biting (Boyd *et al.*, 1965). Self-mutilation behavior following caffeine overdose has been forwarded as a relevant model for the Lesch–Nyhan syndrome of self-mutilation in children who suffer from a deficiency in hypoxanthine-guanine phosphoribosyltransferase (HGPRTase). In a recent study by Minana *et al.* (1984), the administration to rats of up to 8 gm/kg caffeine in drinking water, leading to as much as 32 mg/kg of caffeine in the brain, was associated with concentration-related increases in HGPRTase activity, in contrast to the decreases seen in Lesch–Nyhan syndrome. There must be, therefore, serious doubt about the basis of a relationship between caffeine-induced mutilation in rats and Lesch–Nyhan syndrome in children. Further, sympathomimetic amines such as amphetamine also produce self-mutilation in rats (Mueller *et al.*, 1982). Minana *et al.* (1984) suggest that the bulk of available evidence relates self-injurious behavior induced by both caffeine and sympathomimetic amines to altered dopamine transmission.

The concrete conclusion that can be drawn from the above sections regarding the effects of dietary caffeine on behavior is that the effects are modest and, most often, inconsequential. Undesirable effects tend to be related to timing rather than to the effects themselves. Insomnia at 3 PM is usually advantageous while insomnia at 3 AM may be a problem.

C.   Caffeinism and Anxiety

The symptoms of caffeinism are given in the DSM III of the American Psychiatric Association (1980) as anxiety, irritation, agitation, muscle tremor, and sensory disturbances. Although 500–600 mg caffeine/day has been cited as representing a significant health risk (James and Stirling, 1983), such levels of intake clearly do not produce those symptoms reliably. Most of the available reports utilize subjective and often misleading self-reports of consumption and of state of well-being. Objective measures definitively associated with anxiety in human subjects either have not been developed or simply are not used.

A report by Greden (1974) based on three case histories pointed out that physiological and behavioral consequences of caffeine intake in excess of 1000 mg/day might be mistaken for symptoms of anxiety disorder. In a follow-up evaluation of questionnaires submitted by 83 inpatients, Greden *et al.* (1978) reported that high levels of caffeine consumption were more likely to be associated with anxiety and depression than were low to moderate levels of consumption. Greden *et al.* (1978) quite correctly warned that their findings in male psychiatric inpatients could not be generalized to other groups (not even to *female* psychiatric inpatients), that confounding variables including medications, smoking, and hospital life-style were not excluded, and that causality could not be inferred from their survey data. By and large, subsequent reports also have provided anecdotal accounts which indicate some deleterious effects of caffeine in various psychiatric disorders (see Couper-Smartt and Couper-Smartt, 1984). Recently, Boulenger *et al.* (1984) and Charney *et al.* (1985) have studied the effects of dietary consumption of caffeine in patients with diagnosed panic disorder. They conducted a self-report survey in 53 patients and controls and found that patients with panic disorder reported themselves as more susceptible to symptoms related to the putative "anxiogenic" effects of caffeine than were patients with depressive disorders or healthy subjects. Details in the report, however, are questionable or uncomfortably vague. For example, patients recruited their own controls, the effects of a single cup of coffee are compared between patient and control groups through retrospective self-report, and patients with panic disorder rated themselves more depressed than did patients with diagnosed depression. The conclusions of this preliminary investigation must await confirmation. It may be speculated that patients with anxiety disorders should tend to consume less caffeine than do other people. The evidence, however, is not conclusive. In a study of 43 patients with anxiety disorders and 124 other inpatients, Lee *et al.* (1985) found that 84% of the former and only 41% of the latter took less than 250 mg/day (Lee *et al.*, 1985). In contrast, Boulenger *et al.* (1984) found that patients with panic or depressive disorders reported average daily caffeine consumption that was clearly within a standard deviation of the average consumption reported by matched control groups. Charney *et al.* (1985) confirmed the similar consumption of caffeine by patients with panic disorder or agoraphobia and by healthy subjects and, additionally, compared the effects of orally administered 10 mg/kg caffeine and of placebo on self-rated psychiatric and somatic symptomatology, steroid levels, and catecholamine metabolite levels. Although they employed rating scales that involved subjectively defined parameters to assess anxiety, the magnitude of effects in their data are impressive and compel attention. Caffeine produced similar plasma caffeine levels ($\sim$8 mg/liter) and similar increases in plasma cortisol in patients and healthy subjects without altering MHPG levels; however, psychiatric patients reported a greater severity in self-rated anxiety and nervousness and in somatic symptoms related to anxiety, and fully 71% reported that the effects were similar to those suffered in panic attack. Clearly, studies such as those discussed herein demonstrate that caffeine may pose a hazard to certain psychiatric patients in hospital. Such subjects, bereft of normal employment and confined within a restricted environment, may develop rather stereotyped activities that have as an integral component the ingestion of continuously available coffee. Such repeated patterns of behavior can lead much more easily to excessive intakes than occur under normal free-living circumstances.

Findings such as those discussed in the above paragraphs have prompted speculation that dietary consumption of caffeine might contribute similar symptoms in the population at large. The evidence does not support such speculation. Increases in self-rated anxiety and nervousness and in somatic symptoms following po administration of 10 mg/kg caffeine to healthy subjects in the report by Charney *et al.* (1985) were minor and not related to plasma caffeine levels. Other recent studies have yielded only ambiguous or negative findings. Veleber and Templer (1984), administered placebo or caffeine (150 or 300 mg) to a group of 171 normal volunteers who filled out checklists designed to measure anxiety, depression, and hostility, and found that scores for all three measures correlated positively with dose of caffeine. However, their tabulated data illustrate nicely the dangers of utilizing subjective self-reports as measures of drug effect: the range of scores following different doses overlap greatly, and the mean scores do not change much and not systematically as a function of dose. In the absence of dose–effect relations, the proposed correlations can be given little weight. Eaton and McLeod (1984) also examined the correlation between self-reported consumption of caffeine and self-rated symptoms of anxiety. In a sample of 3854 respondents, they found absolutely no indication of a positive correlation between symptoms and daily consumption of none to seven or more cups of coffee. Some 94% of the respondents reported daily consumption of five or fewer cups of coffee, that is, less than approximately 500 mg caffeine. As Eaton and McLeod (1984) suggest, it appears that caffeine intake is a self-limiting phenomenon in the normal population, that is, that consumption tends to slow or stop before levels that produce overt symptoms are reached. This idea receives some limited support from a recent report in which 20 of 30 patients with panic disorder reported discontinuing coffee consumption altogether (Uhde *et al.*, 1984). Regrettably, there is no indication in the report of whether patients discontinued coffee as a consequence of symptoms of anxiety, insomnia, tremor, or other potentially unpleasant drug effects.

In human subjects, caffeine has been reported to attenuate performance decrements due to diazepam (Mattila and Nuotto, 1983) or to lorazepam (File *et al.*, 1982). At 500 mg, caffeine also attenuated the reported anxiety-reducing effects of lorazepam (File *et al.*, 1982). Experiments in laboratory animals, however, do not support ''anxiogenic'' effects of dietary caffeine in normal subjects. Benzodiazepines and other drugs that are used clinically in the treatment of anxiety regularly produce characteristic effects in certain well-defined laboratory situations. For example, a benzodiazepine such as diazepam leads to increased occurrences of behavioral activities that have been suppressed by noxious consequences (Sepinwall and Cook, 1980). Caffeine may augment rather than antagonize such effects of benzodiazepines (Coffin and Spealman, 1985) and may even have benzodiazepine-like effects when given alone (Beer *et al.*, 1972).

In summary, then, although it appears to be reasonable to limit caffeine intake among institutionalized individuals suffering certain psychiatric disorders, especially panic disorders, usual dietary consumption of caffeine in the normal population appears to pose little hazard to psychiatric well-being. This conclusion is especially warranted in light of the tolerance which is known to develop to most of the effects of reasonable doses of caffeine and in view of the self-limiting nature of caffeine consumption.

D. Effects of Caffeine in Juveniles

Until recent years it was commonly accepted that juveniles were more susceptible to the behavioral effects of caffeine than were adults (Goodman and Gilman, 1975) and more likely, perhaps, to suffer toxic consequences of dietary consumption. Most recent investigations in children have focused on the effects of caffeine in hyperactivity disorders in the hope of discovering a new medicament without the side effects of methylphenidate (for review, see Elkins *et al.*, 1981). Although therapeutic effects of caffeine were disappointing, the results suggested clearly that the hyperactive children were no more susceptible to caffeine than were normal adults. The same conclusion has been reached from the results of studies in normal juveniles. Direct comparison of dose-related effects of caffeine showed some differences in juveniles and in adults, but the juveniles were not generally more susceptible (Elkins *et al.*, 1981; Rapoport, 1982–1983). Some of the differences were that juveniles tended to report greater sensitivity to the effects of acutely—but not repeatedly—administered caffeine on performance-based measures including motor activity and reaction time, while adults tended to report greater sensitivity to caffeine's subjectively measured effects involving, for example, alterations in mood. However, as Rapoport (1982–1983) points out, these findings may reflect simply the differences in the conceptualization of drug effects by juveniles and adults rather than differences in the biological effects of caffeine in the two groups.

A difference has been reported in the effects of caffeine on children who regularly consume less and children who regularly consume more dietary caffeine. Rapoport *et al.* (1981) studied the effects of placebo and of 5 mg/kg caffeine administered twice daily to children who in an earlier screen had reported low daily consumption of caffeine (<1 mg/kg) or, in a second group, a high level of daily consumption (>10 mg/kg). Upon repeated administration, the effects of caffeine on reaction time disappeared. Side effects, though more striking in the group with normally low intake, were reliably reported by both groups. Of special interest, during a week-long baseline period preceding the administration of placebo or caffeine and in which presumably normal caffeine intake occurred in both groups, high consumers presented a profile of effects similar to that seen in hyperactive children; that is, they reported greater nervousness and irritability and were found to have a less reactive skin conductance than were low consumers. In a follow-up investigation 798 grade-school children completed a questionnaire on caffeine consumption in the preceding 24 hr (Rapoport *et al.*, 1984). Nineteen subjects reporting more than 500 mg intake and 19 reporting less than 50 mg were selected for further study. While the general findings on effective differences between groups reporting high or low intakes described above were confirmed, there was a striking finding on results of diary assessments of intakes. At the time of the definitive study a week-long diary of caffeine intake was obtained. The subjects reporting more than 500 mg intake in the 24-hr screen (mean 641 mg) actually took in an average of only 42 mg/day in the 7-day record, with high standard deviation, so that there must have been substantial overlap of the two groups in their 7-day reports. As the authors point out, (high-consuming) subjects might have reduced their intake as a result of being selected as high consumers, although a 15-fold reduction would entail a substantial change in life-style. Such uncertainties emphasize the desirability of objective assessments of intakes, as by assays of salivary caffeine levels which were used by these workers. Unfortunately, the frequency and timing of the caffeine assays did not permit the levels to be related to the reported intakes. In reviewing the findings, Rapoport (1982–1983) notes that the influence of high levels of caffeine consumption on reported side effects or on academic scores were no different than the influence of low levels of caffeine, but that "high consumers were more likely than low consumers to be rated hyperactive by their teachers . . ." (p. 189). As discussed earlier, correlative survey findings do not establish causality. Reports of high levels of caffeine consumption in the present context may reflect increased rates of a variety of behaviors that result in (or are produced by) hyperactivity or, simply, may indicate a possibly unwitting attempt by hyperactive juveniles to self-medicate. The possibility of some sort of relationship between high levels of caffeine intake and hyperactivity in juveniles remains to be clarified.

VII. CONCLUSION

The evidence available provides ample assurance that sane dietary intakes of caffeine have no substantial deleterious effects on health. Reports and allegations of serious bad effects have consistently failed to be sustained by careful further examination. The task of assessing whether there are slight and inconstant deleterious effects of dietary caffeine on health or performance is difficult because assessment of all slight effects in people is difficult. Work is continuing. The task is probably endless, as advances in medical science continuously make new studies conceivable and feasible.

ACKNOWLEDGMENTS

The preparation of this manuscript was supported in part by USPHS Grants DA03774, DA00499, MH07658, and RR00168. The authors thank Ms. K. McDonald for her assistance in the preparation of this manuscript.

REFERENCES

Aeschbacher, H. U., Milon, H., and Wurzner, H. P. (1978). Caffeine concentrations in mice plasma and testicular tissue and the effect of caffeine on the dominant lethal test. *Mutat. Res.* **57**, 115–118.

American Psychiatric Association (1980). "Diagnostic and Statistical Manual of Mental Disorders," 3rd ed. APA, Washington, D.C.

Aranda, J. V., Cook, C. E., Gorman, W., Collinge, J. M., Loughnan, P. M., Outerbridge, E. W., Aldridge, A., and Neims, A. H. (1979). Pharmacokinetic profile of caffeine in the premature newborn infant with apnea. *Pediatr. Pharmacol. Ther.* **94**, 663–668.

Banner, W. J., and Czajka, P. A. (1980). Acute caffeine overdose in the neonate. *Am. J. Dis. Child.* **134**, 495–498.

Barnes, C. D., and Eltherington, L. G. (1973). "Drug Dosage in Laboratory Animals: A Handbook." Univ. of California Press, Berkeley.

Batirbaygil, Y., Quinby, G. E., and Nakamoto, T. (1985). Effects of oral caffeine intubation on bones in protein–energy malnourished newborn rats. *Biol. Neonate* **48**, 29–35.

Battig, K., Buzzi, R., Martin, J. R., and Feierabend, J. M. (1984). The effects of caffeine on physiological functions and mental performance. *Experientia* **40**, 1218–1223.

Beer, B., Chasin, M., Clody, D. E., Vogel, J. R., and Horowitz, Z. T. (1972). Cyclic adenosine monophosphodiesterase in brain: Effects on anxiety. *Science* **176**, 428–430.

Berglund, B., and Hemmingsson, P. (1982). Effects of caffeine ingestion on exercise performance at low and high altitudes in cross-country skiers. *Int. J. Sports Med.* **3**, 234–236.

Berkowitz, G. S., Kelsey, J. L., LiVolsi, V. A., Holford, T. R., Merino, M. J., Ort, S., O'Connor, T. Z., and White, C. (1985). Risk factors for fibrocystic breast disease and its histopathologic components. *JNCI, J. Natl. Cancer Inst.* **75**, 43–50.

Blinks, J. R., Olson, C. B., Jewell, B. R., and Braveny, P. (1972). Influence of caffeine and other methylxanthines on mechanical properties of isolated mammalian heart msucle. *Circ. Res.* **30**, 367–392.

Boulenger, J. P., Uhde, T. W., Wolff, E. A., and Post, R. M. (1984). Increased sensitivity to caffeine in patients with panic disorders. *Arch. Gen. Psychiatry* **41**, 1067–1071.

Boyd, E. M. (1959). The acute oral toxicity of caffeine. *Toxicol. Appl. Pharmacol.* **1**, 250–257.

Boyd, E. M., Dolman, M., Knight, L. M., and Sheppard, E. P. (1965). The chronic oral toxicity of caffeine. *Can. J. Physiol. Pharmacol.* **43**, 995–1007.

Brezinova, V. (1974). Effect of caffeine on sleep: EEG study in late middle age people. *Br. J. Clin. Pharmacol.* **1**, 203–208.

Broverman, D. M., and Casagrande, E. (1982). Effect of caffeine on performances of a perceptual-restructuring task at different stages of practice. *Psychopharmacology* **78**, 252–255.

Bryant, J. (1981). Letter. *Arch. Pathol. Lab. Med.* **105**, 685–686.

Butcher, R. E., Vorhees, C. V., and Wootten, V. (1984). Behavioral and physical development of rats chronically exposed to caffeinated fluids. *Fundam. Appl. Toxicol.* **4**, 1–13.

Callahan, M. M., Rohovsky, M. W., Robertson, R. S., and Yesair, D. W. (1979). The effect of coffee consumption on plasma lipids, lipoproteins, and the development of aortic atherosclerosis in rhesus monkeys fed an atherogenic diet. *Am. J. Clin. Nutr.* **32,** 834–845.

Campbell, D. E. S., and Richter, W. (1967). An observational method estimating toxicity and drug actions in mice applied to 68 reference drugs. *Acta Pharmacol. Toxicol.* **25,** 245–363.

Charney, D. S., Heninger, G. R., and Jatlow, P. I. (1985). Increased anxiogenic effects of caffeine in panic disorders. *Arch. Gen. Psychiatry* **42,** 233–243.

Clusin, W. T. (1985). Do caffeine and metabolic inhibitors increase free calcium in the heart? Interpretation of conflicting intracellular calcium measurements. *J. Mol. Cell. Cardiol.* **17,** 213–220.

Coffin, V. L., and Spealman, R. D. (1985). Modulation of the behavioral effects of chlordiazepoxide by methylzanthines and analogs of adenosines in squirrel monkeys. *J. Pharmacol. Exp. Ther.* **235,** 724–728.

Collins, T. F. X., Welsh, J. J., Black, T. N., and Collins, E. V. (1981). A study of the teratogenic potential of caffeine given by oral intubation to rats. *Regul. Toxicol. Pharmacol.* **1,** 355–378.

Couper-Smartt, J., and Couper-Smartt, I. (1984). Caffeine consumption: A review of its use, intake, clinical effects and hazards. *Food Technol. Aust.* **36,** 131–134.

Curatolo, P. W., and Robertson, D. (1983). The health consequences of caffeine. *Ann. Intern. Med.* **98,** 641–653.

Davis, H. H., Simons, M., and Davis, J. B. (1964). Cystic disease of the breast: Relationship to carcinoma. *Cancer (Philadelphia)* **17,** 957–976.

DeBacker, G., Jacobs, D., Prineas, R., Crow, R., Vilandre, J., Kennedy, H., and Blackburn, H. (1979). Ventricular premature contractions: A randomized non-drug intervention trial in normal men. *Circulation* **59,** 762–769.

Dews, P. B. (1972). Assessing the effects of drugs. *In* "Methods of Pyschobiology" (R. D. Myers, ed.), pp. 83–124. Academic Press, New York.

Dews, P. B. (1982). Caffeine. *Annu. Rev. Nutr.* **2,** 323–341.

Dews, P. B. (1984a). Caffeine, exercise, and catecholamines in macaques. *In* "Neuronal and Extraneuronal Events in Autonomic Pharmacology" (W. W. Fleming *et al.,* eds.), pp. 231–239. Raven Press, New York.

Dews, P. B. (1984b). Behavioral effects of caffeine. *In* "Caffeine" (P. B. Dews, ed.), pp. 86–106. Springer-Verlag, Berlin and New York.

Dews, P. B., and Wenger, G. R. (1979). Testing for behavioral effects of agents. *Neurobehav. Toxicol.* **1,** 119–127.

Dobmeyer, D. J., Stine, R. A., Leier, C. V., Greenberg, R., and Schaal, S. F. (1983). The arrhythmogenic effects of caffeine in human beings. *N. Engl. J. Med.* **308,** 814–816.

Eaton, W. W., and McLeod, J. (1984). Consumption of coffee or tea and symptoms of anxiety. *Am. J. Public Health* **74,** 66–68.

Eichler, O., ed. (1976). "Kaffee und Coffein, "2nd ed. Springer-Verlag, Berlin and New York.

Elkins, R. N., Rapoport, J. L., Zahn, T. P., Buchsbaum, M. S., Weingartner, H., Kopin, I. J., Langer, D., and Johnson, C. (1981). Acute effects of caffeine in normal prepubertal boys. *Am. J. Psychiatry* **138,** 178–183.

Ernster, V. L. (1984). Epidemiologic studies of coffee and breast disease. *Banbury Rep.* **17,** 167–176.

Ernster, F. L., Mason, L., Goodson, W. H., Sickles, E. A., Sacks, S. T., Selvin, S., Dupuy, M. E., Hawkinson, J., and Hunt, T. K. (1982). Effects of caffeine-free diet on benign breast disease: A randomized trial. *Surgery (St. Louis)* **91,** 263–267.

File, S. E., Bond, A. J., and Lister, R. G. (1982). Interaction between effects of caffeine and lorazepam in performance tests and self-ratings. *J. Clin. Psychopharmacol.* **2,** 102–106.

Forde, O. H., Knutsen, S. F., Arnesen, E., and Thelle, D. S. (1985). The Tromso Heart Study:

Coffee consumption and serum lipid concentrations in men with hypercholesterolaemia: A randomised intervention study. *Br. Med. J.* **290**, 893–895.

Gilliland, K., and Andress, D. (1981). Ad lib caffeine consumption, symptoms of caffeinism, and academic performance. *Am. J. Psychiatry* **138**, 512–514.

Goldstein, A., Warren, R., and Kaizer, S. (1965). Psychotropic effects of caffeine in man. I. Individual differences in sensitivity to caffeine-induced wakefulness. *J. Pharmacol. Exp. Ther.* **149**, 156–159.

Goodman, L. S., and Gilman, A., eds. (1975). "The Pharmacological Basis of Therapeutics," 5th ed. Macmillan, New York.

Gordon, N. F., Myburgh, J. L., Kruger, P. E., Kempff, P. G., Cilliers, J. F., Moolman, J., and Grobler, H. C. (1982). Effects of caffeine ingestion on thermoregulatory and myocardial function during endurance performance. *S. Afr. Med. J.* **62**, 644–647.

Gould, L., Venkataraman, K., Goswami, M., and Gomprecht, R. F. (1973). The cardiac effects of coffee. *Angiology* **24**, 455–463.

Greden, J. F. (1974). Anxiety or caffeinism: A diagnostic dilemma. *Am. J. Psychiatry* **131**, 1089–1092.

Greden, J. F., Fontaine, P., Lubetsky, M., and Chamberlin, K. (1978). Anxiety and depression associated with caffeinism among psychiatric inpatients. *Am. J. Psychiatry* **135**, 963–966.

Greenblatt, E. N., and Osterberg, A. C. (1961). Correlations of activating and lethal effects of excitatory drugs in grouped and isolated mice. *J. Pharmacol. Exp. Ther.* **131**, 115–119.

Gresham, S. C., Webb, W. B., and Williams, R. L. (1963). Alcohol and caffeine: Effect on inferred visual dreaming. *Science* **140**, 1226–1227.

Heinonen, O. P., Slone, D., and Shapiro, S. (1977). "Birth Defects and Drugs in Pregnancy," pp. 366–494. PSG Publishing Company, Inc., Littleton, Massachusetts.

Heyden, S., and Muhlbaier, L. H. (1984). Prospective study of "fibrocystic breast disease" and caffeine consumption. *Surgery (St. Louis)* **96**, 479–483.

Heyden, S., DeMaria, W., Johnston, W. W., and O'Fallon, W. M. (1969). Caffeine effects on cholesterol and development of aortic and coronary atherosclerosis in rabbits. *J. Chronic Dis.* **21**, 677–685.

Heyden, S., Tyroler, H. A., Heiss, G., Hames, C. G., and Bartel, A. (1978). Coffee consumption and mortality. *Arch. Intern. Med.* **138**, 1472–1475.

James, J. E., and Stirling, K. P. (1983). Caffeine: A survey of some of the known and suspected deleterious effects of habitual use. *Br. J. Addict.* **78**, 251–258.

Jick, H., Miettinen, O. S., Neff, R. K., Shapiro, S., Heinonen, O. P., and Slone, O. (1973). Coffee and myocardial infraction. *N. Engl. J. Med.* **289**, 63–67.

Karacan, I., Thornby, J. I., Anch, A. M., Booth, G. H., Williams, R. L., and Salis, P. J. (1976). Dose-related sleep disturbances induced by coffee and caffeine. *Clin. Pharmacol. Ther.* **20**, 682–689.

Klatsky, A. R., Pettiti, D. B., Armstrong, M. A., and Friedman, G. D. (1985). Coffee, tea and cholesterol. *Am. J. Cardiol.* **55**, 577–578.

Konishi, M., Kurihara, S., and Sakai, T. (1984). The effects of caffeine on tension development and intracellular calcium transients in rat ventricular muscle. *J. Physiol. (London)* **355**, 605–618.

Lee, M. A., Cameron, O. G., and Greden, J. F. (1985). Anxiety and caffeine consumption in people with anxiety disorders. *Psychiatry Res.* **15**, 211–217.

McGee, M. B. (1980). Caffeine poisoning in a 19-year old female. *J. Forensic Sci.* **25**, 29–32.

Maloney, A. H. (1935). Contradictory actions of caffeine, coramine, and metrazol. *Q. J. Exp. Physiol.* **25**, 155–166.

Marangos, P. J., Martino, A. M., Paul, S. M., and Skolnick, P. (1981). The benzodiazepines and inosine antagonize caffeine-induced seizures. *Psychopharmacology* **72**, 269–273.

Mattila, M. J., and Nuotto, E. (1983). Caffeine and theophylline counteract diazepam effects on man. *Med. Biol.* **61**, 337–343.

Minana, M. D., Portoles, M., Jorda, A., and Grisolia, S. (1984). Lesch–Nyhan syndrome, caffeine model: Increase of purine and pyrimidine enzymes in rat brain. *J. Neurochem.* **43,** 1556–1560.

Minton, J. P., Foecking, M. K., Webster, D. J. T., and Matthews, R. H. (1979a). Caffeine, cyclic nucleotides, and breast disease. *Surgery (St. Louis)* **86,** 105.

Minton, J. P., Foecking, M. K., Webster, D. J. T., and Matthews, R. H. (1979b). Response of fibrocystic disease to caffeine withdrawal and correlation of cyclic nucleotides with breast disease. *Am. J. Obstet. Gynecol.* **135,** 157.

Mitoma, C., Lombrozo, L., Le Valley, S. E., and Dehn, F. (1969). Nature of the effect of caffeine on the drug-metabolizing enzymes. *Arch. Biochem. Biophys.* **134,** 434–441.

Mohr, U., Althoff, J., Ketkar, M. B., Conradt, P., and Morgareidge, K. (1984). The influence of caffeine on tumour incidence in Sprague–Dawley rats. *Food Chem. Toxicol.* **22,** 377–382.

Mueller, K., Saboda, S., Palmour, R., and Nyhan, W. L. (1982). Self-injurious behavior produced in rats by daily caffeine and continuous amphetamine. *Pharmacol., Biochem. Behav.* **17,** 613–617.

Nicholson, A. N., and Stone, B. M. (1977). Studies on the sleep of the young adult after caffeine. *Proc. Br. Pharmacol. Soc.* **59,** 48.

Nicholson, A. N., and Stone, B. M. (1980). Heterocyclic amphetamine derivatives and caffeine on sleep in man. *Br. J. Clin. Pharmacol.* **9,** 195–203.

Palm, P. E., Arnold, E. P., Nick, M. S., Valentine, J. R., and Doerfler, T. E. (1984). Two-year toxicity/carcinogenicity study of fresh-brewed coffee in rats initially exposed in utero. *Toxicol. Appl. Pharmacol.* **74,** 364–382.

Paspa, P., and Vassale, M. (1984). Mechanism of caffeine-induced arrhythmias in canine cardiac purkinje fibers. *Am. J. Cardiol.* **53,** 313–319.

Paul, O., Lepper, M. H., Phelan, W. H., Dupertuis, G. W., MacMillan, A., McKean, H., and Park, H. (1963). A longitudinal study of coronary heart disease. *Circulation* **28,** 20–31.

Paulus, W. J., Serizawa, T., and Grossman, W. (1982). Altered left ventricular diastolic properties during pacing-induced ischemia in dogs with coronary stenoses. *Circ. Res.* **50,** 214–227.

Powers, S. K., and Dodd, S. (1985). Caffeine and endurance performance. *Sports Med.* **2,** 165–174.

Prineas, R. J., Jacobs, D. R., Crow, R. S., and Blackburn, H. (1980). Coffee, tea and VPB. *J. Chronic Dis.* **33,** 66–72.

Rapoport, J. L. (1982–1983). Effects of dietary substance in children. *J. Psychiatry* **17,** 187–191.

Rapoport, J. L., Elkins, R., Neims, A., Zahn, T., and Berg, C. (1981). Behavioral and autonomic effects of caffeine in normal boys. *Dev. Pharmacol. Ther.* **3,** 74–82.

Rapoport, J. L., Berg, C. J., Ismond, D. R., Zahn, T. P., and Neims, A. (1984). Behavioral effects of caffeine in children. *Arch. Gen. Psychiatry* **41,** 1073–1079.

Roberts, J. J. (1984). Mechanism of potentiation by caffeine of genotoxic damage induced by physical and chemical agents: Possible relevance to carcinogenesis. *In* "Caffeine" (P. B. Dews, ed.), pp. 239–254. Springer-Verlag, Berlin and New York.

Robertson, D., Frolich, J. C., Carr, R. K., Watson, J. T., Hollifield, J. W., Shand, D. G., and Oates, J. A. (1978). Effects of caffeine on plasma renin activity, catecholamines and blood pressure. *N. Engl. J. Med.* **298,** 181–186.

Robertson, D., Wade, D., Workman, R., Woosley, R. L., and Oates, J. A. (1981). Tolerance to the humoral and hemodynamic effects of caffeine in man. *J. Clin. Invest.* **67,** 1111–1117.

Robertson, R. M., Tantengco, M. V., Bernard, Y., Gore, T., and Robertson, D. (1985). Effect of caffeine on serum lipids in miniature swine. *Am. Fed. Clin. Res.* (abstr.).

Salant, W., and Rieger, J. B. (1909–1910). The toxicity of caffeine. *J. Pharmacol. Exp. Ther.* **1,** 572–574.

Scott, C. C., and Chen, K. K. (1944). Comparison of the action of 1-ethyl theobromine and caffeine in animals and man. *J. Pharmacol. Exp. Ther.* **82,** 89–97.

Seale, T. W., Johnson, P., Roderick, T. H., Carney, J. M., and Rennert, O. M. (1985). A single gene difference determines relative susceptibility to caffeine-induced lethality in SWR and CBA inbred mice. *Pharmacol., Biochem. Behav.* **23,** 275–278.

Sepinwall, J., and Cook, L. (1980). Mechanism of action of the benzodiazepines: Behavioral aspects. *Fed. Proc., Fed. Am. Soc. Exp. Biol.* **39,** 3024–3031.

Shirlow, M. J., and Mathers, C. D. (1984). Caffeine consumption and serum cholesterol levels. *Int. J. Epidemiol.* **13,** 422–427.

Smith, B., Onrot, J., and Robertson, D. (1985). Significance of caffeine in common preparations. *Physician Patient,* **18,** 18–22.

Smith, J. M., Pearson, S., and Marks, V. (1982). Plasma caffeine concentrations in outpatients. *Lancet* **2,** 985–986.

Sobotka, T. J., Spaid, S. L., and Brodie, R. E. (1979). Neurobehavioral teratology of caffeine exposure in rats. *Neurotoxicology* **1,** 403–416.

Sollman, T., and Pilcher, J. D. (1911). The actions of caffeine on the mammalian circulation. *J. Pharmacol. Exp. Ther.* **3,** 19–92.

Stillner, V., Popkin, M. K., and Pierce, C. M. (1978). Caffeine-induced delirium during prolonged competitive stress. *Am. J. Psychiatry* **135,** 855–856.

Sutherland, D. J., McPherson, D. D., Renton, K. W., Spencer, C. A., and Montague, T. J. (1985). The effect of caffeine on cardiac rate, rhythm, and ventricular repolarization. *Chest* **87,** 319–324.

Temples, T. E., Geoffray, D. J., Nakamoto, T., Hartman, A. D., and Miller, H. I. (1985). Effects of chronic caffeine ingestion on growth and myocardial function. *Proc. Soc. Exp. Biol. Med.* **179,** 388–395.

Thelle, D. S., Arnesen, E., and Forde, O. H. (1983). The Tromso Heart Study. Does coffee raise serum cholesterol? *N. Engl. J. Med.* **308,** 1454–1457.

Turner, J. E., and Cravey, R. H. (1977). A fetal ingestion of caffeine. *Clin. Toxicol.* **3,** 341–344.

Uhde, T. W., Boulenger, J. P., Jimerson, D. C., and Post, R. M. (1984). Caffeine: Relationship to human anxiety, plasma MHPG, and cortisol. *Psychopharmacol. Bull.* **20,** 426–440.

van den Berg, B. J. (1977). Epidemiologic observations of prematurity: Effects of tobacco, coffee and alcohol. *In* "The Epidemiology of Prematurity" (D. M. Freed and F. F. Stanley, eds.). Urban & Schwarzenberg, Baltimore/Munich.

Veleber, D. M., and Templer, D. I. (1984). Effects of caffeine on anxiety and depression. *J. Abnorm. Psychol.* **93,** 120–122.

Vellucci, S. V., and Webster, R. A. (1984). Antagonism of caffeine-induced seizures in mice by Ro15-1788. *Eur. J. Pharmacol.* **97,** 289–293.

Weber, A., and Herz, R. (1968). The relationship between caffeine contracture of intact muscle and the effect of caffeine on reticulum. *J. Gen. Physiol.* **52,** 750–759.

Wharrad, H. J., Birmingham, A. T., Macdonald, I. A., Inch, P. J., and Mead, J. L. (1985). The influence of fasting and of caffeine intake on finger tremor. *Eur. J. Clin. Pharmacol.* **29,** 37–43.

Williams, P. T., Wood, P. D., Vranizan, K. M., Albers, J. J., Garay, S. C., and Taylor, C. B. (1985). Coffee intake and elevated cholesterol and apolipoprotein B levels in men. *JAMA, J. Am. Med. Assoc.* **253,** 1407–1411.

Wilson, J. G., and Scott, W. J. (1984). The teratogenic potential of caffeine in laboratory animals. *In* "Caffeine" (P. B. Dews, ed.), pp. 165–187. Springer-Verlag, Berlin and New York.

Wurzner, H. P., Lindstrom, E., and Vuataz, L. (1977). A 2-year feeding study of instant coffees in rats. I. Body weight, food consumption, haematological parameters and plasma chemistry. *Food Cosmet. Toxicol.* **15,** 7–16.

9

The Toxicology of Dietary Tin, Aluminum, and Selenium

Janet L. Greger and Helen W. Lane

I. TIN

The essentiality of tin is debatable (Schwarz *et al.*, 1970; Schroeder *et al.*, 1964; Underwood, 1977). Currently the primary concern about tin is its toxicity, not its essentiality.

A. Dietary Exposure to Tin

The tin content of typical Western diets has been reported to range from 1 to 38 mg/day (Schroeder *et al.*, 1964; Greger and Baier, 1981; Sherlock and Smart,

223

Copyright © 1987 by Academic Press, Inc.
All rights of reproduction in any form reserved.

1984; Tipton *et al.*, 1969). The differences in the estimates primarily reflect differences in the amounts of canned foods, particularly foods packed in unlacquered cans, included in the diets.

Most foods contain small amounts of tin naturally (Schroeder *et al.*, 1964; Sherlock and Smart, 1984). Furthermore, although stannous chloride is a GRAS food additive and several organotin compounds are used as polymerization aids in plastics, little tin from these compounds actually enters food (Kumpulainen and Koivistoinen, 1977). Hence, most fresh-frozen and bottled foods contain less than 1 µg Sn/gm food.

The tin content of canned foods can vary greatly. Foods packed in cans that are totally coated with lacquer generally contain less than 4 µg Sn/gm food (Greger and Baier, 1981). Foods (e.g., pineapple, grapefruit, and orange juices, applesauce, tomato sauce) that are often packed in cans that are not coated with lacquer have been found to contain 40–150 µg Sn/gm food when the cans were opened (Greger and Baier, 1981; Sherlock and Smart, 1984).

The amount of tin in canned foods can be increased by storage conditions. Canned foods, particularly those with high nitrate and acid levels, accumulate tin when stored for several months (Nagy *et al.*, 1980). Moreover, foods stored in opened cans in the refrigerator for 3–7 days can accumulate very high (>250 µg/g) levels of tin (Greger and Baier, 1981; Capar and Boyer, 1980).

Although most American and Europeans consume a limited amount of canned foods, there are exceptions. Low-income individuals and institutions, such as nursing homes and schools, often select canned fruits, vegetables, and juices because of economy and ease of storage. Mothers sometimes leave juice in opened cans in the refrigerator for their children's snacks. Individuals who routinely consume canned fruits, vegetables, and juices from unlacquered cans could ingest 50 to more than 200 mg tin daily.

B. Metabolism of Inorganic Tin

1. *Excretion*

Hiles (1974) observed that rats absorbed a single dose of tin (II) more efficiently than tin(IV) (2.85 vs. 0.64%). Absorption of tin does not appear to be sensitive to changes in the anion component of tin salts or to the presence of a number of other dietary components (Hiles, 1974; Fritsch *et al.*, 1977). However, Johnson and Greger (1985) observed that a three-fold increase in dietary zinc levels resulted in greater fecal losses of tin when animals were fed 100–200 µg Sn/gm diet. Some tin lost in the feces may be of endogenous origin (Hiles, 1974).

Little tin is excreted in the urine of animals, but urinary losses of tin will reflect large differences in tin intake (Hiles, 1974; Fritsch *et al.*, 1977; Tipton *et al.*, 1969; Johnson and Greger, 1982). Eight human subjects excreted four times as much tin (122 vs. 29 μg Sn/day) when fed 50 mg rather than 0.11 mg Sn/day (Johnson and Greger, 1982).

2. Retention

Although the absorption and overall apparent retention of tin by human subjects in balance studies is low (Calloway and McMullen, 1966; Tipton *et al.*, 1969; Johnson and Greger, 1982), tin has been found in at least trace amounts in most mammalian tissues (Schroeder *et al.*, 1964).

Rats fed diets supplemented with tin have been found to accumulate tin to their tibias, kidneys, and livers in proportion to their dietary intake of tin. Johnson and Greger (1985) found that the concentrations of tin in the tibias of rats fed diets supplemented with tin were more than 5 times greater than the concentrations of tin in kidneys and nearly 20 times greater than the concentrations of tin in livers. Other investigators have also observed that animals accumulated more tin in bone than soft tissues (Hiles, 1974; Greger and Johnson, 1981; Yamaguchi *et al.*, 1980).

C. Toxic Effects of Organic Tin

A variety of organic tin compounds are used commercially; a number are extremely toxic (Kimbrough, 1976). The toxicity of these compounds is depedent on the organic constituents of the tin compounds, the manner of exposure, and the animal species studied. This topic has been reviewed throughly and will be discussed only briefly here.

Trimethyl and triethyltin compounds are the most toxic organotin compounds, partially because they are well absorbed from the gastrointestinal tract (Kimbrough, 1976). However, trimethyltin and triethyltin differ in their effects. Triethyltin causes cerebral edema, myelinopathies, and spongy degeneration of the brain (Squibb *et al.*, 1980). Trimethyltin produces brain damage which is primarily restricted to limbic system structures (Dyer *et al.*, 1982). The liver and thymus are also affected adversely by organotin compounds.

D. Toxic Effects of Inorganic Tin

1. Acute Effects

Animals and humans are fairly resistant to single large oral doses of tin, and reports of acute responses to dietary tin are rare (Warbur *et al.*, 1962; Benoy *et al.*, 1971; Barker and Runte, 1972). Generally, individuals have developed symptoms, including nausea, abdominal cramping, diarrhea, and vomiting, after consuming canned juices or acidic punches prepared in tinned vessels. The levels of tin in the contaminated foods have ranged from 500 to 2000 μg/ml. Other factors in the beverages may have exacerbated the local irritation of the gastrointestinal tract by tin in some cases.

2. *Chronic Effects*

a. Growth Depression and Changes in Cellular Function. Some of the effects of tin on growth and cell function may be indirect and due to interactions between tin and essential minerals such as zinc, copper, iron, and selenium; some of the effects may be direct. McLean *et al.* (1983) have found that *in vitro* tin(II) but not tin(IV) was readily taken up by ovary cells and damaged the DNA in the cells.

Several investigators have observed that the effects of inorganic tin on growth are dependent on the dose and the form of the tin salts fed. Growth of rats was usually depressed when dietary tin levels were elevated above 500 μg/gm (de-Groot, 1973; deGroot *et al.*, 1973; Dreef van der Muelen *et al.*, 1974; Johnson and Greger, 1984).

Ingestion of tin has been demonstrated to depress the activity of serum alkaline phosphatase and serum lactic dehydrogenase (Yamaguchi *et al.*, 1980; Dreef van der Meulen *et al.*, 1974). A single injection of stannous chloride has been found to depress hepatic azo-reductase and aromatic hydroxylase activity (Burba, 1983). In contrast, injections of tin have been found to induce heme oxygenase activity in the kidneys of rats (Kappas and Maines, 1976).

Chiba *et al.* (1980) have demonstrated that animals injected with tin had decreased activity of blood δ-aminolevulinic dehydratase (δ-ALAD). Johnson and Greger (1985) demonstrated that very high levels of dietary tin ($>$2000 μg Sn/gm diet), but not moderate levels of dietary tin ($\approx$200 μg Sn/gm diet), inhibited blood δ-ALAD activity in rats. Zinc partially reversed *in vitro* the inhibition of δ-ALAD by tin (Chiba and Kikuchi, 1984), but ingesting additional zinc did not counteract the effect of tin on δ-ALAD activity in rats.

Only a limited amount of work has been done on the effects of tin on immune function. Dimitrov *et al.* (1981) found that a single injection of stannic chloride decreased the formation of plaque-forming cells in mice. Levine and Sowinski (1983) observed marked proliferation of plasma cells and Russell body cells in draining lymph nodes of Lewis rats inoculated once with metallic tin. Prior administration of tin chloride in drinking water, but not pretreatment with immunosuppressive drugs, prevented plasma cell hyperplasia in response to the single injected dose of tin.

b. Interactions with Zinc and Selenium. Potentially some of the effects of tin on growth, enzyme levels, and even immune function can be explained on the basis of interactions between tin and zinc or selenium. It is well established that growth depression is a common symptom of zinc deficiency (Underwood, 1977). Several of the enzymes affected by tin are zinc metalloproteins. Moreover immune function is sensitive to changes in the nutritional status of both zinc and selenium (Beisel, 1982).

Rats fed 500 μg or more of tin per gram of diet have depressed levels of zinc in bone and soft tissues (Greger and Johnson, 1981; Johnson and Greger, 1984). Tibia zinc levels are even sensitive to moderate doses of tin (100–200 μg Sn/gm diet). At least part of this effect is due to the effect of dietary tin on apparent absorption of zinc. Johnson *et al.* (1982) found that human subjects lost an additional 2 mg of zinc daily in the feces when fed 50 mg Sn/day rather than 0.1 mg Sn/day; this resulted in significantly poorer overall retention of zinc by these subjects. Valberg *et al.* (1984) confirmed these results and found inorganic tin depressed the absorption of humans of ^{65}Zn from zinc chloride and from a turkey test meal. However, Solomons *et al.* (1983) could not demonstrate a tin–zinc interaction in subjects fed loading doses of both tin and zinc.

The mechanism by which tin affects zinc absorption appears to depend on the dose. When rats were fed high levels of tin ($\simeq$2000 μg Sn/gm diet) their gastrointestinal tracts were hypertrophied and endogenous losses of zinc in the feces were significantly increased (Johnson and Greger, 1984). When moderate levels of tin ($\simeq$200 and 500 μg Sn/gm diet) were fed, endogenous losses of zinc in the feces were constant but the true absorption of zinc tended to be depressed.

Less is known about the interaction between tin and selenium. Hill and Matrone (1970) showed that high dietary levels of tin depressed the apparent absorption of selenium from chick intestinal segments. Greger *et al.* (1982) demonstrated that human subjects fed 500 mg versus 0.11 mg Sn/day apparently absorbed significantly less selenium.

c.   Anemia and Interactions with Copper and Iron.   The ingestion of high level of dietary tin can induce anemia in rats (deGroot, 1973; deGroot *et al.*, 1973; Dreef van der Meulen *et al.*, 1974). One potential mechanism involves copper. Generally dietary tin did not depress tissue levels of iron in rats, but ingestion of 200 μg or more of tin per gram of diet usually depressed copper levels in soft tissues (Greger and Johnson, 1981; Johnson and Greger, 1985). The plasma copper levels of animals fed high levels of tin (500 and 2000 μg Sn/gm diet) were depressed to less than 20% of the levels found in control animals. It is well established that copper deficiency can induce anemia (Underwood, 1977). Moreover, deGroot (1973) demonstrated that the addition of copper to the diets of rats eliminated the anemia induced by feeding 150 μg Sn/gm diet.

Ingestion of high levels of dietary tin (>1000 μg Sn/gm diet), but probably not moderate levels of tin, may induce anemia in other ways too (Johnson and Greger, 1985). Tin can alter the activity of at least two enzymes involved in heme metabolism, δ-ALAD and heme oxygenase (Kappas and Maines, 1976; Chiba *et al.*, 1980).

Although all of these factors may affect the development of anemia in laboratory animals that are fed high levels of tin, their significance to humans fed moderate levels of tin is questionable. Johnson *et al.* (1982) found that the addition of 50 mg Sn/day (equivalent to ~100 μg Sn/gm dry diet) to the diets of human subjects for 20 days had no effect on the apparent absorption of copper or iron or on plasma copper, ceruloplasmin, or ferritin levels. Similarly, no changes in copper or iron metabolism were observed in rats fed only 100 μg Sn/gm diet (Johnson and Greger, 1985).

d.   Changes in Calcium and Bone Metabolism. A group of Japanese workers have reported that the ingestion of tin reduced the calcium content of bone, reduced the calcium levels of serum, and increased kidney calcium levels (Yamaguchi *et al.*, 1980, 1981; Yamamoto *et al.*, 1976). They found that even dietary levels of tin as low as 50 μg/gm diet had significant effects on the calcium content of the femoral epiphysis (Yamaguchi *et al.*, 1981). Johnson and Greger (1985) also observed that low levels of dietary tin ($\approx$100 μg Sn/gm diet) depressed the calcium content of bone but observed no changes in plasma calcium levels. The addition of 50 mg Sn/day to the diets of humans had no effects on calcium or magnesium excretion or retention (Johnson and Greger, 1982; Johnson *et al.*, 1982). Differences between studies may be due to difference in how tin was administered, the dietary levels of calcium and phosphorus, and the size of animals.

Ogoshi *et al.* (1981) have observed that compressive strength of femurs of rats given tin (300 μg Sn/ml) in their drinking water was significantly decreased. Yamaguchi *et al.* (1982) also observed that collagen synthesis was depressed in bones of rats orally dosed with tin.

e.   Conclusion. Exposure to high dietary levels of tin would chiefly be important to those individuals who consume low levels of essential elements (e.g., zinc, copper, and perhaps calcium) and who are already in marginal nutritional status in regard to these elements. For example, many elderly individuals and some children routinely consume less than two-thirds of the Recommended Dietary Allowances (RDA) for zinc (Hambidge *et al.*, 1976; Sandstead *et al.*, 1982). Most women in the United States consume less than two-thirds of the RDA for calcium (Science and Education Administration, 1980). For these individuals the routine consumption of foods packed in unlacquered cans may result in excessive exposure to tin.

II.   ALUMINUM

Aluminum is the third most abundant element in the earth's crust. However, there is no conclusive evidence that aluminum is essential for growth, reproduction, or health of humans and animals (Underwood, 1977). Thus, as with tin, the primary concern about aluminum is in regard to its toxicity.

A. Dietary Exposure to Aluminum

Most Americans probably consume 20–40 mg aluminum in food and beverages daily. A few may consume as little as 3 mg daily, and a few may consume as much as 100 mg aluminum daily (Greger, 1985).

Most foods contain some aluminum naturally; a few foods, such as tea and herbs, contain very high levels of aluminum (Sorenson *et al.*, 1974; Schlettwein-Gsell and Mommsen-Straub, 1973). However, the amount of aluminum from natural sources in the daily diets of Americans is small (i.e., 2–10 mg/day), because herbs are consumed in small quantities and most aluminum in tea leaves is insoluble (Greger, 1985).

Food additives are generally the major dietary source of aluminum. In 1982 approximately 4.0 million pounds of aluminum were used in food additives in the United States (Committee on Food Additives Survey Data, 1984). This means that the average U.S. citizen theoretically consumed 21.5 mg aluminum daily in food additives. Average figures such as this can be misleading. The Committee on the GRAS List Survey—Phase III (1979) estimated that 5% of adult Americans consumed more than 95 mg aluminum daily in food additives. Those foods which contributed the greatest amounts of aluminum in food additives to the diets of Americans were baked goods prepared with chemical leavening agents and processed cheeses.

Generally, investigators have found that most foods stored or cooked in aluminum pans, trays, or foil accumulated some aluminum (Greger *et al.*, 1985b; Ondreička *et al.*, 1971; Poe and Leberman, 1949: Lione, 1984). The amounts of aluminum that accumulated in foods during preparation depended on the pH of the foods, the length of the cooking periods, the type of utensils, and how they had been used previously. The few foods that accumulated more than 0.2 mg Al/100 gm of food during preparation and storage were tomato products. Servings (100-gm) of tomato sauce cooked for several hours in aluminum pots accumulated 3–6 mg of aluminum (Lione, 1984; Greger *et al.*, 1985b).

B. Pharmacological Exposure to Aluminum

The quantities of aluminum in foods are small compared to the amounts of aluminum that can be ingested in pharmaceutical products, such as antacids, buffered analgesics, antidiarrheals, and certain antiulcer drugs. Lione (1983) estimated that 840–5000 mg aluminum and 126–728 mg aluminum were possible daily doses of aluminum in antacids and in buffered analgesics, respectively.

C. Metabolism of Aluminum

1. *Excretion*

When human subjects were fed pharmacological doses of aluminum ($\approx$2000 mg Al/day), fecal losses of aluminum generally were less than aluminum intake

(Clarkson *et al.*, 1972; Cam *et al.*, 1976; Gorsky *et al.*, 1979). However, when subjects were fed 5–125 mg Al/day, aluminum losses in the feces approximated dietary intake (Tipton *et al.*, 1969; Cam *et al.*, 1976; Gorsky *et al.*, 1979; Greger and Baier, 1983a). This does not mean that aluminum absorption did not occur in this range, but it suggests that balance techniques were not sensitive enough to detect these differences.

A variety of factors may influence aluminum absorption. Children may absorb aluminum more efficiently than adults. Dietary levels of fluoride, magnesium, and boron may alter aluminum absorption (Ondreička *et al.*, 1971; Nielsen, 1984). However, Feinroth *et al.* (1982) reported that aluminum absorption in rat everted gut sacs was not influenced by renal failure or changes in parathyroid hormone levels. Furthermore, they believed that aluminum absorption from the rat jejunum was energy-dependent and carrier-mediated.

Generally humans excrete less than 100 μg Al/day in urine (Greger and Baier, 1983a; Kaehny *et al.*, 1977; Recker *et al.*, 1977). However, urine, not bile, appears to be the major excretory route for injected aluminum (Kovalchik *et al.*, 1978). Moreover, urinary aluminum levels do reflect changes in dietary intake. Subjects excreted three times as much aluminum in urine when they were fed 125 mg rather than 5 mg Al/day (Greger and Baier, 1983a).

2. *Retention of Aluminum in Tissues*

Aluminum, at least in trace amounts, has been found in most tissues of humans and animals (Underwood, 1977; Sorenson *et al.*, 1974). Usually more aluminum has been found to accumulate in bone than in soft tissues (Ondreička *et al.*, 1971; Greger *et al.*, 1985a, 1986; Slanina *et al.*, 1984, 1985). However, the response of tissue levels of aluminum to changes in aluminum intake have not been found to be always directly proportional to intake levels or length of exposure.

Many investigators have reported that aluminum accumulated in the tissues of renal dialysis patients. For example, Alfrey *et al.* (1976) found that dialysis patients who were the most severely affected by aluminum toxicity—that is, those with dialysis encephalopathy syndrome—accumulated 10 times the normal levels of aluminum in bone. Dialysate fluids were probably the major source of aluminum exposure for many of the patients during the 1960s and 1970s (King *et al.*, 1981). Several groups of investigators have since reported the accumulation of aluminum in tissues, particularly bone, of uremic patients who were dialyzed with aluminum-free fluids (Heaf and Nielsen, 1984; Salusky *et al.*, 1984) and in tissues of children who were not dialyzed (Andreoli *et al.*. 1984; Nathan and Pederson, 1980; Griswold *et al.*, 1983; Freundlich *et al.*, 1985). Generally the source of this aluminum was aluminum-containing phosphate binders; however, in one situation infant formula was the reported source of the aluminum (Freundlich *et al.*, 1985).

Patients receiving iv solutions have also been found to accumulate aluminum in their tissues when the solutions contained aluminum, as in casein-hydrolysate solutions for total parenteral nutrition (TPN) (Klein *et al.*, 1982; deVernejoul *et al.*, 1985). Some ulcer patients also have been found to accumulate aluminum in bone (Recker *et al.*, 1977). Generally these patients have accumulated less aluminum than dialysis patients.

Aluminum levels tend to increase in tissues, including brain, with age (McDermott *et al.*, 1979; Markesbery *et al.*, 1981). Some experts (Crapper *et al.*, 1976; Perl and Brody, 1980; Crapper-McLachlan *et al.*, 1983), but not all experts (McDermott *et al.*, 1979; Markesbery *et al.*, 1981), found increased aluminum levels in the brains of patients with Alzheimer's disease. Brain aluminum levels are also elevated sometimes in patients with amyotrophic lateral sclerosis and parkisonnism dementia (ALS-PD) in Guam (Traub *et al.*, 1981; Perl *et al.*, 1982; Garruto *et al.*, 1984).

D. Toxic Effects of Aluminum

Although some of the symptoms of aluminum toxicity are caused by the direct interaction of aluminum with nucleic acids and membranes (Haug, 1984), many of the toxic effects of aluminum are at least partially ascribable to interactions of aluminum with essential minerals. Because Haug (1984) has reviewed extensively the molecular aspects of aluminum toxicity, they will not be discussed here.

1. Interactions with Essential Minerals

Several investigators have observed that large oral doses of aluminum interfered with phosphorus absorption and lowered tissue phosphorus levels (Ondreička *et al.*, 1971; Valdivia *et al.*, 1982; Clarkson *et al.*, 1972; Cam *et al.*, 1976). The bone pain and fractures observed in patients who have used large doses of aluminum-containing antacids for years has been related to a phosphorus depletion syndrome (Lotz *et al.*, 1968; Dent and Winter, 1974; Insogna *et al.*, 1980). The effect of moderate doses of aluminum on phosphorus metabolism is less clear. Although the additions of 120 mg of aluminum to the daily diets of young adults depressed phosphorus absorption initially, subjects appeared to adjust so that no effect could be observed after 2 weeks (Greger and Baier, 1983b). Similarly, rats fed about 1000 μg Al/gm diet for 30 days absorbed phosphorus less efficiently than control rats, but the effect was not observed after 60 days (Greger *et al.*, 1986).

The interactions between aluminum and calcium are complex. Spencer *et al.* (1982) observed that subjects fed low dietary levels of calcium excreted more calcium in the feces when antacids containing aluminum and magnesium salts were administered. Valdivia *et al.* (1982) observed that sheep apparently absorbed calcium less efficiently when fed 2000 μg Al/gm diet. Greger *et al.* (1985c) observed that rats fed about 260 or about 1000 μg Al/gm diet for 30 days, but not 60 days, apparently absorbed less calcium than control animals. Other investigators have found that oral administration of aluminum did not affect calcium absorption or tissue levels of calcium (Greger *et al.*, 1985a, 1986; Valdivia *et al.*, 1978, 1982; Greger and Baier, 1983b). The elevation of urinary and serum calcium levels observed in patients given pharmaceutical doses of aluminum have sometimes been attributed to changes in phosphorus metabolism induced by aluminum (Spencer *et al.*, 1982: Insogna *et al.*, 1980). Parathyroid hormone may also play a role in these interactions (Cannata *et al.*, 1983; Cournot-Witmer *et al.*, 1981).

It is well documented that dietary aluminum will depress fluoride absorption (Said *et al.*, 1977; Spencer *et al.*, 1980). The effects of aluminum on magnesium, iron, zinc, and copper metabolism is less consistent (Valdivia *et al.*, 1978, 1982; Rosa *et al.*, 1982; Greger *et al.*, 1985a,c; Skikne *et al.*, 1981). The differences in results may reflect differences in the measures of mineral retention (i.e., absorption or tissue levels), the length of the studies, and the general composition of the diets. It might be anticipated that aluminum hydroxide because of its acid-neutralizing capacities might affect the absorption of minerals, particularly iron, more than other aluminum-containing compounds, but this has not been documented (Greger *et al.*, 1985a).

2. Clinical Symptoms

The two main tissues in which the effects of aluminum toxicity have been documented in humans are bone and brain. As already noted, aluminum has been found to accumulate in the bones of patients dialyzed with aluminum-contaminated fluids, patients dosed with aluminum-containing phosphate binders and ulcer medications, and patients treated with aluminum-containing TPN solutions. Clinical symptoms include bone pain and an increased rate of fractures and resistance to vitamin D therapy (King *et al.*, 1981).

Aluminum accumulated in the bones of these patients at the interface between the thickened osteoid and calcified bone (Cournot-Witmer *et al.*, 1981). Possible mechanisms of aluminum toxicity are changes in vitamin D and parathyroid hormone metabolism, phosphorus depletion, and direct (but undefined) toxic actions of aluminum (Drüeke, 1980). However, several investigators believe that the primary action of aluminum toxicity is probably not via interference with vitamin D metabolism (Drüeke, 1980; Chan *et al.*, 1983). Aluminum probably reduces osteoblast numbers in bone both directly and through reduced parathyroid hormone action (Dunstan *et al.*, 1984).

As already noted, several neurological conditions—dialysis encephalopathy, amyotrophic lateral sclerosis and parkinsonism dementia (ALS-PD) on Guam, and *perhaps* Alzheimer's disease—are associated with elevated levels of aluminum in brain tissues. The symptoms of dialysis encephalopathy include speech difficulties, motor abnormalities, dementia, and eventually coma and death (King *et al.*, 1981). Moreover, behavioral changes have been reported in animals fed very high levels of aluminum (Bowdler *et al.*, 1979). Thus, clinical symptoms of these syndromes and those in animal models may appear similar, but histological and chemical analyses of brains have revealed differences.

Patients with dialysis encephalopathy have found to accumulate aluminum in most tissues, not just brain (King *et al.,* 1981; Heaf and Nielsen, 1984; Salusky *et al.,* 1984). Patients with Alzheimer's disease do not have elevated serum aluminum levels (Shore *et al.,* 1980). However, the two uremic infants who died after consuming aluminum-contaminated formulas exhibited elevated brain, but not bone, aluminum levels (Freudlich *et al.,* 1985).

The site of aluminum deposition within cells also differs between syndromes. The aluminum contents of the nuclear and heterochromatin fractions were elevated in brains from patients with Alzheimer's disease or with ALS-PD in Guam but not in those with dialysis encephalopathy (Crapper *et al.,* 1980; Perl *et al.,* 1982). DeBoni *et al.* (1976) found that rabbits injected sc with aluminum developed neurofibrillary degeneration, with aluminum being concentrated in the brain's nuclear chromatin.

Furthermore, the activity of choline acetyltransferase has been found to be reduced by 60–90% in the cerebral cortex and hippocampus formations of brains of patients with Alzheimer's disease (Coyle *et al.,* 1983). Hertnarski *et al.* (1980) observed that rabbits injected with aluminum developed neurofibrillary degeneration, but the activity of choline acetyltransferase in brain samples was unaltered.

The mechanism by which aluminum induces neurological damage in animal models and patients with dialysis encephalopathy and the pathogenic mechanism causing Alzheimer's disease and ALS-PD in Guam are unknown, but several possible mechanisms have been advanced. Banks and Kastin (1983) observed that aluminum increased the permeability of the blood–brain barrier to peptides such as β-endorphin. Gajdusek (1985) hypothesized that anything (trauma, aluminum, or subviral pathogens) that interfered with the slow axonal transport of neurofilaments down the axons of nerve cells could lead to amyloid accumulations and degeneration of the central nervous system. Obviously much work is needed.

3. Conclusions

At this time dietary exposure to aluminum does not appear to have adverse effects on healthy individuals. However, the long-term consequences of chronic use of pharmacological doses of aluminum by sensitive individuals (i.e., those with impaired kidney function, including the elderly and low-birthweight infants) need further evaluation.

III. SELENIUM

Selenium is an essential nutrient for animal and human health as well as a toxic element (Underwood, 1977).

A. Dietary Exposure to Selenium

The selenium content of human diets varies from 30 to 1000 μg/day (Keshan Disease Research Group, 1979; Thomson and Robinson, 1980; Yang *et al.*, 1983; Helzlsouer *et al.*, 1985), depending on the region of the world. Both the lowest and the highest dietary selenium levels exist in China. Generally, North Americans consume between 50 and 200 μg Se/day (Thompson *et al.*, 1975; Welsh *et al.*, 1981; Snook *et al.*, 1983; Lane *et al.*, 1983b). Unlike China, there are no reports in the United States of selenium toxicity when humans ingested all their selenium in foods.

Selenium concentration has been determined in a wide variety of foods and feeds (Morris and Levander, 1970; Thompson *et al.*, 1975; Lane *et al.*, 1983a; Olson and Palmer, 1984; Wolinsky *et al.*, 1986). In general, food selenium concentrations vary with soil selenium concentrations, soil types, climatic conditions, and types of plant. Thus, geographical regions have significant effects on food selenium concentration. Processing and treatment of foods also affect the final selenium concentration of foods (Higgs *et al.*, 1972). As a consequence of these various factors, it is difficult to generalize about selenium concentrations in foods.

However, selenium is generally associated with the protein fraction of the foods and thus, foods with low concentrations of protein frequently have low concentrations of selenium (Burk, 1978; Lane *et al.*, 1983a). Such foods are fruits, high-lipid and sugar-containing foods such as orange juice, salad dressing, cola drinks, and sugar cookies.

B. Metabolism of Selenium

1. *Gastrointestinal Absorption*

Generally apparent absorption of selenium is greater than the apparent absorption of most minerals by animals and humans (Thomson and Stewart, 1973; Whanger *et al.*, 1976; Stewart *et al.*, 1978; Robinson *et al.*, 1978; Levander *et al.*, 1981; Greger and Marcus, 1981; Swanson *et al.*, 1983).

A limited amount of work has been done on mechanisms of selenium absorption. McConnell and Cho (1965) were unable to demonstrate active transport of DL-selenocysteine. Canolty and Nasset (1975) found methionine and selenomethionine were equally wll absorbed, suggesting that absorption of selenomethionine is controlled by factors that control amino acids, not inorganic selenium absorption. McConnell and Cho (1965) on the basis of their studies with hamster intestine believed selenite absorption occurred by simple diffusion. Whanger *et al.* (1976) noted selenite was absorbed better from the duodenum than other intestinal segments. Wolfram *et al.* (1985) have observed that selenate was absorbed much faster than selenite and that selenate absorption occurred mainly in the lower small intestine by a saturable transport mechanism. Ardüser *et al.* (1985) suggested that a common transport mechanism exists for selenate and sulfate. Thus the gut does not appear to regulate selenium absorption per se.

A number of dietary factors, including the form of dietary selenium (i.e., selenite or selenomethionine) and dietary levels of sulfate and methionine, can affect the absorption of selenium (Lane *et al.*, 1979; Cantor *et al.*, 1981; Sunde *et al.*, 1981). The complexity of these interactions is further complicated by the fact that selenium bioavailability can be quite different from selenium "absorption." For example, Thomson and Stewart (1973) demonstrated that DL-selenomethionine disappeared from rat intestinal tracts slightly faster than selenite, but Whanger *et al.* (1976) observed no difference in selenium incorporation into tissues of animals dosed with selenite and selenomethionine. Furthermore, selenite prevents exudative diathesis more effectively than selenoamino acids, but selenomethionine prevents pancreatic fibrosis in chickens more effectively than selenite (Cantor *et al.*, 1981). DL-Selenoamino acids were used in these studies. Competition between the D- and L-forms may be one reason that selenoamino acids sometimes result in poorer nutritional status in regard to selenium than selenite.

2. *Selenium Excretion*

Burk (1978) has stated that "selenium homeostasis is accomplished by the production of excretory metabolites." Ganther and Hsieh (1974) proposed that inorganic salts of selenium were rapidly reduced in tissues of animals to selenotrisulfides, selenopersulfides, hydrogen selenide, di- and trimethyl selenide, and probably other low molecular weight metabolites and protein derivatives by the pathway shown in Fig. 1.

When toxic levels of selenite are fed, the excess selenium can be expelled in the breath as dimethyl selenide (Burk, 1978). However, urine is the major excretory route of excess selenium, and trimethylselenonium is a major metabolite (Kraus *et al.*, 1985). Previous nutritional status in regard to selenium may affect urinary excretion of standardized doses of selenium (Robinson *et al.*, 1985).

3. *Glutathione Peroxidase Activity*

Glutathione peroxidase (GSH-Px) is a selenium-containing enzyme and in fact is the only known mammalian function for selenium (Sunde and Hoekstra, 1980). Most mammalian tissues contain GSH-Px. The enzyme has a molecular weight of about 80,000, with 4 atoms of selenium per mole of enzyme.

C. Toxic Effects of Selenium

Levels of selenium that induce toxicity depend on form and route of administration of selenium and the species studied. To obtain a 40–50% death rate by iv injections, 3 and 1.5 mg Se/kg was required for rats and rabbits, respectively

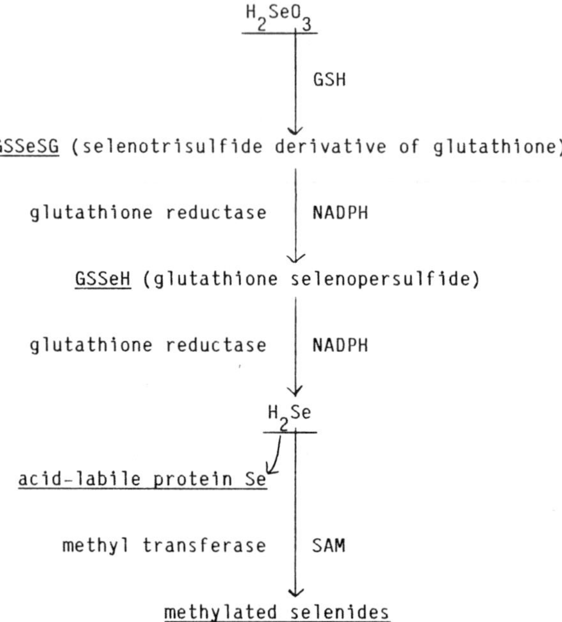

Fig. 1. Proposed mechanism of metabolism and excretion of inorganic selenium salts (Ganther and Hsieh, 1974).

(Wilber, 1980). The LD$_{50}$ values for rats of selenium as selenocystine, selenomethionine, and dimethyl selenide were 4, 4.3, and 1600 mg Se/kg body weight. Thompson and co-workers (1984) found hepatotoxicity among rats fed 6 µg Se/gm diet as selenomethionine but not among those fed selenite. Selenium toxicity has been a practical problem in domestic livestock and has been well reviewed elsewhere (Wilber, 1980; Goehring *et al.*, 1984; Mahan and Moxon, 1984; Lo and Sandi, 1980; El-Begearmi and Combs, 1982). This review will focus on human selenium toxicity and on recent reports on the environmentally disastrous selenium contamination to the Kesterson National Wildlife Refuge.

1. *Dental Caries*

Hadjimarkos and co-workers (1952) demonstrated a higher incidence of dental caries in children with urinary selenium levels above 0.07 ppm than in children with lower urinary levels. Although the mechanism of this toxicity is unknown, animal studies have confirmed the observation (Britton *et al.*, 1980; Bowen, 1972).

2. *Cataracts*

Ostadalova *et al.* (1979) found that sc administration of 30 µg Se as selenite per kilogram body weight to suckling rat pups resulted in increased permanent lens cataracts. Premature weaning protected rats against selenium-induced cataracts (Babicky and Ostadalova, 1982). The mechanism for cataract formation has not been elucidated, but Bunce *et al.* (1983) has suggested that both selenium and GSH may be involved. The potential importance of this form of selenium toxicity to human premature neonates given selenium in TPN solutions has not been adequately assessed.

3. *Wildlife Selenium Toxicity*

In 1985 an acute selenium toxicity outbreak in wildlife living in the Kesterson National Wildlife Refuge (a region of the San Joaquin Valley in California) received a great deal of attention in the popular press (Beno, 1985; Smith, 1984). The U.S. Department of Interior, Fish and Wildlife Service reported that the selenosis was caused by specific agricultural water management practices that concentrated selenium and other minerals in water. Water runoff from the mountains was used for irrigation, then recaptured by drain tiles layered under the agriculture fields and used for grasslands and wetlands. The water eventually drained into the San Joaquin River.

Water in the Kesterson ponds contained 0.0089–0.3143 μg Se/ml (Smith, 1984). The U.S. Environmental Protection Agency water quality criterion for these ponds is less than 0.035 μg Se/ml. Between 1972 and 1981 there was a significant increase in selenium concentrations in Sacramento blackfish—from 0.131 to 1.17 μg/gm (Smith, 1984). Ohlendorf *et al.* (1986) reported that waterfowl in this area had increased congenital defects, such as abnormal eyes. legs, and feet, stilts, and wings, and exencephaly. Liver selenium concentrations of these birds ranged from 21 to 63 μg/gm, while eggs contained 34–110 μg Se/gm. Normal levels are less than 2 μg Se/gm.

Human toxicities have not been reported, probably because the local residents have been warned to reduce drastically their consumption of fish and birds from the Kesterson ponds. It is logical to assume that a selenium buildup in the food chain could occur in other regions where water is recycled in a similar manner.

4. *Human Selenium Toxicity in China*

An outbreak of acute human selenosis in Enshi County of Hubei Province, China, was confirmed in 1961–1964 (Yang *et al.*, 1983). Although several regions of China had high soil selenium levels, acute selenosis occurred only in this region. Selenosis probably occurred in Enshi County because soil selenium was more available for incorporation into plants after the application of lime to the fields. The lime increased soil pH and may have oxidized the soil selenium into a more soluble form.

Acute selenosis affected 49.2% of the 248 residents in the Enshi region. This selenosis was characterized primarily by loss of hair and nails, skin lesions, tooth decay, and several neurological symptoms. Neurological problems occurred in 18 residents and included the following: peripheral anesthesia, acroparesthesia, pain in the extremities, hyperreflexia of the tendon, some numbness, convulsion, motor disturbances, and paralysis. Removal of the residents from the selenosis

TABLE I

Comparison of Average Selenium Concentrations in Blood, Hair, and Urine of Subjects from Regions with High Soil and Water Selenium Levels in China and the United States

	Exposure estimates (mg/day)	Whole blood[c] (μg/ml)	Hair[c] (μg/gm)	Urine[c] (μg/ml)
China[a]				
Patients with selenosis	4.99	3.2	32.2	2.68
		(1.3–7.5)	(4.1–100)	(0.88–6.63)
Subjects from "adequate"				
Se area	0.12	0.10	0.36	0.03
United States[b]				
Subjects from "high" Se area	0.54	0.17	0.46	0.08
		(0.13–0.25)	(0.02–2.0)	(0.02–0.20)

[a]Yang *et al.* (1983).
[b]Valentine *et al.* (1978).
[c]Range in parentheses.

district resulted in immediate reversal of all symptoms except those of the nervous system. Neurological symptoms eventually reversed in 17 patients.

Table I compares the levels of selenium in samples from Chinese control subjects (with no exposure to high-selenium areas), U.S. subjects consuming water containing high selenium levels (Valentine *et al.*, 1978), and patients with selenosis. The Chinese patients with selenosis had significantly higher selenium levels in blood, hair, and urine than the other subjects, suggesting that any of these three measures could be useful indices of high selenium exposure.

5. Human Selenium Toxicity in the United States

Acute selenosis was reported in 13 individuals (Helzlsouer *et al.*, 1985) consuming tablets containing from 27 to more than 2000 mg Se/day over 1 day to 2.5 months. All the individuals experienced nausea and some experienced abdominal pain and diarrhea. Similar to the selenosis found in China, other symptoms included nail and hair changes, peripheral neuropathy, fatigue, and irritability. A 57-year-old female who consumed nearly 2000 mg selenium had nail loss and alopecia; her serum selenium level was 0.53 μg/ml (Jensen and Clossen, 1984). Typical human selenosis is shown in Figs. 2–3. Helzlsouer and co-workers reported rapid reversal of the symptoms when subjects stopped ingesting the supplements.

6. Conclusions

Human selenosis is rare and depends on consumption of excessive levels of selenium, greater than 1 mg/day. However, human selenosis can occur. Condi-

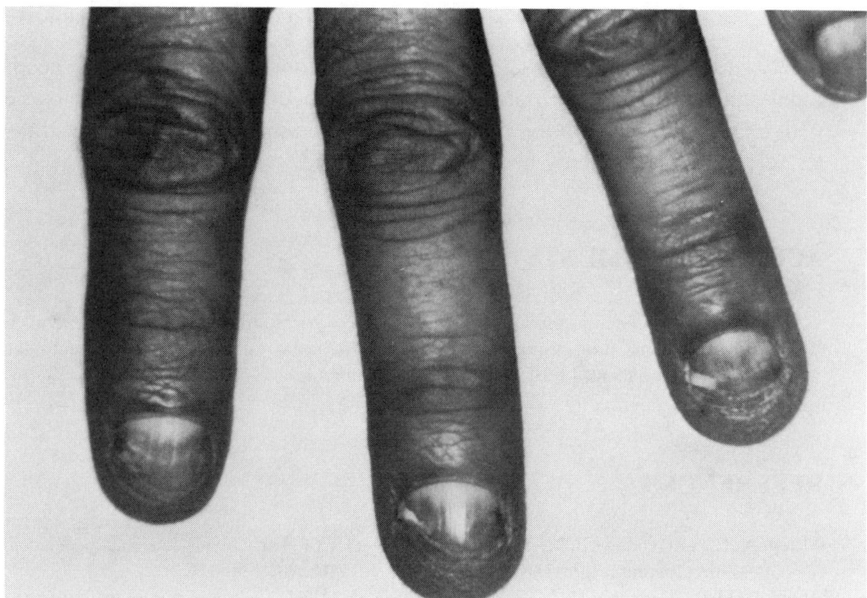

Fig. 2. Nail changes in a middle-aged man who had consumed a selenium-containing supplement for a 2-week period. Total dose was calculated to be 1500 mg selenium (50 tablets). Nails developed white streaks, separated from the nailbed, and sloughed off. New nails can be seen forming.

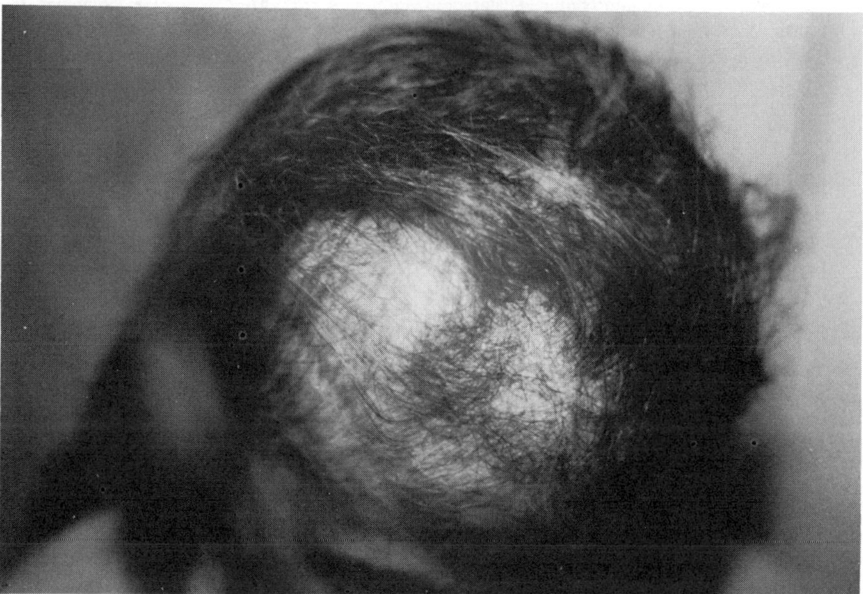

Fig. 3. Partial alopecia in a 57-year-old woman who had consumed a selenium-containing supplement that contained 30 mg per tablet. She consumed this supplement for a period of 77 days, one tablet per day (total dose 2310 mg selenium). Hair was dry and brittle, leading to breakage.

tions that lead to increased selenium concentrations in the food supply need to be monitored. In the United States, the greatest potential for human selenosis exists with excessive consumption of selenium-containing tablets; thus over-the-counter selenium supplements need to be monitored.

ACKNOWLEDGMENTS

The authors appreciate the support of the College of Agriculture and Life Sciences, University of Wisconsin—Madison, project no. 2623, and the Alabama Agricultural Experiment Station at Auburn. The authors thank Dr. R. Jacobs for supplying the photographs.

REFERENCES

Alfrey, A. C., LeGendre, G. R., and Kaehny, W. D. (1976). The dialysis encephalopathy syndrome: Possible aluminum intoxications. *N. Engl. J. Med.* **294,** 184–188.

Andreoli, S. P., Bergstein, J. M., and Sherrard, D. J. (1984). Aluminum intoxication from aluminum-containing phosphate binders in children with azotemia not undergoing dialysis. *N. Engl. J. Med.* **310,** 1079–1084.

Ardüser, F., Wolfgram, S., and Scharrer, E. (1985). Active absorption of selenate by rat. *J. Nutr.* **115,** 1203–1208.

Babicky, A., and Ostadalova, I. (1982). Protective effect of premature weaning against the appearance of selenium induced cataract in young rats. *IRCS Med. Sci.: Libr. Compend.* **10,** 464.

Banks, W. A., and Kastin, A. J. (1983). Aluminum increases permeability of the blood–brain barrier to labeled DSIP and β-endorphin: Possible implications for senile and dialysis dementia. *Lancet* **2,** 1127–1229.

Barker, W. H., Jr., and Runte, V. (1972). Tomato juice-associated gastroenteritis, Washington and Oregon, 1969. *Am. J. Epidemiol.* **96,** 219–226.

Beisel, W. R. (1982). Single nutrients and immunity. *Am. J. Clin. Nutr.* **35,** 417–468.

Beno, M. (1985). What price water? *Ducks Unlimited* **49,** 83, 116–118.

Benoy, C. J., Hooper, P. A., and Schneider, R. (1971). The toxicity of tin in canned fruit juices and solid foods. *Food Cosmet. Toxicol.* **9,** 645–656.

Bowdler, N. C., Beasley, D. S., Fritze, E. C., Goulette, A. M., Hatton, J. D., Hession, J., Ostman, D. L., Rugg, D. J., and Schmittdiel, C. J. (1979). Behavioral effects of aluminum ingestion on animal and human subjects. *Pharmacol., Biochem. Behav.* **10,** 505–512.

Bowen, W. H. (1972). The effects of selenium and vanadium on caries activity in monkeys (*M. irus*). *Ir. Dent. Assoc.* **18,** 83–89.

Britton, J. L., Shearer, T. R., and DeSart, D. J. (1980). Cariostasis by moderate doses of selenium in the rat model. *Arch. Environ. Health* **35,** 74–76.

Bunce, G. E., Wisthoff, F., and Hess, J. L. (1983). Lens metabolic changes which precede cataract in selenite-injected young rats. *Fed. Proc., Fed. Am. Soc. Exp. Biol.* **42,** 928.

Burba, J. V. (1983). Inhibition of hepatic azo-reductase and aromatic hydroxylase by radiopharmaceuticals containing tin. *Toxicol. Lett.* **18,** 269–272.

Burk, R. F. (1978). Selenium in nutrition. *World Rev. Nutr. Diet.* **30,** 88–106.

Calloway, D. H., and McMullen, J. J. (1966). Fecal excretion of iron and tin by men fed stored canned foods. *Am. J. Clin. Nutr.* **18,** 1–5.

Cam, J. M., Luck, V. A., Eastwood, J. B., and deWardener, H. E. (1976). The effect of aluminum hydroxide orally on calcium, phosphorus and aluminum metabolism in normal subjects. *Clin. Sci. Mol. Med.* **51**, 407–414.

Cannata, J. B., Junor, B. J. R., Briggs, J. D., Fell, G. S., and Beastall, G. (1983). Effect of acute aluminum overload on calcium and parathyroid hormone metabolism. *Lancet* **1**, 501–503.

Canolty, N. L., and Nasset, E. S. (1975). Intestinal absorption of free and protein-bound methionine in the rat. *J. Nutr.* **105**, 867–877.

Cantor, A. H., Moorhead, P. D., and Musser, M. A. (1981). Biological availability of selenium in selenium compounds and feed ingredients. *In* "Selenium in Biology and Medicine" (J. E. Spallholz, J. L. Martin, and H. E. Ganther, eds.), pp. 192–202. Avi Publ. Co., Westport, Connecticut.

Capar, S. G., and Boyer, K. W. (1980). Multielement analysis of foods stored in their opened cans. *J. Food Saf.* **2**, 105–118.

Chan, Y. L., Alfrey, A. C., Posen, S., Lissner, D., Hills, E., Dunstan, C. R., and Evans, R. A. (1983). Effect of aluminum on normal and uremic rats: Tissue distribution, vitamin D metabolites and quantitative bone histology. *Calcif. Tissue Int.* **35**, 344–351.

Chiba, M., and Kikuchi, M. (1984). The in vitro effects of zinc and manganese on δ-aminolevulinic acid dehydratase activity inhibited by lead or tin. *Toxicol. Appl. Pharmacol.* **73**, 388–394.

Chiba, M., Ogihara, K., and Kikuchi, M. (1980). Effect of tin on porphyrin biosynthesis. *Arch. Toxicol.* **45**, 189–195.

Clarkson, E. M., Luck, V. A., Hynson, W. V., Bailey, R. R., Eastwood, J. B., Woodhead, J. S., Clements, V. R., O'Riordan, J. L. H., and deWardener, H. E. (1972). The effect of aluminum hydroxide on calcium, phosphorus and aluminum balances, the serum parathyroid hormone concentration and the aluminum content of bone in patients with chronic renal failure. *Clin. Sci.* **43**, 519–531.

Committee on Food Additives Survey Data (1984). "Poundage Update of Food Chemicals, 1982," PB 84-16214. Natl. Acad. Press, Washington, D.C.

Committee on the GRAS List Survey—Phase III (1979). "The 1977 Survey of Industry on the Use of Food Additives," pp. 1786, 1789, 1973, 1918, 1922, 1923, 1955. Natl. Acad. Sci., Washington, D.C.

Cournot-Witmer, G., Zingraff, J., Plachot, J. J., Escaig, F., Lefevre, R., Boumati, P., Bourdeau, A., Garabedian, M., Galle, P., Bourdon, R., Drueke, T., and Balsan, S. (1981). Aluminum localization in bone from hemodialyzed patients: Relationship to matrix mineralization. *Kidney Int.* **20**, 375–385.

Coyle, J. T., Price, D. L., and DeLong, M. R. (1983). Alzheimer's disease: A disorder of cortical cholinergic innervation. *Science* **219**, 1184–1190.

Crapper, D. R., Krishnan, S. S., and Quittkat, S. (1976). Aluminum neurofibrillary degeneration and Alzheimer's disease. *Brain* **99**, 67–80.

Crapper, D. R., Quittkat, S., Krishnan, S. S., Dalton, A. J., and DeBoni, U. (1980). Intranuclear aluminum content in Alzheimer's disease, dialysis encephalopathy, and experimental aluminum encephalopathy. *Acta Neuropathol.* **50**, 19–24.

Crapper-McLachlan, D. R., Farnell, B., Galin, H., Karlik, S., Eichhorn, G., and DeBoni, U. (1983). Aluminum in human brain disease. *In* "Biological Aspects of Metals and Metal-Related Disease" (B. Sarkar, ed.), pp. 209–219. Raven Press, New York.

DeBoni, V., Otvos, A., Scott, J. W., and Crapper, D. R. (1976). Neurofibrillary degeneration induced systemic aluminum. *Acta Neuropathol.* **35**, 285–294.

deGroot, A. P. (1973). Subacute toxicity of inorganic tin as influenced by dietary levels of iron and copper. *Food Cosmet. Toxicol.* **11**, 955–962.

deGroot, A. P., Feron, V. J., and Til, H. P. (1973). Short-term toxicity studies on some salts and oxides of tin in rats. *Food Cosmet. Toxicol.* **11**, 19–30.

Dent, C. E., and Winter, C. S. (1974). Osteomalacia due to phosphate depletion from excessive aluminum hydroxide ingestion. *Br. Med. J.* **1**, 551–552.

deVernejoul, M. C., Messing, B., Modrowski, D., Bielakoff, J., Buisine, A., and Miravet, L. (1985). Multifactoral low remodeling bone disease during cyclic total parenteral nutrition. *J. Clin. Endocrinol. Metab.* **60,** 109–112.

Dimitrov, N. V., Meyer, C., Nakhas, F., Miller, C., and Averill, B. A. (1981). Effect of tin on immune responses of mice. *Clin. Immunol. Immunopathol.* **20,** 39–48.

Dreef van der Meulen, H. C., Feron, V. J., and Til, H. P. (1974). Pancreatic atrophy and other pathological changes in rats following feeding of stannous chloride. *Pathol. Eur.* **9,** 185–192.

Drüeke, T. (1980). Dialysis osteomalacia and aluminum intoxication. *Nephron* **26,** 207–210.

Dunstan, C. R., Evans, R. A., Hills, E., Wong, S. Y. P., and Alfrey, A. C. (1984). Effect of aluminum and parathyroid hormone on osteoblasts and bone mineralization in chronic renal failure. *Calcif. Tissue Int.* **36,** 133–138.

Dyer, R. S., Walsh, T. J., Wonderlin, W. F., and Bercegeay, M. (1982). The trimethyltin syndrome in rats. *Neurobehav. Toxicol. Teratol.* **4,** 127–133.

El-Begearmi, M. M., and Combs, G. F., Jr. (1982). Dietary effects on selenite toxicity in the chick. *Poult. Sci.* **61,** 770–776.

Feinroth, M., Feinroth, M. V., and Berlyne, G. M. (1982). Aluminum absorption in the rat everted gut sac. *Miner. Electrolyte Metab.* **8,** 29–35.

Freundlich, M., Abitbol, C., Zilleruelo, G., Strauss, J., Faugere, M. C., and Mallucke, H. H. (1985). Infant formula as a case of aluminum toxicity in neonatal uremia. *Lancet* **2,** 527–529.

Fritsch, P., deSaint Blanquat, G., and Derache, R. (1977). Effect of various dietary components on absorption and tissue distribution of orally administered inorganic tin in rats. *Food Cosmet. Toxicol.* **15,** 147–149.

Gajdusek, D. C. (1985). Hypothesis, interference with axonal transport of neurofilament as a common pathogenetic mechanism in certain diseases of the central nervous system. *N. Engl. J. Med.* **312,** 714–719.

Ganther, H. E., and Hsieh, M. S. (1974). Mechanisms for the conversion of selenite to selenides in mammalian tissues. *In* "Trace Element Metabolism in Animals-2" (W. G. Hoekstra, J. W. Suttie, H. E. Ganther, and W. Mertz eds.), pp. 339–353. University Park Press, Baltimore, Maryland.

Garruto, R. M., Fukatsu, R., Yanagihara, R., Gajdusek, D. C., Hook, G., and Fiori, C. E. (1984). Imaging of calcium and aluminum in neurofibrillary tangle-bearing neurons in parkinsonism-dementia of Guam. *Proc. Natl. Acad. Sci. U.S.A* **81,** 1875–1879.

Goehring, T. B., Palmer, I. S., Olsen, O. E., Libal, G. W., and Wahlstrom, R. C. (1984). Toxic effects of selenium on growing swine fed corn–soybean meal diets. *J. Anim. Sci.* **59,** 733–737.

Gorsky, J. E., Dietz, A. A., Spencer, H., and Osis, D. (1979). Metabolic balance of aluminum studies in six men. *Clin. Chem. (Winston. Salem, N.C.)* **25,** 1739–1743.

Greger, J. L. (1985). Aluminum content of the American diet. *Food Technol.* **39,** 73, 74, 76, 78–80.

Greger, J. L., and Baier, M. (1981). Tin and iron content of canned and bottled food. *J. Food Sci.* **46,** 1751–1754, 1765.

Greger, J. L., and Baier, M. J. (1983a). Excretion and retention of low or moderate levels of aluminum by human subjects. *Food Chem. Toxicol.* **21,** 473–477.

Greger, J. L., and Baier, M. J. (1983b). Effect of dietary aluminum on mineral metabolism of adult males. *Am. J. Clin. Nutr.* **38,** 411–419.

Greger, J. L., and Johnson, M. A. (1981). Effect of dietary tin on zinc, copper, and iron utilization by rats. *Food Cosmet. Toxicol.* **19,** 163–166.

Greger, J. L., and Marcus, R. E. (1981). Effect of dietary protein, phosphorus and sulfur amino acids on selenium metabolism of adult males. *Ann. Nutr. Metab.* **25,** 97–108.

Greger, J. L., Smith, S. A., Johnson, M. A., and Baier, M. J. (1982). Effects of dietary tin and aluminum on selenium utilization by adult males. *Biol. Trace Elem. Res.* **4,** 269–278.

Greger, J. L., Bula, E. N., and Gum, E. T. (1985a). Mineral metabolism of rats fed moderate levels of various aluminum compounds for short periods of time. *J. Nutr.* **115,** 1708–1716.

Greger, J. L., Goetz, W., and Sullivan, D. (1985b). Aluminum levels in foods cooked and stored in aluminum pans, trays and foil. *J. Food Prot.* **48,** 772–777.

Greger, J. L., Gum, E. T., and Bula, E. N. (1986). Mineral metabolism of rats fed various level of aluminum hydroxide. *Biol. Trace Elem. Res.* **9,** 67–77.

Griswold, W. R., Reznik, V., Mendoza, S. A., Trauner, D., and Alfrey, A. C. (1983). Accumulation of aluminum in a nondialyzed uremic child receiving aluminum hydroxide. *Pediatrics* **71,** 56–58.

Hadjimarkos, D. M., Storvick, C. A., and Remmert, L. F. (1952). Selenium and dental caries. An investigation among school children of Oregon. *J. Pediatr.* **40,** 451–455.

Hambidge, K. M., Walravens, P. A., Brown, R. M., Webster, J., White, S., Anthony, M., and Roth, M. L. (1976). Zinc nutrition of preschool children in the Denver Head Start Program. *Am. J. Clin. Nutr.* **29,** 734–738.

Haug, A. (1984). Molecular aspects of aluminum toxicity. *CRC Crit. Rev. Plant Sci.* **1,** 345–373.

Heaf, J. G., and Nielsen, L. P. (1984). Serum aluminum in hemodialysis patients: Relation to osteodystrophy, encephalopathy and aluminum hydroxide consumption. *Miner. Electrolyte Metab.* **10,** 345–350.

Helzlsouer, K., Jacobs, R., and Morris, S. (1985). Acute selenium intoxication in the United States. *Fed. Proc., Fed. Am. Soc. Exp. Biol.* **44,** 1670 (Abstr. 7366).

Hetnarski, B., Wisniewski, H. M., Iqbal, K., Dziedzic, J. D., and Lajtha, A. (1980). Central cholinergic activity in aluminum-induced neurofibrillary degeneration. *Ann. Neurol.* **7,** 489–490.

Higgs, D. J., Morris, V. C., and Levander, O. A. (1972). Effect of cooking on selenium content of foods. *J. Agric. Food Chem.* **20.** 678–680.

Hiles, R. A. (1974). Absorption, distribution and excretion of inorganic tin in rats. *Toxicol. Appl. Pharmacol.* **27,** 366–379.

Hill, C. H., and Matrone, G. (1970). Chemical parameters in the study on in vivo and in vitro interactions of transition elements. *Fed. Proc., Fed. Am. Soc. Exp. Biol.* **29,** 1474–1481.

Insogna, K. L., Bordley, D. R., Caro, J. F., and Lockwood, D. H. (1980). Osteomalacia and weakness from excessive antacid ingestion. *JAMA, J. Am. Med. Assoc.* **244,** 2544–2546.

Jensen, R., and Clossen, W. (1984). Selenium intoxication—New York, *JAMA, J. Am. Med. Assoc.* **251,** 1938.

Johnson, M. A., and Greger, J. L. (1982). Effects of dietary tin on tin and clacium metabolism of adult males. *Am. J. Clin. Nutr.* **35,** 655–660.

Johnson, M. A., and Greger, J. L. (1984). Absorption, distribution and endogenous excretion of zinc by rats fed various dietary levels of inorganic tin and zinc. *J. Nutr.* **114,** 1843–1852.

Johnson, M. A., and Greger, J. L. (1985). Tin, copper, iron and calcium metabolism of rats fed various dietary levels of inorganic tin and zinc. *J. Nutr.* **115,** 615–624.

Johnson, M. A., Baier, M. J., and Greger, J. L. (1982). Effects of dietary tin on zinc, copper, iron, manganese and magnesium metabolism of adult males. *Am. J. Clin. Nutr.* **35,** 1332–1338.

Kaehny, W. D., Hegg, A. P., and Alfrey, A. C. (1977). Gastrointestinal absorption of aluminum from aluminum-containing antacids. *N. Engl. J. Med.* **296,** 1389–1390.

Kappas, A., and Maines, M. D. (1976). Tin: A potent inducer of heme oxygenase in kidney. *Science* **192,** 60–62.

Keshan Disease Research Group (1979). Epidemiological studies on the etiological relationship of selenium on the etiological relationship of selenium and Keshan disease. *Chin. Med. J.* **92,** 471–472.

Kimbrough, R. D. (1976). Toxicity and health effects of selected organotin compounds: A review. *Environ. Health Perspect.* **14,** 51–56.

King, S. W., Savory, J., and Wills, M. R. (1981). The clinical biochemistry of aluminum. *CRC Crit. Rev. Clin. Lab. Sci.* **14,** 1–20.

Klein, G. L., Alfrey, A. C., Miller, N. L., Sherrard, D. J., Hazlet, T. K., Ament, M. E., and

Coburn, J. W. (1982). Aluminum loading during total parenteral nutrition. *Am. J. CLin. Nutr.* **35**, 1425–1429.

Kovalchik, M. T., Kaehny, W. D., Hegg, A. P., Jackson, J. T., and Alfrey, A. C. (1978). Aluminum kinetics during hemodialysis. *J. Lab. Clin. Med.* **92**, 712–720.

Kraus, R. J., Foster, S. J., and Ganther, H. E. (1985). Analysis of trimethyl-selenonium ion in urine by high performance liquid chromatography. *Anal. Biochem.* **147**, 432–436.

Kumpulainen, J., and Koivistoinen, P. (1977). Advances in tin compound analysis with special reference to organotin pesticide residues. *Residue Rev.* **66**, 1–18.

Lane, H. W., Shirley, R. L., and Cerda, J. J. (1979). Glutathione peroxidase activity in intestinal and liver tissues of rats fed various levels of selenium, sulfur, and α-tocopherol. *J. Nutr.* **109**, 444–452.

Lane, H. W., Taylor, B. J., Stool, E., Servance, D., and Warren, D. C. (1983a). Selenium content of selected foods. *J. Am. Diet. Assoc.* **82**, 24–28.

Lane, H. W., Warren, D. C., Taylor, B. J., and Stool, E. (1983b). Blood selenium and glutathione-peroxidase levels and dietary selenium of free-living and institutionalized elderly subjects. *Proc. Soc. Exp. Biol. Med.* **173**, 87–95.

Levander, O. A., Sutherland, B., Morris, V. C., and King, J. C. (1981). Selenium balance in young men during selenium depletion and repletion. *Am. J. Clin. Nutr.* **34**, 2662–2669.

Levine, S., and Sowinski, R. (1983). Tin salts prevent the plasma cell response to metallic tin in Lewis rats. *Toxicol. Appl. Pharmacol.* **68**, 110–115.

Lione, A. (1983). The prophylactic reduction of aluminum intake. *Food Chem. Toxicol.* **21**, 103–109.

Lione, A. (1984). Letters to the editor. *Nutr. Rev.* **42**, 31.

Lo, M., and Sandi, E. (1980). Selenium: Occurrence in foods and its toxicological significance—a review. *J. Environ. Pathol. Toxicol.* **4**, 193–218.

Lotz, M., Zisman, E., and Bartter, F. C. (1968). Evidence for a phosphorus-depletion syndrome in man. *N. Engl. J. Med.* **278**, 409–415.

McConnell, K. P., and Cho, G. J. (1965). Transmucosal movement of selenium. *Am. J. Physiol.* **208**, 1191–1195.

McDermott, J. R., Smith, I., Igbal, K., and Wisniewski, H. M. (1979). Brain aluminum in aging and Alzheimer disease. *Neurology* **29**, 809–814.

McLean, J. R. N., Blakey, D. H., Douglas, G. R., and Kaplan, J. G. (1983). The effect of stannous and stannic (tin) chloride on DNA in Chinese hamster ovary cells. *Mutat. Res.* **119**, 195–201.

Mahan, D. C., Moxon, A. L. (1984). Effect of inorganic selenium supplementation on selenosis in postweaning swine. *J. Anim. Sci.* **58**, 1216–1221.

Markesbery, W. R., Ehmann, W. D., Hossain, T. I. M., Alauddin, M., and Goodin, D. T. (1981). Instrumental neutron activation analysis of brain aluminum in Alzheimer disease and aging. *Ann. Neurol.* **10**, 511–516.

Morris, V. C., and Levander, O. A. (1970). Selenium content of foods. *J. Nutr.* **100**, 1383–1388.

Nagy, S., Rouseff, R., and Ting, S. V. (1980). Effects of temperature and storage on the iron and tin contents of commercially canned single-strength orange juice. *J. Agric. Food Chem.* **28**, 1166–1169.

Nathan, E., and Pederson, S. E. (1980). Dialysis encephalopathy in a non-dialyzed uremic body treated with aluminum hydroxide orally. *Acta Paediatr. Scand.* **69**, 793–796.

Nielsen, F. H. (1984). Effect of boron nutriture on the response of rats to high dietary aluminum. *In* "Trace Substances in Environmental Health–XVIII" (D. D. Hemphill, ed.), pp. 47–52. University of Missouri, Columbia.

Ogoshi, K., Kurumatani, N., Aoki, Y., Moriyama, T., and Nanzai, Y. (1981). Decrease in compressive strength of the femoral bone in rats administered stannous chloride for a short period. *Toxicol. Appl. Pharmacol.* **58**, 331–332.

Ohlendorf, M. M., Hoffman, D. J., Saiki, M. K., and Aldrich, T. W. (1986). Embryonic mortality and abnormalities of aquatic birds: Apparent impacts by selenium from irrigation drainwater. *Sci. Total Environ.* **52,** 49–63.

Olson, O. E., and Palmer, I. E. (1984). Selenium in foods purchased or produced in South Dakota. *Food Sci.* **49,** 446–452.

Ondreička, R., Kortus, J., and Ginter, E. (1971). Aluminum, its absorption, distribution and effects on phosphorus metabolism. *In* "Intestinal Absorption of Metal Ions, Trace Elements, and Radionuclides" (S. C. Skoryna and D. Waldron-Edward, eds.), pp. 293–305. Permagon, Oxford.

Ostadalova, I., Babicky, A., and Obenberger, J. (1979). Cataractogenic and lethal effect of selenite in rats during postnatal ontogenesis. *Physiol. Bohemoslov.* **28,** 393–397.

Perl, D. P., Gajdusek, D. C., Garruto, R. M., Yanagihara, R. T., and Gibbs, C. J., Jr. (1982). Intraneuronal aluminum accumulation in amyotrophic lateral sclerosis and Parkinsonism-dementia of Guam. *Science* **217,** 1053–1055.

Perl, D. P., and Brody, A. R. (1980). Alzheimer's disease: X-ray spectrometric evidence of aluminum accumulation in neurofibrillary tangle-bearing neurons. *Science* **208,** 297–299.

Poe, C. F., and Leberman, J. M. (1949). The effect of acid foods on aluminum cooking utensils. *Food Technol.* **3,** 71–74.

Recker, R. R., Blotcky, A. J., Leffler, J. A., and Rack, E. P. (1977). Evidence for aluminum absorption from the gastrointestinal tract and bone deposition by aluminum carbonate ingestion with normal renal function. *J. Lab. Clin. Med.* **90,** 810–815.

Robinson, J. R., Robinson, M. F., Levander, O. A., and Thomson, C. D. (1985). Urinary excretion of selenium by New Zealand and North American human subjects on differing intakes. *Am. J. Clin. Nutr.* **41,** 1023–1031.

Robinson, M. F., Rea, H. M., Friend, G. M., Stewart, R. D. H., Snow, P. C., and Thomson, C. D. (1978). On supplementing the selenium intake of New Zealanders. *Br. J. Nutr.* **39,** 589–599.

Rosa, I. V., Henry, P. R., and Ammerman, C. B. (1982). Interrelationship of dietary phosphorus, aluminum and iron on performance and tissue mineral composition in lambs. *J. Anim. Sci.* **55,** 1231–1240.

Said, A. N., Slagsvold, P., Bergh, H., and Laksesvela, B. (1977). High fluorine water to wether sheep maintained in pens. *Nord. Veterinaer Med.* **29,** 172–180.

Salusky, I. B., Coburn, J. W., Paunier, L., Sherrard, D. J., and Fine, R. N. (1984). Role of aluminum hydroxide in raising serum aluminum levels in children undergoing continuous ambulatory peritoneal dialysis. *J. Pediatr.* **105,** 717–720.

Sandstead, H. H., Henriksen, L. K., Greger, J. G., Prasad, A., and Good, R. A. (1982). Zinc nutritive in the elderly in relation to taste acuity, immune response and wound healing. *Am. J. Clin. Nutr.* **36,** 1046–1059.

Schlettwein-Gsell, D., and Mommsen-Straub, S. (1973). Spurenelemente in Lebensmitteln. XII. Aluminium. *Int. J. Vitam. Nutr. Res.* **43,** 251–263.

Schroeder, H. A., Balassa, J. J., and Tipton, I. H. (1964). Abnormal trace metals in man: Tin. *J. Chronic. Dis.* **17,** 483–502.

Schwarz, K., Milne, D. B., and Vinyard, E. (1970). Growth effects of tin compounds in rats maintained in a trace element-controlled environment. *Biochem. Biophys. Res. Commun.* **40,** 22–29.

Science and Education Adminstration (1980). "Nationwide Food Consumption Survey 1977–78, "Prelim. Rep. No. 2., p. 75. U.S. Dept. of Agriculture, Washington, D.C.

Sherlock, J. C., and Smart, G. A. (1984). Tin in foods and the diet. *Food Addit. Contam.* **1,** 277–282.

Shore, D., Millson, M., Holtz, J. L., King, S. W., Bridge, T. P., and Wyatt, R. J. (1980). Serum aluminum in primary degenerative dementia. *Biol. Psychol.* **15,** 971–977.

Skikne, B. S., Lynch, S. R., and Cook, J. D. (1981). Role of gastric acid in food iron absorption. *Gastroenterology* **81,** 1068–1071.

Slanina, P., Falkiborn, Y., Frech, W., and Cedergren, A. (1984). Aluminum concentrations in the brain and bone of rats fed citric acid, aluminum citrate or aluminum hydroxide. *Food Chem. Toxicol.* **22,** 391–397.

Slanina, P., Frech, W., Bernhardson, A., Cedergren, A., and Mattsson, P. (1985). Influence of dietary factors on aluminum absorption and retention in the brain and bone of rats. *Acta Pharmacol. Toxicol.* **56,** 331–336.

Smith, F. E. (1984). A discussion—selenium sources and associated problems in the San Joaquin Valley (personal communication).

Snook, J. T., Palmquist, D. L., Moxon, A. L., Cantor, A. H., and Vivian, V. M. (1983). Selenium status of a rural (predominantly Amish) community living in a low-selenium area. *Am. J. Clin. Nutr.* **38,** 620–630.

Solomons, N. W., Marchini, J. S., Duarte-Favaro, R. M., Vannuchi, H., and Dutra de Oliveira, J. E. (1983). Studies on the bioavailability of zinc in humans: Intestinal interaction of tin and zinc. *Am. J. Clin. Nutr.* **37,** 566–571.

Sorenson, J. R. J., Campbell, I. R., Tepper, L. B., and Lingg, R. D. (1974). Aluminum in the environment and human health. *Environ. Health Perspect.* **8,** 3–95.

Spencer, H., Kramer, L., Norris, C., and Wiatrowski, E. (1980). Effect of aluminum hydroxide on fluoride metabolism. *Clin. Pharmacol. Ther.* **28,** 529–535.

Spencer, H., Kramer, L., Norris, C., and Osis, D. (1982). Effect of small doses of aluminum-containing antacids on calcium and phosphorus metabolism. *Am. J. Clin. Nutr.* **36,** 32–40.

Squibb, R. E., Carmichael, N. G., and Tilson, H. A. (1980). Behavioral and neuromorphological effects of triethyl tin bromide in adult rats. *Toxicol. Appl. Pharmacol.* **55,** 188–197.

Stewart, R. D. H., Griffiths, N. M., Thomson, C. D., and Robinson, M. F. (1978). Quantitative selenium metabolism in normal New Zealand women. *Br. J. Nutr.* **40,** 45–54.

Sunde, R. A., and Hoekstra, W. G. (1980). Structure, synthesis and function of glutathione peroxidase. *Nutr. Rev.* **38,** 265–273.

Sunde, R. A., Gutzke, G. E., and Hoekstra, W. G. (1981). Effect of dietary methionine on the biopotency of selenite and selenomethionine in the rat. *J. Nutr.* **111,** 76–86.

Swanson, C. A., Reamer, D. C., Veillon, C., King, J. C., and Levander, O. A. (1983). Quantitative and qualitative aspects of selenium utilization in pregnant and non-pregnant women: An application of stable isotope methodology. *J. Nutr.* **38,** 169–180.

Thompson, J. N., Erdody, P., and Smith, P. C. (1975). Selenium content of food consumed by Canadians. *J. Nutr.* **105,** 274–277.

Thompson, M. J., Meeker, L. D., and Kokoska, S. (1984). Effect of an inorganic and organic form of dietary selenium on the promotional stage of mammary carcinogenesis in the rat. *Cancer Res.* **44,** 2803–2806.

Thomson, C. D., and Robinson, M. F. (1980). Selenium in human health and disease with emphasis on those aspects peculiar to New Zealand. *Am. J. Nutr.* **33,** 303–323.

Thomson, C. D., and Stewart, R. D. M. (1973). Metabolic studies of [^{75}Se]selenomethionine and [^{75}Se]selenite in the rat. *Br. J. Nutr.* **30,** 139–147.

Tipton, I. H., Steward, P. L., and Dickson, J. (1969). Patterns of elemental excretion in long-term balance studies. *Health Phys.* **16,** 455–462.

Traub, R. D., Rains, T. C., Garruto, R. M., Gajdusek, D. C., and Gibbs, C. J., Jr. (1981). Brain destruction alone does not elevate brain aluminum. *Neurology* **31,** 986–990.

Underwood, E. J. (1977). ''Trace Elements in Human and Animal Nutrition.'' Academic Press, New York.

Valberg, L. S., Flanagan, P. R., and Chamberlain, M. J. (1984). Effects of iron, tin, and copper on zinc absorption in humans. *Am. J. Clin. Nutr.* **40,** 536–541.

Valdivia, R., Ammerman, C. B., Wilcox, C. J., and Henry, P. R. (1978). Effect of dietary aluminum on animal performance and tissue mineral levels in growing steers. *J. Anim. Sci.* **47,** 1351–1356.

Valdivia, R., Ammerman, C. B., Henry, P. R., Feaster, J. P., and Wilcox, C. J. (1982). Effect of dietary aluminum and phosphorus on performance, phosphorus utilization and tissue mineral composition in sheep. *J. Anim. Sci.* **55,** 402–410.

Valentine, J. L., Kang, H. K., and Spivey, G. H. (1978). Selenium levels in human blood, urine, and hair in response to exposure via drinking water. *Environ. Res.* **17,** 347–355.

Warburton, S., Udler, W., Ewert, R. M., and Haynes, W. S. (1962). Outbreak of foodborne illness attributed to tin. *Public Health Rep.* **77,** 798–800.

Welsh, S. O., Holden, J. M., Wolf, W. R., and Levander, O. A. (1981). Selenium in self-selected diets of Maryland residents. *J. Am. Diet. Assoc.* **79,** 277–285.

Whanger, P. D., Pedersen, N. D., Hatfield, J., and Weswig, P. M. (1976). Absorption of selenium and selenomethionine from digestive tract segments in rats. *Proc. Soc. Exp. Biol. Med.* **153,** 295–297.

Wilber, C. G. (1980). Toxicology of selenium: A review. *Clin. Toxicol.* **17,** 171–230.

Wolfram, S., Ardüser, F., and Scharrer, E. (1985). In vivo intestinal absorption of selenate and selenite by rats. *J. Nutr.* **115,** 454–459.

Wolinsky, I., Lane, H. W., Warren, D. C., and Whaley, B. S. (1986). Zinc, selenium levels in selected and ethnic/regional foods. *J. Am. Diet. Assoc.* (in press).

Yamaguchi, M., Saito, R., and Okada, S. (1980). Dose–effect of inorganic tin on biochemical indices in rats. *Toxicology* **16,** 267–273.

Yamaguchi, M., Sugii, K., and Okada, S. (1981). Inorganic tin in the diet affects the femur in rats. *Toxicol. Lett.* **9,** 207–209.

Yamaguchi, M., Sugii, K., and Okada, S. (1982). Inhibition of collagen synthesis in the femur of rats orally administered stannous chloride. *J. Pharm. Dyn.* **5,** 388–393.

Yamamoto, T., Yamaguchi, M., and Sato, H. (1976). Accumulation of calcium in kidney and decrease of calcium in serum of rats treated with tin chloride. *J. Toxicol. Environ. Health* **1,** 749–756.

Yang, G., Wang, S., Zhou, R., and Sun, S. (1983). Endemic selenium intoxication of humans in China. *Am. J. Clin. Nutr.* **37,** 872–881.

10

Toxicology of Pesticide Residues in Foods

Joel R. Coats

I. INTRODUCTION

The usage of chemical pesticides has increased dramatically over the last 30 years. Today, very few food crops are produced on an economically competitive basis without some type of pesticide input. Insects, weeds, and pathogens are responsible for most pesticide needs. The role of insecticides, herbicides, and fungicides in protecting food plants and animals from death, injury, disease, or competition for resources has become well established on a worldwide basis. The chemicals may be applied before growth of the food product, during its growth, or after it has been harvested or processed. Other types of compounds also are used in agricultural production and storage of foodstuffs: rodenticides, molluscicides, acaricides, growth regulators, soil sterilants, fumigants, antibiotics, repellents, and synergists, among others. By design, most of them possess marked biological activity at very low concentrations. Impurities that occur in commercial preparations of these chemicals may also have significant impact on living

249

Copyright © 1987 by Academic Press, Inc.
All rights of reproduction in any form reserved.

systems. Even some of the "inert" ingredients (adjuvants) of certain formulated products, such as surfactants, solvents, and aerosol propellants, are capable of inducing deleterious effects.

This chapter will address the types of acute toxic effects, as well as types of chronic and delayed effects, but will not attempt to catalog all the known toxic effects of pesticides. Although many can cause toxic symptoms alone, some chemicals may generate harmful effects only in combination with certain other compounds. Such interactions are very difficult to predict and impossible to screen for during normal safety evaluations by virtue of the limitless number of combinations possible. Mechanisms of action will be discussed to the depths of current understanding. Factors that influence the toxicology of the chemicals in our diet and drinking water include biotransformation, elimination, and environmental parameters such as movement and persistence. This discussion will examine documented effects in humans, as well as those that have been demonstrated in model organisms, primarily other warm-blooded animals.

II.   MECHANISMS OF TOXICITY

The modes of action for many of the earlier, inorganic pesticides have been determined through decades of research. Among the organic chemicals, both synthetic and natural, some mechanisms of action are well known while others have not been elucidated. In those cases, the leading theories will be presented. Various types of effects elicited by the pesticides, impurities, metabolites, or adjuvants will be discussed, and relevant examples will be cited for each type of effect.

The route of entry of toxicants bears considerably on the type, timing, and severity of effects. The inhalation route usually is the most rapid mechanism of uptake and most direct route to the bloodstream. Immediate and dire effects can result when certain types of vapors are inhaled. However, the general population seldom is exposed to dangerous airborne concentrations of pesticidal compounds for any extended time; also, an olfactory warning frequently alerts us to such a hazard before we suffer deleterious consequences.

The dermal route of absorption of pesticides is important primarily through occupational types of exposure, for example, manufacturing and applying the pesticides. Many organic insecticides of relatively high water solubility penetrate the skin readily and can be toxic by this route, including some organophosphorus and carbamate insecticides. Chemicals with relatively low water solubilities are not as easily absorbed through the skin. The resultant hazard of a dermal exposure is always a composite of penetration rate plus the distribution and potency of the toxicant once inside the body.

The oral route of entry is the one of greatest concern to a large segment of the population. Most pesticides are more acutely toxic via the oral route compared with dermal exposure. Also, low-level residues that occur in foods and beverages are virtually unavoidable components of our diet. It therefore is critical that we perceive and understand the potential toxic manifestations of ingested pesticides.

A. Acute Effects

Acute toxic effects are those that typically occur within minutes or hours of ingestion. The time of response depends on the sensitivity of the site of action, dose level, and the toxicokinetics of the chemical, that is, absorption, distribution, biotransformation, and elimination from the body. The severity of the intoxication is directly related to the amount of toxicant at the site of action at a given time, which is determined by the dose and the toxicokinetics of the chemical in the body.

1. *Neurotoxins*

The nervous system is considered to be the most sensitive site of toxic action in mammals. Indeed, the basic morphology and physiology of nerves do not vary appreciably throughout the animal kingdom. Pesticides targeted at disrupting insect nerve function therefore are quite potent poisons in the mammalian nervous systems. Some selectivity is gained via capabilities to degrade the compounds enzymatically, but much of the ''safety margin'' still relies on preventing toxic quantities of the chemical from entering our bodies. The modes of action for most groups of neurotoxic insecticides have been investigated in mammalian systems, partly toward understanding possible gains to be made in selectivity.

2. *Cholinesterase Inhibitors*

Two major groups of insecticides, organophosphorus compounds and carbamates, exert toxic effects through inhibition of acetylcholinesterase. The poisonous organic esters of phosphorus were first produced as nerve gases for the purpose of chemical warfare. The origins of the carbamate esters lie in the calabar or ordeal bean and its ''trial-by-poison'' uses in West Africa. Both classes of chemicals were further developed for medicinal uses, including treatment for conditions such as myasthenia gravis and glaucoma. Insecticidal uses initially were developed in the 1940s and 1950s after they were well known for their powerful effects on the human nervous system.

A partial list of types of organophosphorus esters (OPs) is presented in Fig. 1. A more complete discussion of the classification of OPs can be found in Eto's book (1974). The most commonly used kinds today are the phosphorothionates and the phosphorodithioates.

The most common types of carbamate insecticides–acaricides are shown in Fig. 2. The carbamic esters are structurally more similar to the transmitter

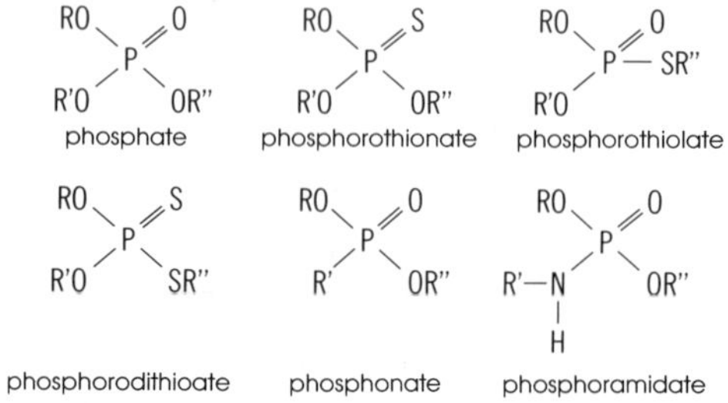

Fig. 1.   Common classes of toxic organophosphorus esters.

substance acetylcholine (Fig. 3). Kuhr and Dorough (1976) present a thorough treatment of carbamates.

Valuable sources for detailed discussions of the toxicology of cholinesterase inhibitors are Matsumura (1985), O'Brien (1967, 1976), O'Brien *et al.* (1974), and Eto (1974).

The site of action is the same for both OPs and carbamates: nerve synapses, in both the autonomic and somatic nervous systems. The basic mechanism is similar for both: inhibition of acetylcholinesterase, the enzyme responsible for deactivating the transmitter substance (acetylcholine) that chemically conveys the neural message across a synapse. The result is an accumulation of excess acetylcholine, which causes a repetitive firing of the postsynaptic nerve.

When acetylcholine binds with acetylcholinesterase, it is rapidly hydrolyzed, and turnover time is very short. The OPs and carbamates are competitive inhibitors that bind to the enzyme in much the same way. The process occurs in three steps, each with a distinct set of kinetics and determining factors. The initial step is the alignment of an inhibitor molecule with the enzyme. The rate is dependent on the affinity of the inhibitor for the active site on the enzyme as determined by optimal steric fit and electronic charge distribution. The next step is covalent bonding of the P, or carbonyl C, to a serine hydroxyl at the esteratic site of the enzyme, that is, the site that is instrumental in hydrolyzing the acetate ester linkage in acetylcholine. The formation of the bond (called phosphorylation or carbamylation) is accompanied by a simultaneous loss of one ''leaving group,'' usually the largest, most electronegative substitutent. The third step is the regeneration of the enzyme through the release of the bound group.

One standard measurement of potency of the OP and carbamate inhibitors is the I_{50} value, a molar concentration of inhibitor that effects a 50% inhibition of

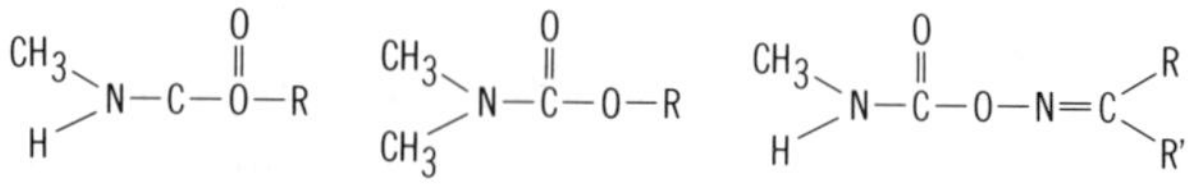

Fig. 2.   Common classes of toxic esters of carbamic acid.

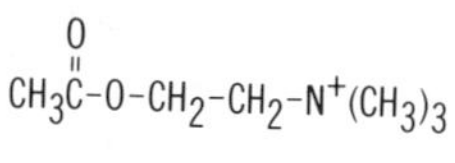

$$CH_3\overset{\overset{\text{O}}{\|}}{C}-O-CH_2-CH_2-N^+(CH_3)_3$$

Fig. 3. Acetylcholine.

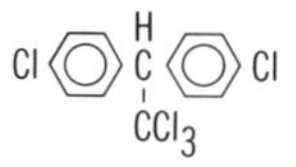

Fig. 4. DDT.

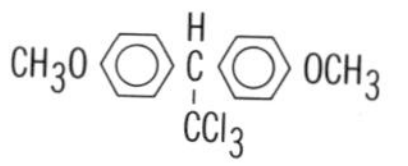

Fig. 5. Methoxychlor.

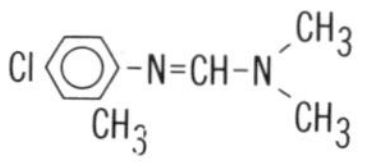

Fig. 6. Permethrin.

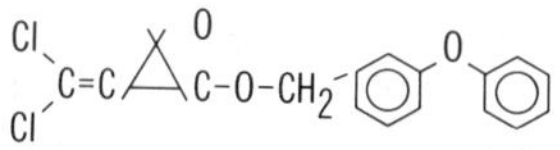

Fig. 7. Chlordimeform.

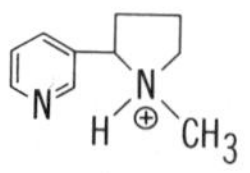

Fig. 8. Nicotine.

cholinesterase. Many insecticidal OPs and carbamates produce I_{50} values in the range of 10^{-6} to 10^{-8} M. The OPs that possess the thiono arrangement (P=S) are poorer inhibitors than the P=O types, but *in vivo* activation to the P=O form improves their I_{50} values by several orders of magnitude.

The effectiveness of the OPs and carbamates also is partly dependent on the electron-withdrawing or -donating properties of the substituents on the leaving group (e.g., substituted phenyl rings). The OP compounds are more potent inhibitors if substituents are electron-withdrawing (Fukuto, 1971), that is, with a positive Hammett σ value. Such substituents as halogens, nitro, sulfinyl, sulfonyl, or carboxyl groups create a stronger δ^+ on the P atom and enhance binding (phosphorylation) to the cholinesterase molecule at the esteratic sites.

Carbamates typically are stronger inhibitors when lipophilic groups such as alkyl, alkoxy, and alkylthio are attached. Some electron-donating moieties must be in optimal steric positions, which probably reflects the importance of fit and hydrophobic attractions in the carbamate molecule's affinity for cholinesterase. The carbonyl cannot harbor as potent a δ^+ charge as a phosphorus atom can; the steric and lipophilic factors therefore override electron-withdrawing effects, and electronegative groups actually cause a reduction in inhibitory capability of a carbamate (Metcalf, 1971).

The most important difference between OPs and carbamates lies in the rates at which the phosphoryl and carbamoyl groups are released from the active site of cholinesterase. The release step, which occurs, of course, very quickly with the natural substrate acetylcholine (milliseconds), proceeds at a moderate rate for carbamate inhibitors (seconds or minutes), but only at extremely low rates for OP inhibitors (hours or days). Carbamate poisoning is caused by a reversible inhibitor, while OP poisoning is the result of an essentially irreversible inhibition. Although the toxicosis may reach a crisis phase rapidly with either type of insecticide, the finite rate of spontaneous recovery of acetylcholinesterase can contribute somewhat to survival of a carbamate-poisoned mammal.

Poisonings caused by cholinesterase inhibitors can be treated by commercially available antidotes. Atropine is effective against either type of inhibitor as it binds to the postsynaptic acetylcholine receptors and protects them from the excess acetylcholine that accumulates at the synapse. Another class of antidotes, the aldoximes (e.g., 2-PAM or pyridine-2-aldoximomethiodide), can aid in recover of OP-inhibited enzyme by artificially increasing the rate of hydrolysis of the phosphoryl moiety off the cholinesterase molecule (Matsumura, 1985; Hayes, 1975).

The importance of the R substituents on an OP is twofold. Considerable mammalian selectivity is gained with methyl substituents if compared with ethyl and isopropyl groups due to easier metabolic attack by glutathione-dependent alkyltransferases. In addition, the rate of recovery of cholinesterase is affected by the type of R group: increasing the alkyl chain length from methyl to ethyl to propyl or isopropyl decreases rate of regeneration from slow to negligible. This is thought to be the result of more rapid "aging" of the phosphorylated enzyme, or loss of an alkyl to the enzyme, for the larger alkyl groups. The des-alkyl phosphorylated enzyme will not recover at all.

The spectrum of esterases inhibited differ for OPs and carbamates, and the OPs generally affect a greater variety of other enzymes (Eto, 1974; Kuhr and Dorough, 1976).

Human poisoning by OPs or carbamates is typified by headache, nausea, constricted pupils, excess salivation, lacrimation, and perspiration, followed by more serious symptoms such as tremors, convulsions, and cardiovascular problems. Death can occur as a result of respiratory failure (Matsumura, 1985). Effects of parathion on the mammalian nervous system have been summarized by Woolley *et al.* (1979).

3.   *Chlorinated Insecticides*

A large group of insecticides developed in the late 1940s and early 1950s were called chlorinated hydrocarbons or organochlorines. Major categories of those chemicals included the chlorinated bicyclodienes (or cyclodienes), hexachlorocyclohexanes (or BHC after incorrect assumption that they were benzene hexachlorides), toxaphene (from the chlorination of the natural terpene, camphene), and the DDT group, which will be discussed in a separate section.

The cyclodienes include aldrin, dieldrin, chlordane, heptachlor, endrin, and endosulfan. The one important hexachlorocyclohexane is lindane (γ-BHC). Toxaphene is a complex mixture of chlorination isomers that also possess the bicylcic cagelike form of the cyclodienes. A total of 177 components were identified (Casida *et al.*, 1974; Nelson and Matsumura, 1975), but only three possess high neurotoxic activity (Turner *et al.*, 1975; Matsumura *et al.*, 1975).

The mechanism of toxic action probably is similar for the cyclodienes, lindane, and toxaphene because all have the same general effect on mammalian nerves. The excitatory effect on the central nervous system (CNS) has been attributed to the stimulation of neurotransmitter release from the presynaptic terminal (Uchida *et al.*, 1978; Shankland, 1979). The transmitter substance, acetylcholine, is contained in vesicles within the presynaptic terminal, and release of excessive quantities can be induced by this group of insecticides. The biochemical mechanism for triggering the release lies in Ca^{2+} availability. During normal nerve function, rapid increases in Ca^{2+} in the presynaptic terminal cause transmitter release. Cyclodienes inhibit certain Ca^{2+}-ATPases, decreasing their capacity for binding Ca^{2+}, and therefore stimulating the release of excess acetylcholine (Yamaguchi *et al.*, 1979).

These chlorinated hydrocarbons also inhibit γ-aminobutyric acid (GABA)-activated Cl^{-} uptake in nerves, which results in destabilized, more easily stimulated nerve membranes. The chemicals bind competitively at the same site at which picrotoxinin binds to prevent GABA activation of the chloride channels (Matsumura, 1983, 1985; Casida and Lawrence, 1985).

Several biotransformation products, most notable aldrin *trans*-diol, also have been demonstrated to induce toxic effects (Narahashi, 1976), but there is not general agreement that such products are necessary for intoxication (Shankland, 1982).

Most compounds in this category are of moderate acute toxicity (oral LD_{50}s of 50–500 mg/kg) to mammals, but a few are highly toxic (e.g., endrin). Acute symptoms in mammals are tremors, headache, nausea, dizziness, and convulsions (Matsumura, 1985; Frank and Braun, 1984). A summary of chlorinated hydrocarbon structures, actions, and metabolism was published by Brooks (1974).

4. *DDT-Type Insecticides*

DDT was the first highly insecticidal synthetic organic chemical and was widely acclaimed for its safety margin (Fig. 4). After its spectacular successes in ending typhus epidemics during World War II and in suppression of malaria-transmitting mosquitoes, it was hailed as one of the most remarkable chemicals ever invented. Indeed, uses that involved intimate human contact with the compound resulted in no symptoms of toxicity nor reports of death. Over the years, it became evident that DDT had serious drawbacks: it became less effective as resistance developed in pests, it was very persistent in the environment, reproductive failures were reported for some vertebrate species exposed to relatively low levels over long periods, low-level residues were ubiquitous in food, organisms at higher trophic levels in food chains were observed to accumulate higher levels, and human adipose tissue and human milk contained concentrations in excess of maximum tolerable amounts in marketed beef or dairy products. No reproductive nor any other serious effects were even demonstrated or observed in human beings. However, the effects in other species and the uncertainty of possible future consequences of residues stored in the human body precipitated a nearly total ban on DDT in many countries. Worldwide, millions of pounds still are used each year in public health and crop protection, primarily because of its low cost and lack of acute toxicity to humans.

The mode of action of DDT and its derivatives has not been elucidated totally despite 40 years of research in that area. The action in mammals is on the nerve axon, causing a hyperexcitability and repetitive firing of the nerve. Two theories currently predominate: (1) the DDT molecule acts to alter physically the nerve membrane permeability to Na^+ and/or K^+ ions, thus promoting constant or repetitive depolarizations; (2) DDT inhibits ATPase(s) in the nerve membrane, thus affecting the Na^+, K^+, or even Ca^{2+} equilibria therein. The effects on ionic channels in the nerve membrane have been summarized by Narahashi (1979), and on ATPases by Cutkomp *et al.* (1982) and Matsumura (1983).

A saclike receptor has been proposed for either site of action. Dimensions of the receptor sac have been described (Holan, 1969). Bidirectional elasticity (Metcalf *et al.*, 1971) and, subsequently, tridirectional flexibility (Coats *et al.*, 1977) have been demonstrated among analogs of DDT. Stereospecificity of the site also have been reported (Brown *et al.*, 1981). Steric and electronic structure–activity relationships have been reviewed by Coats (1982).

The acute mammalian toxicity of DDT is in the range of 100–500 mg/kg, depending on species. Derivatives that can be more easily degraded biologically are considerably less toxic, such as methoxychlor (Fig. 5).

5. *Pyrethroids*

This class includes the natural insecticide pyrethrum (extracted from certain chrysanthemums) as well as any derivative or analog with a similar structure. The characteristic feature of the pyrethroid molecule is the presence of a cyclopropyl carboxylic acid moiety (Fig. 6), although a few recently developed analogs do not contain that group. Although the insecticidal properties were long known to natives of western Asia, the structures of the major components of pyrethrum were not determined until more recently (reviewed by Elliott and Janes, 1973). These compounds are primarily of low toxicity to mammals, especially by oral or dermal routes of exposure. Studies in experimental animals reveal them to be highly toxic if administered by iv injection. Pyrethroids are quite toxic at the site of action but normally undergo rapid and extensive biological degradation before high concentrations can accumulate at that site. Most modern analogs have retained that large degree of mammalian safety, although a few fall in the moderately toxic category. The properties of pyrethrum have been summarized by Casida (1973), and the synthetic pyrethroids by Elliott (1977). The acute toxicity of pyrethroids to mammals has been discussed by James (1980).

Three theories on pyrethroid mode of action prevail currently. Axonal excitability is observed, with the Na^+ channels affected in much the same way as the DDT-type insecticides act to induce overstimulation (Lund, 1984; Narahashi, 1982). Another mechanism proposed is the inhibition of Ca- and Ca,Mg-ATPases, which leads to excessive Ca-induced neurotransmitter release at nerve synapses (Clark and Matsumura, 1982). In addition, the GABA receptor site complex is also affected by pyrethroids, inhibiting Cl^- uptake and thereby destabilizing the nerve membrane (Lawrence and Casida, 1983; Casida and Lawrence, 1985). Both the central and peripheral nervous systems are affected, including these specific sites: spinal reflex arcs, sensory axons, and neuromuscular junctions (Miller and Adams, 1982). The CNS effects seem to be most important in test mammals (van den Bercken, 1980).

6. *Formamidines*

This class of pesticides has been shown to have a wide variety of biochemical and neurotoxic actions in mammals, including inhibition of monoamine oxidases, inhibition of prostaglandin synthesis, uncoupling of oxidative phosphorylation, abnormal carbohydrate metabolism, as well as axonic and neuromuscular junction effects. Various sublethal, behavioral, and acutely toxic symptoms have been observed, corresponding to the different modes of action. The neurotoxic effects have been reviewed by Lund *et al.* (1979). The most recent view is that they may mimic biogenic amines in the nervous system, such as octopamine or epinephrine, and act as agonists of these substances (Hollingworth and Murdock, 1980; Hollingworth and Lund, 1982). Chlordimeform (Fig. 7) is the most widely studied pesticide of this class, but the des-methyl derivative of it is much more potent in induction of toxicity. Vertebrate effects have been addressed by Knowles (1982).

7. *Nicotine*

The neurotoxic effects of nicotine (Fig. 8), one of the earliest Western Hemisphere insecticides, have been known for more than two centuries. It acts at the synapses but not as an inhibitor of acetylcholinesterase. Rather, it acts as an agonist of acetylcholine, resulting in overstimulation of all mammalian cholinergic junctions (Matsumura, 1985). The mammalian toxicity of nicotine and related chemicals is moderate to high, depending on route of exposure, causing uses to be restricted in recent years. The ingestion route is a less hazardous route of exposure than the inhalation and dermal absorption routes.

8. *Metabolic Inhibitors*

Relatively few modern insecticides are inhibitors of primary metabolic functions, but a large number of earlier pesticides do act at that level. Greater potential for selectivity can be obtained with the neurotoxic agents already discussed if the mammalian system can eliminate or degrade them quickly enough.

9. *Arsenicals*

The arsenite, As^{3+}, pesticides possess very little selectivity and are toxic to most types of organisms. They inhibit the acetylation of pyruvate by acetyl coenzyme A and also prevent the conversion of α-ketoglutarate to succinate in the Krebs cycle. They are very toxic to mammals.

Arsenate, As^{5+}, possesses a little more selectivity than arsenite, with mammalian LD_{50} values in the range of 30–150 mg/kg. In glycolysis, arsenate can inhibit phosphorylation of glucose to G6P and fructose 6-phosphate to fructose 1,6-diphosphate. Arsenate also is an uncoupler of oxidative phosphorylation.

Residues on food and in soil and general lack of selectivity have contributed to decreased use and increased restrictions on the arsenical pesticides. Properties are discussed by Metcalf *et al.* (1962) and Matsumura (1985).

10. *Rotenoids*

This group, which includes rotenone, is of botanical origin, extracted from the roots of several legumes from South America and Southeast Asia. They are of moderate toxicity to mammals, but are very quickly degraded and pose little residue problem. The primary action is ostensibly on the electron transport system, by blocking the reduction of flavoprotein and/or ubiquinone (Corbett, 1984). Acute mammalian toxicity varies widely with species.

11. *Inorganic Fluorides*

The inorganic fluorides act by inhibiting the oxidation of 3-phosphoglutaraldehyde in glycolysis. Sodium fluoride has a human oral LD_{50} of 75 mg/kg while fluoroaluminates and fluorosilicates are somewhat safer.

12. *Fluoroacetate*

This rodenticide is quite toxic to most mammals (e.g., dog LD_{50} is 0.05 mg/kg; rat LD_{50} is 5 mg/kg). It enters the TCA cycle and is converted to fluorocitrate, which binds, irreversibly, with *cis*-aconitase.

13. *Phenols*

DNOC (or dinitro-*o*-cresol) and pentachlorophenol are among the least selective pesticides used. Mammalian oral LD_{50} values range from 20 to 80 mg/kg. This class of primitive synthetic organics has been used as insecticides, herbicides, fungicides, and molluscicides, among other uses. The mode of action is the uncoupling of oxidative phosphorylation. The fungicides hexachlorobenzene and pentachloronitrobenzene are considered to act via the same action following metabolic conversion to a phenolic derivative. They are, however, considerably less toxic to mammals and other nontarget species.

14. Cyanide

Hydrogen cyanide fumigant inhibits cytochrome c oxidase ($I_{50} = 10^{-8} M$), thus preventing the utilization of oxygen in the electron transport system (Isom and Way, 1976). It is one of the most toxic pesticides to mammals, with an oral LD_{50} to dog of 1.6 mg/kg. Sodium thiosulfate is a proved antidote for cyanide poisoning (Pettersen and Cohen, 1985).

15. Organotins

Trisubstituted tin hydroxides (trialkyl, tricycloalkyl, triaryl) are used as acaricides. They act as inhibitors of oxidative phosphorylation. The cycloalkyl ones are of notably less toxicity than the normal alkyl ones.

16. Haloalkane Fumigants

Chloropicrin, methyl bromide, ethylene dibromide, and related fumigants act primarily by inhibiting the conversion of succinate to fumarate in the TCA cycle through binding with sulfhydryl groups in succinic dehydrogenase and other enzymes. The CNS is most dramatically affected (Honma *et al.*, 1985), and severe CNS depression can be fatal (Letz *et al.*, 1984; Alexeeff *et al.*, 1985).

17. Paraquat and Diquat

The class of herbicides known as the bipyridiliums include these two chemicals, which are, unlike most herbicides, toxic to mammals (LD_{50} values of 100–250 mg/kg). The mode of action is through their potent oxidative capability. Paraquat generates peroxides, which in mammals cause a slow but irreversible fibrosis of lung tissue (McEwen and Stephenson, 1979). The lung damage seems to be primarily the result of effects on the type II alveolar epithelial cells (Pratt *et al.*, 1980). Mechanisms have recently been studied utilizing cell culture techniques (Wong and Stevens, 1985).

B. Chronic and Delayed Effects

In addition to acute toxic effects, some pesticides can induce other types of deleterious changes in biological systems. Chronic effects are those caused over longer periods as a result of continuous or repeated exposures to subacute doses. The toxic symptoms may be severe or relatively subtle. They may commence soon after initial exposures or sometimes can be cumulative, not being manifested until weeks, months, or years later. In some cases, a single dose can induce a delayed response.

A number of effects will be discussed with examples given, but this discussion is not intended to serve as comprehensive list of all pesticidal chemicals that can cause such effects.

1. Neurotoxicity

One particularly debilitating response caused by certain organophosphorus esters is called delayed neurotoxicity and is primarily the result of degeneration of myelin and axons. The major group of OPs that can cause the phenomenon are the phenylphosphonothioates (Abou-Donia, 1979a,b; Johnson, 1984). Single sublethal doses of 10–500 mg/kg or repeated doses of 0.1–50 mg/kg can elicit the response, characterized by ataxia and paralysis (Abou-Donia and Graham, 1979; El-Sebae *et al.*, 1980; Abou-Donia *et al.*, 1986). The onset of irreversible nerve damage occurs at 10 or more days after initial exposure in most cases. Species differences are extreme among warm-blooded animals: humans, sheep, cats, dogs, pigs, water buffalo, ducks, pheasants, and chickens are sensitive; mice, rats, guinea pigs, rabbits, partridge, and quail are resistant to the effects (Francis *et al.*, 1980; Hollingshaus *et al.* 1981; Abou-Donia *et al.*, 1983). Leptophos, desbromoleptophos, cyanofenphos, EPN, and S-Seven (EPBP) demonstrate potency in sensitive species.

The action of delayed neurotoxic OPs has been postulated to be the inhibition of a "neurotoxic esterase" (Johnson, 1975; Lotti *et al.*, 1985). Effects on microtubule involvement in spindle formation have contributed toward a hypothesis that phosphorylation of a protease inhibits or disrupts synthesis of microtubules (Seifert and Casida, 1982).

Another effect of certain OPs, and especially impurities in some commercial-grade products, is that of a simple delayed toxicity whereby rats die at 4–22 days after a single oral dose (Umetsu *et al.*, 1981). O,O,S-Trimethyl phosphorothioate and related isomers are potent at 15–90 mg/kg, with little known about the mode of toxic action.

Kepone, or chlordecone, causes various nervous system effects as a result of low-level chronic exposures. The ability of chlordecone to inhibit ATPases may be responsible for changes in neurotransmitter release and uptake (Chang-Tsui and Ho, 1979). Alternatively, the mammalian tremor that typifies chlordecone poisoning (Gerhart *et al.*, 1983) may be due to an effect on biogenic amine levels (Chen *et al.*, 1985). Human effects have been discussed by Taylor *et al.* (1978).

The rodenticide Vacor can cause severe neurotoxicity in humans, possibly through suppression of norepinephrine release (LeWitt, 1980).

Alkyl mercury compounds (e.g., methylmercury) cause severe nervous disorders in mammals in response to very low-level chronic exposures. CNS effects include tremors, emotional instability, incoordination, and paralysis. Cell body damage and alteration of the blood–brain barrier are important factors in the toxicity of alkyl mercury (Hammond and Beliles, 1980).

2. Mutagenicity

Numerous pesticides have shown potency as mutagenic agents in various screening techniques (Ames *et al.*, 1975; Marshall *et al.*, 1976; Shiau *et al.*, 1981; Moriya *et al.*, 1983). Mechanisms of changing genetic information include alkylation, substitution of base analogs, intercalations, as well as chromosome breakage and cross-linking. Some pesticides (e.g., toxaphene) are innately mutagenic (Hooper *et al.*, 1979), while others require activation to a degradation product or a derivative, such as the *N*-nitroso derivative of carbofuran (Nelson *et al.*, 1981).

3. Carcinogenicity

Many of the same mechanisms responsible for mutagenesis also cause cancer in mammals. Thus, many mutagenic pesticides also are carcinogenic. Mutagenesis and carcinogenesis are highly correlated in some assays, but questions always remain with regard to the examples that are carcinogenic and not mutagenic or vice versa. In addition, assay systems sometimes produce false positive or false negative responses that make extrapolation from bacterial or cell culture tests to humans even more uncertain. Tests with greater predictive value and accuracy are still needed (Bishun *et al.*, 1978).

Many types of organochlorine pesticides cause malignant tumors in mammals (Reuber, 1979; Epstein, 1977). Nitrosamine impurities in nitroaniline herbicides have caused concern (Ross *et al.*, 1977). A degradation product of ethylene bisdithiocarbamate fungicides (e.g., nabam, zineb) is the very potent oncogen ethylene thiourea (Lewerenz *et al.*, 1977). Mirex has also been demonstrated to be carcinogenic (Innes *et al.*, 1969), as has aminotriazole (Steinhoff *et al.*, 1983).

4. Teratogenicity

Effects on development of an embryo or fetus, as a result of maternal exposure, have been demonstrated for a wide range of pesticidal chemicals (Longo, 1980). Types of effects include abnormal growth rates of offspring, incomplete development, skeletal, visceral, and biochemical anomalies, as well as abortions.

Certain chlorinated hydrocarbons have demonstrated teratogenic activity: mirex (Khera *et al.*, 1976), Kepone (Chernoff and Rogers, 1976), and DDT (Dean *et al.*, 1980), among others. One of the most potent teratogens known is 2,3,7,8-tetrachlorodibenzodioxin (TCDD), an impurity in 2,4,5-T herbicide (Courtney and Moore, 1971). Although 2,4,5-T has been reported to be teratogenic at high doses (Hood *et al.*, 1979), controversy persists primarily in regard to the low levels of the dioxin in the product (Hanify *et al.*, 1981; Hay, 1982).

Organophosphates have shown some effects—for example, dimethoate (Khera, 1979), monocrotophos (Jaffee and Mitrosky, 1979), methylparathion (Gupta *et al.*, 1985), and others (Misawa *et al.*, 1982)—but are implicated less commonly than the more persistent chlorinated hydrocarbons. The mercurial fungicides and ethylenethiourea can induce developmental abnormalities (Lewerenz and Bleyl, 1980). Mechanisms usually are considered to be identical or similar to those for mutagenic and carcinogenic effects.

5. Reproductive Effects

Detrimental influences on reproduction, aside from teratogenicity, can result from exposure to some pesticides. The types of effects include decreased number, size, and growth rate of offspring, fetotoxicity, lowered sperm count, as well as behavioral abnormalities such as decreased libido.

Chlorinated hydrocarbons have been shown to affect reproduction in many species. Estrogenic effects are caused by *o,p'*-DDT (an impurity in DDT), Kepone, methoxychlor, and two of its phenolic degradation products, seemingly acting directly as an estrogen (Kupfer and Bulger, 1976; Bulger *et al.*, 1985). Acephate decreases luteinizing hormone in mice (Rattner and Michael, 1985). Aldrin, dieldrin, hexachlorobenzene, and DDE (a degradation product of DDT) all induce some symptoms of reproductive dysfunction (Matsumura, 1985; McEwen and Stephenson, 1979). The fumigant dibromochloropropane (DBCP) has caused azoospermia and abnormal hormone levels in factory workers and experimental animals (Sandifer *et al.*, 1979; Kluwe *et al.*, 1983b; Rao *et al.*, 1983). The mechanism of toxic action may be through alkylation of certain proteins by an oxidative metabolite of DBCP (Kato *et al.*, 1980; Kluwe *et al.*, 1983a). Carbaryl has been associated with abnormal sperm shapes in occupationally exposed men (Wyrobek *et al.*, 1981). Benomyl fungicide has been shown to have deleterious effects on the male reproductive system in rats (Carter *et al.*, 1984), as do triphenyltin compounds (Snow and Hays, 1983).

6. Behavioral Effects

Behavioral toxicology studies have demonstrated that mammalian behavior is extremely sensitive to xenobiotic chemicals. Very low exposure levels can cause decreased learning and memory function, hyperactivity, altered aggressive and defensive behavior, or abnormal courtship, resulting indirectly in reduced reproduction. Some instances of pesticide effects on vertebrate behavior include changes in schedule-controlled responding induced by chlordimeform (Leander and MacPhail, 1980), and decamethrin (McPhail *et al.*, 1981); flavor aversions caused by chlordimeform (MacPhail and Leander, 1980); errors in discrimination and problem solving caused by toxaphene and endrin (Kreitzer, 1980); impaired swimming in neonatal offspring of mothers dosed with dieldrin (Olson *et al.*, 1980). Mirex and Kepone also have been shown to affect behavior of rats

(Reiter *et al.*, 1977; Dietz and McMillan, 1979), as have permethrin and deltamethrin (Bloom *et al.*, 1983).

7. Enzyme Induction

Pesticide-induced increases in enzymatic activity have been reported for numerous species. Different types of enzymes may be affected, but the most commonly observed effects involve the mixed-function oxidases (MFOs) (Hayes, 1975; Madhukar and Matsumura, 1979). Possible mechanisms may include increased biosynthesis of enzymes, decreased degradation rates of enzymes, or increased activation of enzymes (Nigg *et al.*, 1976). Many chlorinated hydrocarbon pesticides are capable of inducing enzyme activity: DDT, toxaphene, hexachlorobenzene, chlordane, Kepone, mirex, dieldrin, and endosulfan (Kinoshita *et al.*, 1966; Iverson, 1976; Brimfield and Street, 1981; Fabacher and Hodgson, 1976; Tyagi *et al.*, 1984; Carpenter *et al.*, 1985). Enzyme induction can cause abnormally high rates of degradation of endogenous substances (e.g., steroids) or of intentionally introduced substances (e.g., drugs), thereby reducing their physiological effects; enhanced enzyme activity also can increase the rates of formation of certain deleterious metabolites of xenobiotics, including acutely toxic ones and carcinogenic products.

8. Growth, Assimilation, and Respiration

The slowing of growth may occur through various mechanisms and frequently involves a subchronic effect, rather than a toxic effect per se (e.g., causing normal physiological functions to proceed at an abnormal rate). Some chlorinated aromatic organophosphorus insecticides (e.g., ronnel, chlorpyrifos-methyl, and leptophos) increase growth rates (Rumsey *et al.*, 1975; Rumsey, 1979; Johnson *et al.*, 1947); ronnel also increases efficiency of feed utilization (Trankina *et al.*, 1981, 1982).

Chronic oral exposure of monkeys to DDT resulted in changes in intestinal brush border membrane, including altered structure, enzyme activities, and rates of uptake of glucose, leucine, and glycine (Mahmood *et al.*, 1979).

A photodegradation product of mirex, called photomirex, caused several types of abnormalities in the ultrastructure of liver cells in rats fed doses as low as 0.05 ppm in the diet (Singh *et al.*, 1981).

Electron transport system enzymes from beef heart mitochondria were affected by a number of pesticides. DDT and its degradation products and chlorinated acaricides (e.g., chlorobenzilate) inhibited NADH-oxidase and succinoxidase systems. Carbamate insecticides were less potent inhibitors, although some of their phenolic degradation products were active (Pardini *et al.*, 1980). The fungicide dichlone caused inhibition of glycolysis in rat livers (Pritsos *et al.*, 1985).

9. *Interactions*

Although many types of pesticide interactions have been demonstrated, the number of potential interactions of pesticides with the tens of thousands of other chemical and biochemical agents is astronomical. Premarket screening for all possible interactions is clearly impractical. Although many mechanisms of action for combination effects are poorly understood, those mechanisms may provide the only predictive capabilities for early warning against certain types of interactions. A true toxic interaction is the result of greater-than-additive toxicity for a combination that enhances the deleterious effect, and is termed synergism or potentiation. An interaction that renders the substance(s) less toxic is termed antagonism.

a. Combination Effects from Exposure to More Than One Pesticide. Quite often a potentiation can result from an inhibition of degradative enzymes by one or both chemicals, rendering a larger-than-usual dose of intact toxicant circulating in the bloodstream. Common enzyme systems affected include the MFOs and various esterases. Potentiation may be induced by chemicals within the same class [e.g., the cholinesterase inhibitors EPN and malathion (Murphy and Dubois, 1957; Frawley *et al.*, 1957)] or by unrelated pesticides such as thiuram and chlorfenvinphos (Wysocka-Paruszewska *et al.*, 1980). Mirex and chlordecone have been demonstrated to enhance hepatotoxicity of chloroform (Hewitt *et al.*, 1983) and carbon tetrachloride (Bell and Mehendale, 1985).

b. Drugs or Synergists. Many pharmaceutical products exert an enhanced potency in mammalian systems when present in combination with a pesticide, either through the combination of two biochemical stresses on the system or through the inhibition or induction of degradative enzymes (Udall, 1975; O'Reilly *et al.*, 1980). Synergists are sometimes formulated with insecticides to promote greater potency against target pests. Tissue distribution may change when a drug or synergist is present (Aldous *et al.*, 1983). Piperonyl butoxide is the most widely used commercial synergist and acts by inhibiting MFO activity. Other synergists also exert potentiating effects by inhibition of degradative enzymes (Wilkinson, 1976a,b).

c. Impurities. Chemical reagents and by-products in technical or formulated preparations also can have biological consequences. Certain impurities in malathion can cause delayed toxic effects while others in the mixture provide an antagonistic safening effect (Umetsu *et al.*, 1981; Toia *et al.*, 1980). Formulations of the herbicide 2,3,5-T can contain very small quantities of the very potent 2,3,7,8-tetrachlorodioxin, causing considerable controversy in recent years (Hanify *et al.*, 1981; Chapman and Schiller, 1985).

d.   Adjuvants. The solvents, carriers, emulsifiers, and surfactants have traditionally been considered to be inert ingredients in formulated pesticide products. Recently, the biological implications of aromatic hydrocarbon solvents (Muralidhara and Krishnakumari, 1980; Wood *et al.*, 1983), surfactants (Crocker *et al.*, 1976; Marks and Ledoux, 1982; David, 1982), and asbestos-containing talc (Rohl and Langer, 1974) have been examined more closely.

e.   Viruses. Interactions between a chemical stress (pesticide or emulsifier) and a viral infection have been investigated (Pollack, 1979; Crocker *et al.*, 1976; Krzystyniak *et al.*, 1985).

f.   Immune Response. Some pesticides can cause either depression or stimulation of the immune response of vertebrates, depending on the type of chemical, duration of exposure, size of dose, and specific response monitored (Dandliker *et al.*, 1980; McCorkle *et al.*, 1980; Street, 1981; Allen *et al.*, 1983). Allergic reactions also can develop in individuals who become sensitized to specific pesticides or the adjuvants contained in the formulated products (Cushman and Street, 1982, 1983).

III.   FACTORS AFFECTING THE TOXICOLOGY OF PESTICIDES IN FOOD

In addition to the direct action of the toxicants discussed, many other factors influence the impact of pesticides on a mammalian system. The biotransformations that a foreign chemical undergoes can greatly influence the degree and duration of intoxication that the substance inflicts on an organism. The elimination of the xenobiotic from the body also is a crucial process in protecting the system from a toxic lesion or in lessening the duration of that effect. For a pesticide applied on or near food, the environmental persistence of the compound is a primary factor relating to the levels of residues present in produce. The movement of a chemical in the environment also is of particular interest inasmuch as it determines the availability of that pesticide for consumption. Some principles pertaining to each of these four factors will be presented.

A.   Biotransformation

The processes that an organism utilizes for degrading foreign substances are generally enzymatic but also can include purely chemical reactions (e.g., acid hydrolysis in the stomach) and changes wrought by the microbial flora in the alimentary tract. The sum total of the transformations that occur in the organism is sometimes termed the "metabolism" of the chemical in question. The biochemical "strategy" of the organism is to alter the foreign molecule such that (1) it is likely to be less toxic, and/or (2) it can be more readily eliminated from the body. The types of products formed depend on the structure of the chemical, as well as its toxicokinetic behavior in the body, especially the assimilation, transport, and distribution in organs and tissues. The liver is the primary site of enzymatic biotransformation, although cells at many other sites also possess some capability for metabolizing organic chemicals.

Although the pesticide degradation products are less toxic in most cases, a number of instances have been observed in which the resultant molecules are actually of greater toxicity. Such "activation" reactions are common among the organophosphorus insecticides (Spencer, 1976).

The types of products formed fall into two general categories: degradative and synthetic (or conjugation). The former involves a direct enzymatic attack on the molecule to yield an altered (e.g., oxidized) derivative, while the latter entails the enzymatic bonding of another moiety to the molecule to form a conjugate (e.g., xenobiotic bonded to glucuronic acid).

1. Degradations

    a. *Oxidation by MFO Systems.* This group of extremely important enzymes require oxygen, NADPH, and cytochrome $P\text{-}_{450}$ to convert a chemical to an oxidized form. They are located in the smooth endoplasmic reticulum of cells and are capable of a variety of reactions, all characterized by a net gain in the number of oxygens relative to the number of hydrogens present: (1) aromatic ring hydroxylation, (2) side-chain oxidation, (3) epoxidation, (4) desulfuration, (5) sulfur oxidation, (6) O-dealkylation, (7) N-dealkylation, and (8) S-dealkylation.

    b. Oxidation by FAD-containing monooxygenases

    c. Reduction by reductases

    d. Reductive dehalogenation

    e. Hydrolysis by (1) carboxylesterases, (2) phosphatases, (3) amidases, and (4) MFOs

    f. Dehydrochlorination

The topic has been reviewed by Nakatsugawa and Morelli (1976), Dauterman (1976), Jakoby *et al.* (1982), and Matsumura (1985).

2. Synthetic Reactions

The conjugation of a molecule of a sugar, an inorganic ion, or other group serves mainly to enhance water solubility of a chemical, but also inactivates a molecule that could potentially induce a toxic effect by binding to a critical receptor site.

The four functional groups that can easily be conjugated are (1) R-OH, (2) R-COOH, (3) $R\text{-}NH_2$, and (4) R-SH.

Some groups that can be attached to the xenobiotic include (1) glucuronic acid, (2) glucose, (3) ribose, (4) ribose 5-phosphate, (5) glutathione, (6) sulfate ion, (7) phosphate ion, (8) acetyl, (9) methyl, and (10) a fatty acid. The last three examples generally result in products of decreased water solubility, but with altered biological activity. Yang (1976) provides a summary of insecticide conjugation, while Jakoby (1981) discusses conjugation reactions of drugs.

B. Elimination

The removal of pesticides from the body proceeds via two major pathways. The products of metabolism in the liver accumulate in the bile and subsequently are emptied into the intestine. Metabolites of relatively high water solubility collect in the urine. Exhalation is a route of elimination of little importance for most pesticides, but may be significant with hydrocarbon solvents or the volatile fumigants.

The key to elimination is mobility via the bloodstream. The more water-soluble compounds are thus more easily excreted, while highly lipophilic substances remain sequestered in fatty tissues or bound to membranes or blood proteins. Their low mobility renders these molecules much less available to the liver, kidneys, or lungs.

C. Environmental Persistence

The stability of a pesticide residue in the environment (e.g., on a plant, in soil, in water, in animal feed) is a function of the chemical makeup of that compound, the activity of degradative agents present (light, moisture, temperature, pH, oxygen, and organisms), and the availability of the substance to the degradative agents.

Certain chemical groups are difficult to remove or alter, physically, chemically, or biologically. A pesticide molecule containing many halogens (e.g., DDT, mirex) is quite resistant to degradation, while ones containing groups such as $-OCH_3$, $-SCH_3$, or carboxy esters are readily attacked by environmental agents. Cagelike, bicyclic (triplanar), and highly branched-chain molecules are more recalcitrant than are ones of a straight-chain configuration.

The conditions that typically favor rapid breakdown of pesticides are intense light, moisture, warm temperature, extremes in pH (alkaline pH is especially important for OPs, carbamates, and pyrethroids), adequate oxygen, and rich microbial flora. Anaerobic degradation is a very different situation, yielding products of reductive reactions; examples include bovine rumens and sediment in the bottoms of low-oxygen bodies of water.

D. Movement of Residues

Pesticides are all mobile, to different degrees, in the environment. Physical and biological processes are responsible for such movements, and they may transport a chemical further away from or closer to a human food source. Major physical factors include mobility into soil, surface runoff from soil, leaching downward through soil, binding to soil (and subsequent transport by wind or water), spray drift, and volatilization, resulting in residues being deposited in "reservoirs" such as the soil, surface water, groundwater, or the air, in addition to the originally intended location. Biological movement can include uptake and translocation of some pesticides by plants as well as bioaccumulation through food chains.

Movement of pesticide residues invariably depends on the specific molecular structure and the associated physical properties. For example, the more water-soluble pesticides tend to dissolve in water and move easily in water (i.e., leaching, runoff, uptake by plants). The less soluble types tend to bind to soil or vegetation, thus being physically less mobile (Elgar, 1983). However, hydrophobicity also provides some potential for a chemical to accumulate in lipid "reservoirs" such as adipose tissue in animals, or oils and oily products from plants. A lipophilic compound will accumulate to a great level only if it also is resistant to degradation. Long exposure times in biological systems subject even a lipophilic chemical to repeated enzymatic challenges, and only a relatively nonbiodegradable substance can resist biotransformation effectively enough to be sequestered in large quantities in plant or animal lipids. In summary, a pesticide can bioaccumulate significantly only if it is of high lipid solubility, of low water solubility (not easy to excrete), persistent (not easily degraded *in vivo*), and stable enough in the environment to allow adequate uptake into biological components. General discussions of environmental kinetics of pesticides can be found in McEwen and Stephenson (1979).

IV. OCCURRENCE OF PESTICIDE RESIDUES IN FOOD

The presence of some residual levels of pesticides in produce has long been confirmed and accepted as nearly unavoidable in light of widespread use of insecticides, herbicides, and fungicides in agriculture. The study of pesticide residues takes several different approaches: (1) focus on a specific chemical in one product—for example, pentachloronitrobenzene in peanut butter (Heikes, 1980), monosodium methanearsonate in blackberries (Anderson *et al.*, 1980), or diazinon in spinach (Cairns *et al.*, 1985); (2) examination of one pesticide in a variety of crops—for example, ethoprop in vegetables (Hunt *et al.*, 1981) or acephate in vegetables and fruits (Frank *et al.*, 1984); (3) investigation of the effects of processing on pesticide residues—for example, DDT in cooked, canned beef (Hearnsberger *et al.*, 1976); (4) consideration of a wide variety of produce ingested by consumers and extensive analysis of a large number of commonly used pesticides, called the market basket survey—for example, examining the diet of an age group (Johnson *et al.*, 1979) or a national population

(Smith, 1971; Smith *et al.*, 1973). The overall purposes of residue analyses are to locate reservoirs, or sinks, in which certain pesticides may accumulate to higher than expected levels (e.g., fats and oils, taproots, fruits), and to understand the factors that contribute to the persistence and accumulation of residues.

Residues in the human body also are of concern (Wassermann *et al.*, 1974; Mes *et al.*, 1977), as are those pesticides present in human milk (Kodric-Smit *et al.*, 1980; Macy *et al.*, 1979; Curley and Kimbrough, 1969; Al-Omar *et al.*, 1985). The levels of some chlorinated hydrocarbons in human milk may exceed the legal limits allowed in cows' milk.

The significance of low-level residues in human milk or in any dietary intake can only be surmised in many cases because of the dearth of knowledge on the long-term effects of complex mixtures of chemicals on humans. Any decision to abstain from such foods entails the weighing of any potential deleterious effects of the residues against the nutritional value of the food.

Just as personal decisions of that type must be made, based on available knowledge, similar judgments must be derived at regulatory and advisory levels toward the protection of the general populace. In some cases, the significance of an ingested pesticide is immediately obvious, as in cases of aldicarb poisoning from eating hydroponic cucumbers (Goes *et al.*, 1980) or watermelons (Marshall, 1985). In most cases, any impact of a chemical is more subtle, requiring more careful analysis of the consequences (Poulsen, 1978). National regulatory agencies (e.g., United States Environmental Protection Agency) establish tolerances, that is, acceptable levels of a chemical in various foodstuffs, based on toxicological data on a chemical, average daily intake of a food, and a built-in "safety factor." The risk–benefit analysis involves the weighing of the necessities or advantages of using a particular chemical versus any known risks of its use. The World Health Organization (WHO) and the Food and Agriculture Organization (FAO) of the United Nations provide maximum acceptable daily intake levels for pesticides on a global basis (FAO/WHO, 1972). For a source that examines the complicated process of setting residue limits see Bates (1979).

Sources of drinking water also may contain pesticide residues. Surface sources contain many chemicals from runoff, but even groundwater (well water) can become contaminated with pesticides (Frank *et al.*, 1979; Zoeteman *et al.*, 1980; Awad *et al.*, 1984). The Congressional Research Service published a report that details the extent and mechanisms of groundwater contamination (Gude, 1980).

The methodology available for detection of residues has constantly improved over the years, both in terms of sensitivity (minimum detectable level) and specificity (unambiguous determinations). A standard method in recent years has been gas–liquid chromatography (GLC). It is useful for analyzing picogram (10^{-12} gm) quantities of pesticides that are somewhat heat-stable, nonpolar, and detectable by one of several common detectors. Procedures often are perfected for one commodity in terms of extraction, cleanup, and analytical techniques used (Singmaster, 1980; Reichel *et al.*, 1981), but many require adaptations for suitable use for any other type of produce. The use of high-performance liquid chromatography (HPLC) has increased dramatically in the past few years. It is especially useful for chemicals that are too polar, too heat-labile, or undetectable by GLC methods. It is a nondestructive analytical method and allows repeated recycling of a sample through a column, but typically does not have detection limits as low as GLC (Mourot *et al.*, 1979). Both GLC and HPLC have advantages and are widely used today. Chemical ionization–mass spectrometry methods are also being used for residue analysis (Cairns *et al.*, 1984, 1985). Another method recently employed in pesticide residue analysis is the radioimmunoassay (e.g., Newsome and Shields, 1981; Newsome, 1986; Brimfield *et al.*, 1985). Widespread applications seem probable in the future.

ACKNOWLEDGMENT

This chapter is No. J-10640 of the Iowa Agriculture and Home Economics Experiment Station, Ames, Iowa, Project No. 2306.

REFERENCES

Abou-Donia, M. B. (1979a). Delayed neurotoxicity of *O*-(2,4-dichlorophenyl) *O*-ethyl phenylphosphonothioate (S-seven). *Toxicol. Lett.* **3**, 61–64.

Abou-Donia, M. B. (1979b). Delayed neurotoxicity of phenylphosphonothioate esters. *Science* **205**, 713–715.

Abou-Donia, M. B., and Graham, D. G. (1979). Delayed neurotoxicity of a single oral dose of *O*-ethyl *O*-4-cyanophenyl phenylphosphonothioate in the hen. *Nuerotoxicology (Park Forest South, Ill.)* **1**, 449–466.

Abou-Donia, M. B., Graham, D. G., and Kinnes, C. G. (1983). Sensitivity of the cat to delayed neurotoxicity induced by *O*-ethyl *O*-4-nitrophenyl phenylphosphonothioate. *Toxicol. Appl. Pharmacol.* **68**, 54–65.

Abou-Donia, M. B., Trofatter, L. P., Graham, D. G., and Lapadula, D.M. (1986). Electromyographic, neuropathologic, and functional correlates in the cat as a result of tri-*o*-cresyl phosphate delayed neurotoxicity. *Toxicol. Appl. Pharmacol.* **83**, 126–141.

Aldous, C. N., Chetty, C. S., and Desaiah, D. (1983). Alterations in tissue distribution of chlordecone (Kepone) in the rat following phenobarbital or SKF-525A administration. *J. Toxicol. Environ. Health* **11**, 365–372.

Alexeeff, G. V., Kilgore, W. W., Munoz, P., and Watt, D. (1985). Determination of acute toxic effects in mice following exposure to methyl bromide. *J. Toxicol. Environ. Health* **14**, 109–123.

Allen, A. L., Koller, L. D., and Pollock, G. A. (1983). Effect of toxaphene exposure on immune responses in mice. *J. Toxicol. Environ. Health* **11**, 61–69.

Al-Omar, M. A., Tawfiq, S. J., and Al-Ogaily, N. (1985). Organochlorine residue levels in human milk from Baghdad. *Bull. Environ. Contam. Toxicol.* **35**, 65–67.

Ames, B. N., McCann, J., and Yamasaki, E. (1975). Methods for detecting carcinogens and mutagens with the *Salmonella*/mammalian-microsome mutagenicity test. *Mutat. Res.* **31**, 347–364.

Anderson, A. C., Abdelghani, A. A., Hughes, J., and Mason, J. W. (1980). Accumulation of MSMA in the fruit of the blackberry (*Rubus* sp.). *J. Environ. Sci. Health Part B* **B15**, 247–258.

Awad, T. M., Kilgore, W. W., and Winterlin, W. (1984). Movement of aldicarb in different soil types. *Bull. Environ. Contam. Toxicol.* **32**, 377–382.

Bates, J. A. R. (1979). The evaluation of pesticide residues in food: Procedures and problems in setting maximum residues limits. *J. Sci. Food Agric.* **30**, 401–46.

Bell, A. N., and Mehendale, H. M. (1985). The effect of dietary exposure to a mirex plus chlordecone combination on CCl_4 hepatotoxicity. *Fundam. Appl. Toxicol.* **5**, 679–687.

Bishun, N., Smith, N., and Williams, D. (1978). Mutations, chromosome aberrations and cancer. *Clin. Oncol.* **4**, 251–263.

Bloom, A. S., Staatz, C. G., and Dieringer, T. (1983). Pyrethroid effects on operant responding and feeding. *Neurobehav. Toxicol. Teratol.* **5**, 321–324.

Brimfield, A. A., and Street, J. C. (1981). Microsomal activation of chlordane isomers to derivatives that irreversibly interact with cellular macromolecules. *J. Toxicol. Environ. Health* **7**, 193–206.

Brimfield, A. A., Lenz, D. E., Graham, C., and Hunter, K. W., Jr. (1985). Mouse monoclonal antibodies against paraoxon: Potential reagents for immunoassay with constant immunochemical characteristics. *J. Agric. Food Chem.* **33**, 1237–1242.

Brooks, G. T. (1974). "Chlorinated Insecticides." CRC Press, Cleveland, Ohio.

Brown, D. D., Metcalf, R. L., Sternburg, J. G., and Coats, J. R. (1981). Structure–activity relationships of DDT-type analogs based on *in vivo* toxicity to the sensory nerves of the cockroach *Perplaneta americana* L. *Pestic. Biochem. Physiol.* **15**, 43–57.

Bulger, W. H., Feil, V. J., and Kupfer, D. (1985). Role of hepatic monooxygenases in generating estrogenic metabolites from methoxychlor and from its identified contaminants. *Molec. Pharmacol.* **27**, 115–124.

Cairns, T., Siegmund, E. G., and Savage, T. S. (1984). Persistence and metabolism of aldicarb in fresh potatoes. *Bull. Environ. Contam. Toxicol.* **32**, 274–281.

Cairns, T., Siegmund, E. G., and Froberg, J. E. (1985). Identification of diazinon and its metabolite in spinach by chemical ionization mass spectrometry. *Bull. Environ. Contam. Toxicol.* **35**, 291–295.

Carpenter, H. M., Williams, D. E., and Buhler, D. R. (1985). Hexachlorobenzene-induced porphyria in Japanese quail: Changes in microsomal enzymes. *J. Toxicol. Environ. Health* **15**, 431–444.

Carter, S. D., Hein, J. F., Rehnberg, G. L., and Laskey, J. W. (1984). Effect of benomyl on the reproductive development of male rats. *J. Toxicol. Environ. Health* **13**, 53–68.

Casida, J. E. (1973). Biochemistry of the pyrethrins. *In* "Pyrethrum" (J. E. Casida, ed.), pp. 101–120. Academic Press, New York.

Casida, J. E., and Lawrence, L. J. (1985). Structure–activity correlations for interactions of bicyclophosphorus esters and some polychlorocycloalkane and pyrethroid insecticides with the brain-specific *t*-butylbicyclophosphorothionate receptor. *Environ. Health Perspect.* **61**, 123–132.

Casida, J. E., Holmstead, R. L., Khalifa, S., Knox, J. R., Ohsawa, T., Palmer, K. J., and Wong, R. Y. (1974). Toxaphene insecticide: A complex biodegradable mixture. *Science* **183**, 520–521.

Chang-Tsui, Y. H., and Ho, I. K. (1979). Effects of kepone (chlordecone) on synaptosomal γ-aminobutyric acid uptake in the mouse. *Neurotoxicology* **1**, 357–367.

Chapman, D. E., and Schiller, C. M. (1985). Dose-related effects of 2,3,7,8-tetrachlorodibenzo-*p*-dioxin (TCDD) in C57BL/6J and DBA/2J mice. *Toxicol. Appl. Pharmacol.* **78**, 147–157.

Chen, P. H., Tilson, H. A., Marbury, G. D., Karoum, F., and Hong, J. S. (1985). Effect of chlordecone (Kepone) on the rat brain concentration of 3-methoxy-4-hydroxyphenylglycol: Evidence for a possible involvement of the norepinephrine system in chlordecone-induced tremor. *Toxicol. Appl. Pharmacol.* **77**, 158–164.

Chernoff, N., and Rogers, E. H. (1976). Fetal toxicity of kepone in rats and mice. *Toxicol. Appl. Pharmacol.* **38,** 189–194.

Clark, J. M., and Matsumura, F. (1982). Two different types of inhibitory effects of pyrethroids on nerve Ca- and Ca+Mg-ATPase activity in the squid, *Loligo pealei. Pestic. Biochem. Physiol.* **18,** 180–190.

Coats, J. R. (1982). Structure–activity relationships in DDT analogs. *In* "Insecticide Mode of Action" (J. R. Coats, ed.), pp. 29–43. Academic Press, New York.

Coats, J. R., Metcalf, R. L., and Kapoor, I. P. (1977). Active DDT analogues with altered aliphatic moieties: Isobutanes and chloropropanes. *J. Agric. Food Chem.* **25,** 859–867.

Corbett, J. R. (1984). "The Biochemical Mode of Action of Pesticides," 2nd ed., Academic Press, New York.

Courtney, K. D., and Moore, J. A. (1971). Teratology studies with 2,4,5-trichlorophenoxyacetic acid and 2,3,7,8-tetrachlorodibenzo-*p*-dioxin. *Toxicol. Appl. Pharmacol.* **20,** 396–403.

Crocker, J. F. S., Ozere, R. L., Safe, S. H., Digout, S. C., Rozee, K. R., and Hutzinger, O. (1976). Lethal interaction of ubiquitous insecticide carriers with virus. *Science* **192,** 1351–1353.

Curley, A., and Kimbrough, R. (1969). Chlorinated hydrocarbon insecticides in plasma and milk of pregnant and lactating women. *Arch. Environ. Health* **18,** 156–164.

Cushman, J. R., and Street, J. C. (1982). Allergic hypersensitivty to the herbicide 2,4-D in BALB/c mice. *J. Toxicol. Environ. Health* **10,** 729–741.

Cushman, J. R., and Street, J. C. (1983). Allergic hypersensitivity to the insecticide malathion in BALB/c mice. *Toxicol. Appl. Pharmacol.* **70,** 29–42.

Cutkomp, L. K., Koch, R. B., and Desaiah, D. (1982). Inhibition of ATPases by chlorinated hydrocarbons. *In* "Insecticide Mode of Action" (J. R. Coats, ed.), pp. 45–69. Academic Press, New York.

Dandliker, W. B., Hicks, A. N., Levison, S. A., Stewart, K., and Brawn, R. J. (1980). Effects of pesticides on the immune response. *Environ. Sci. Technol.* **14,** 204–210.

Dauterman, W. C. (1976). Extramicrosomal metabolism of insecticides. *In* "Insecticide, Biochemistry and Physiology" (C. F. Wilkinson, ed.), pp. 149–176. Plenum, New York.

David, D. (1982). Action de la decamethrine de sa solution commerciale, de l'excipient et du xylene sur le potentiel biotique de la caille. Effets sur l'appareil genital embryonnaire. *Arch. Anat. Microsc. Morphol. Exp.* **71,** 159–174.

Dean, M. E., Smeaton, T. C., and Stock, B. H. (1980). The influence of fetal and neonatal exposure to dichlorodiphenyltrichloroethane (DDT) on the testosterone status of neonatal male rat. *Toxicol. Appl. Pharmacol.* **53,** 315–322.

Dietz, D. D., and McMillan, D. E. (1979). Comparative effects of mirex and Kepone on schedule-controlled behavior in the rat. 2. Spaced-responding, fixed-ratio and unsignaled avoidance schedules. *Neurotoxicology* **1,** 387–402.

Elgar, K. E. (1983). Pesticide residues in water—an appraisal. *In* "Pesticide Chemistry: Human Welfare and the Environment" (J. Miyamoto *et al.,* eds.), vol. 3, pp. 33–42. Pergamon, Oxford.

Elliott, M. (1977). Synthetic pyrethroids. *In* "Synthetic Pyrethroids" (M. Elliott, ed.), pp. 1–28. Am. Chem. Soc., Washington, D.C.

Elliott, M., and Janes, N. F. (1973). Chemistry of the natural pyrethrins. *In* "Pyrethrum: The Natural Insecticide" (J. E. Casida, ed.), pp. 56–100. Academic Press, New York.

El-Sebae, A. H., Othman, M. A. S., Hammam, S. M., Tantawy, G., and Soliman, S. A. (1980). Delayed neurotoxicity of cyanofenphos in chickens. *J. Environ. Sci. Health, Part B* **B15,** 267–285.

Epstein, S. S. (1977). The carcinogenicity of organochlorine pesticides. *Cold Spring Harbor Conf. Cell Proliferation* **4,** 243–265.

Eto, M. (1974). "Organophosphorus Pesticides: Organic and Biological Chemistry." CRC Press, Cleveland, Ohio.

Fabacher, D. L., and Hodgson, E. (1976). Induction of hepatic mixed-function oxidase enzymes in adult and neonatal mice by kepone and mirex. *Toxicol. Appl. Pharmacol.* **38,** 71–77.

Food and Agriculture Organization/World Health Organization (FAO/WHO) (1972). Pesticide residues in food. Report of the 1971 joint meeting of the FAO working party of experts on pesticide residues and the WHO expert committee on pesticide residues. *W.H.O. Tech. Rep. Ser.* **502;** *FAO Agric. Stud.* **88.**

Francis, B. M., Hansen, L., and Metcalf, R. L. (1980). Response of Japanese quail (*Coturnix coturnix*) to organophosphorus ester-induced delayed neurotoxicity relative to domestic hens (*Gallus gallus domesticus*). *Bull. Environ. Contam. Toxicol.* **25,** 537–540.

Frank, R., and Braun, H. E. (1984). Lindane toxicity to four-month-old calves. *Bull. Environ. Contam. Toxicol.* **32,** 533–536.

Frank, R., Sirons, G. J., and Ripley, B. D. (1979). Herbicide contamination and decontamination of well waters in Ontario, Canada, 1969–78. *Pestic. Monit. J.* **13,** 120–127.

Frank, R., Ritcey, G., Braun, H. E., and McEwen, F. L. (1984). Disappearance of acephate residues from beans, carrots, celery, lettuce, peppers, potatoes, strawberries, and tomatoes. *J. Econ. Entomol.* **77,** 1110–1115.

Frawley, J. P., Fuyat, H. N., Hagan, E. C., Blake, J. R., and Fitzhugh, O. G. (1957). Marked potentiation in mammalian toxicity from simultaneous administration of two anticholinesterase compounds. *J. Pharmacol. Exp. Ther.* **121,** 96–106.

Fukuto, T. R. (1971). Relationships between the structure of organophosphorus compounds and their activity as acetylcholinesterase inhibitors. *Bull. W.H.O.* **44,** 31–42.

Gerhart, J. M., Hong, J. S., and Tilson, H. H. (1983). Studies on the possible sites of chlordecone-induced tremor in rats. *Toxicol. Appl. Pharmacol.* **70,** 382–389.

Goes, E. A., Savage, E. P., Gibbons, G., Aaronson, M., Ford, S. A., and Wheeler, H. W. (1980). Suspected foodborne carbamate pesticide intoxications associated with ingestion of hydroponic cucumbers. *Am. J. Epidemiol.* **111,** 254–260.

Gude, G. (1980). "Resource Losses from Surface Water, Groundwater, and Atmospheric Contamination: A Catalog." U. S. Govt. Printing Office, Washington, D. C.

Gupta, R. C., Rech, R. H., Lovell, K. L., Welsch, F., and Thornburg, J. E. (1985). Brain cholinergic, behavioral, and morphological development in the rats exposed *in utero* to methylparathion. *Toxicol. Appl. Toxicol.* **77,** 405–413.

Hammond, P. B., and Beliles, R. P. (1980). Metals. *In* "Toxicology, The Basic Science of Poisons" (J. Doull, C. D. Klaassen, and M. O. Amdur, eds.), pp. 409–467. Macmillan, New York.

Hanify, J. A., Metcalf, P., Nobbs, C. L., and Worsley, K. J. (1981). Aerial spraying of 2,4,5-T and human birth malformations: An epidemiological investigation. *Science* **212,** 329–351.

Hay, A. (1982). "The Chemical Scythe: Lessons of 2,4,5T and Dioxin." Plenum, New York.

Hayes, W. J., Jr. (1975). "Toxicology of Pesticides." Williams & Wilkins, Baltimore, Maryland.

Hearnsberger, A. P., Kilgore, L. T., and Rogers, R. W. (1976). Degradation of 1,1,1-trichloro-2,2-bis(*p*-chlorophenyl)ethane (DDT) in beef by canning and cooking. *J. Agric. Food Chem.* **24,** 677–678.

Heikes, D. L. (1980). Residues of pentachloronitrobenzene and related compounds in peanut butter. *Bull. Environ. Contam. Toxicol.* **24,** 338–343.

Hewitt, L. A., Hewitt, W. R., and Plaa, G. L. (1983). Fractional hepatic localization of $^{14}CHCl_3$ in mice and rats treated with chlordecone or mirex. *Fundam. Appl. Toxicol.* **3,** 489–495.

Holan, G. (1969). New halocyclopropane insecticides and the mode of action of DDT. *Nature (London)* **221,** 1025–1029.

Hollingshaus, J. G., Armstron, D., Toia, R. F., McCloud, L., and Fukuto, T. R. (1981). Delayed toxicity and delayed neurotoxicity of phosphorothioate and phosphonothioate esters. *J. Toxicol. Environ. Health* **8,** 619–627.

Hollingworth, R. M., and Lund, A. E. (1982). Biological and neurotoxic effects of amidine pesticides. *In* "Insecticide Mode of Action" (J. R. Coats, ed.), pp. 189–227. Academic Press, New York.

Hollingworth, R. M., and Murdock, L. L. (1980). Formamidine pesticides: Octopamine-like actions in a firefly. *Science* **208,** 74–76.

Honma, T., Miyagawa, M., Sato, M., and Hasegawa, H. (1985). Neurotoxicity and metabolism of methyl bromide in rats. *Toxicol. Appl. Pharmacol.* **81,** 183–191.

Hood, R. D., Patterson, B. L., Thacker, G. T., Sloan, G. L., and Szczech, G. M. (1979). Prenatal effects of 2,4,5-T, 2,4,5-trichlorophenol, and phenoxyacetic acid in mice. *J. Environ. Sci. Health Part C* C**13**(3), 189–204.

Hooper, N. K., Ames, B. N., Saleh, M. A., and Casida, J. E. (1979). Toxaphene, a complex mixture of polychloroterpenes and a major insecticide, is mutagenic. *Science* **205,** 591–593.

Hunt, T. W., Leidy, R. B., Sheets, T. J., and Duncan, H. E. (1981). Residues of ethoprop in eight vegetables. *Bull. Environ. Contam. Toxicol.* **27,** 84–89.

Innes, J. R. M., Ulland, B. M., Valerio, M. G., Petrucelli, L., Fishbein, L., Hart, E. R., Pallotta, A. J., Bates, R. R., Falk, H. L., Gart, J. J., Klein, M., Mitchell, I., and Peters, J. (1969). Bioassay of pesticides and industrial chemicals for tumorigenicity in mice: A preliminary note. *J. Natl. Cancer Inst. (U.S.)* **42,** 1101–1114.

Isom, G. E., and Way, J. L. (1976). Lethality of cyanide in the absence of inhibition of liver cytochrome oxidase. *Biochem. Pharmacol.* **25,** 606–608.

Iverson, F. (1976). Induction of paraxon dealkylation by hexachlorobenzene (HCB) and mirex. *J. Agric. Food Chem.* **24,** 1238–1241.

Jaffee, O. C., and Mitrosky, S. (1979). The effects of an organo-phosphate insecticide (Azodrin) upon cardiovascular development. *Anat. Rec.* **194,** 630.

Jakoby, W. B., ed. (1981). "Detoxication and Drug Metabolism: Conjugation and Related Systems." (Methods in Enzymology, Vol. 77. Academic Press, New York.

Jakoby, W. B., Bend. J. R., and Caldwell, J., eds. (1982). "Metabolic Basis of Detoxication: Metabolism of Functional Groups." Academic Press, New York.

James, J. A. (1980). The toxicity of synthetic pyrethroids to mammals. *Dev. Anim. Vet. Sci.* **6,** 249–255.

Johnson, J. L., Jr., Jones, R. L., Leuck, D. B., Bowman, M. C., and Knox, F. E. (1974). Persistence of chlorpyrifos-methyl in corn silage and effects of feeding dairy cows the treated silage. *J. Dairy Sci.* **57,** 1467–1473.

Johnson, M. K. (1975). Organophosphorus esters causing delayed neurotoxic effects. *Arch. Toxicol.* **34,** 259–288.

Johnson, M. K. (1984). Initiation of organophosphate-induced delayed neuropathy. *Neurobehav. Toxicol. Teratol.* **4,** 759–765.

Johnson, R. D., Manske, D. D., New, D. H., and Podrebarac, D. S. (1979). Pesticides and other chemical residues in infant and toddler. *Pestic. Monit. J.* **13,** 87–98.

Kato, Y., Sato, K., Matano, O., and Goto, S. (1980). Alkylation of cellular macromolecules by reactive metabolic intermediate of DBCP. *J. Pestic. Sci.* **5**(1), 45–53.

Khera, K. S. (1979). Evaluation of dimethoate (cygon 4E) for teratogenic activity in the cat. *J. Environ. Pathol. Toxicol.* **2,** 1283–1288.

Khera, K. S., Villeneuve, D. C., Terry, G., Panopio, L., Nash, L., and Trivett, G. (1976). Mirex: A teratogenicity, dominant lethal and tissue distribution study in rats. *Food Cosmet. Toxicol.* **14,** 25–29.

Kinoshita, F. K., Frawley, J. P., and Dubois, K. P. (1966). Quantitative measurement of induction of hepatic microsomal enzymes by various dietary levels of DDT and toxaphene in rats. *Toxicol. Appl. Pharmacol.* **9,** 505–513.

Kluwe, W. M., Gupta, B. N., and Lamb, J. C. IV (1983a). The comparative effects of 1,2-dibromo-3-chloropropane (DBCP) and its metabolites, 3-chloro-1,3-propanexoide (epichlorohydrin), 3-chloro-1,2-propanediol (alphachlorohydrin) and oxalic acid, on the urogenital system of male rats. *Toxicol. Appl. Pharmacol.* **70**, 67–81.

Kluwe, W. M., Lamb, J. C., IV, Greenwell, A. E., and Harrington, F. W. (1983b). 1,2-Dibromo-3-chloropropane (DBCP)-induced infertility in male rats mediated by a post-testicular effect. *Toxicol. Appl. Pharmacol.* **71**, 294–298.

Knowles, C. O. (1982). Structure–activity relationships among amidine acaricides and insecticides. *In* "Insecticide Mode of Action" (J. R. Coats, ed.), pp. 243–277. Academic Press. New York.

Kodrick-Smit, M., Smit, Z., and Olie, K. (1980). Organochlorine contaminants in human milk from Slavonia province, Yugoslavia, 1978, *Pestic. Monit. J.* **14**, 1–6.

Kreitzer, J. F. (1980). Effects of toxaphene and endrin at very low dietary concentrations on discrimination acquisition and reversal in bobwhite quail, *Colinus virginianus. Environ. Pollut., Ser. A: Ecol. Biol.* **23**, 217–230.

Krzystyniak, K., Hugo, P., Flipo, D., and Fournier, M. (1985). Increased susceptibility to mouse hepatitis virus 3 of peritoneal macrophages exposed to dieldrin. *Toxicol. Appl. Pharmacol.* **80**, 397–408.

Kuhr, R. J., and Dorough, H. W. (1976). "Carbamate Insecticides: Chemistry, Biochemistry, and Toxicology." CRC Press, Cleveland, Ohio.

Kupfer, D., and Bulger, W. H. (1976). Studies on the mechanism of estrogenic actions of o,p'DDT: Interactions with the estrogen receptor. *Pestic. Biochem. Physiol.* **6**, 561–670.

Lawrence, L. J., and Casida, J. E. (1983). Stereospecific action of pyrethroid insecticides on the γ-aminobutryic acid receptor–ionophore complex. *Science* **221**, 139–1401.

Leander, J. D., and MacPhail, R. C. (1980). Effect of chlordimeform (a formamidine pesticide) on schedule-controlled responding of pigeons. *Neurobehav. Toxicol.* **2**, 315–321.

Letz, G. A., Pond, S. M., Osterloh, J. D., Wade, P. L., and Becker, C. E. (1984). Two fatalities after acute occupational exposure to ethylene dibromide. *JAMA, J. Am. Med. Assoc.* **252**, 2428–2431.

LeWitt, P. A. (1980). The neurotoxicity of the rat poison vacor. *N. Engl. J. Med.* **302**, 73–77.

Lewerenz, H. J., and Bleyl, D. W. R. (1980). Postnatal effects of oral administration of ethylenethiourea to rats during late pregnancy. *Arch. Toxicol.* **4**, Suppl., 292–295.

Lewerenz, H. J., Bleyl, D. W. R., Plas, R., and Engst, R. (1977). Toxicology of ethylenethiourea. *Environ. Pollut. Hum. Health., Proc. Int. Symp., 1st, 1975*, pp. 639–660.

Longo, L. D. (1980). Environmental pollution and pregnancy: Risks and uncertainties for the fetus and infant. *Am. J. Obstet. Gynecol.* **137**, 162–173.

Lotti, M., Wei, E. T., Spear, R. C., and Becker, C. E. (1985). Neurotoxic esterase in rooster testis. *Toxicol. Appl. Pharmacol.* **77**, 175–180.

Lund, A. E. (1984). Pyrethroid modification of sodium channel: Current concepts. *Pestic. Biochem. Physiol.* **22**, 161–168.

Lund, A. E., Hollingworth, R. M., and Yim, G. K. W. (1979). The comparative neurotoxicity of formamidine pesticides. *In* "Neurotoxicology of Insecticides and Pheromones" (T. Narahashi, ed.), pp. 119–137. Plenum, New York.

McCorkle, F., Taylor, R., Martin, D., and Glick, B. (1980). The effect of permethrin on the immune response of chickens. *Poult. Sci.* **59**, 1568.

McEwen, F. L., and Stephenson, G. R. (1979), "The Use and Significance of Pesticides in the Environment." Wiley, New York.

MacPhail, R. C., and Leander, J. D. (1980). Flavor aversions induced by chlordimeform. *Neurobehav. Toxicol.* **2**, 363–365.

MacPhail, R. C., Gordon, W. A., and Johnston, M. A. (1981). Behavioral effects of a synthetic pyrethroid insecticide (decamethrin). *Fed. Proc., Fed. Am. Soc. Exp. Biol.* **40**, 678.

Macy, A. M., Kutchinsky, L. E., and Wislocki, A. (1979). A comparative cross sectional study of pesticide residue in human breast milk, cows' milk, canned milk, and infant formula in Colorado. *Clin. Toxicol.* **15**, 482.

Madhukar, B. V., and Matsumura, F. (1979). Comparison of induction patterns of rat hepatic microsomal mixed-function oxidases by pesticides and related chemicals. *Pestic. Biochem. Physiol.* **11**, 301–308.

Mahmood, A., Agarwal, N., Sanyal, S., Dudeja, P. K., and Subrahmanyam, D. (1979). Alterations in the intestinal brush border membrane structure and function in chronic DDT-exposed monkeys. *Pestic. Biochem. Physiol.* **12**, 141–146.

Marks, T. A., and Ledoux, T. A. (1982). Teratogenicity of a commercial xylene mixture in the mouse. *J. Toxicol. Environ. Health* **9**, 97–105.

Marshall, E. (1985). The rise and decline of Temik. *Science* **229**, 1369–1371.

Marshall, T. C., Dorough, H. W., and Swim. H. E. (1976). Screening of pesticides for mutagenic potential using *Salmonella typhimurium* mutants. *J. Agric. Food Chem.* **24**, 560–563.

Matsumura, F. (1983). Influence of chlorinated and pyrethroid insecticides on cellular calcium regulatory mechanisms. *In* "Pesticide Chemistry: Human Welfare and the Environment" (J. Miyamoto *et al.*, eds.), Vol. 3, pp. 3–13. Pergamon, Oxford.

Matsumura, F. (1985). "Toxicology of Insecticides," 2nd ed. Plenum, New York.

Matsumura, F., Howard, R. W., and Nelson, J. O. (1975). Structure of the toxic fraction A of toxaphene. *Chemosphere* **5**, 271–276.

Mes, J., Campbell, D. S., Robinson, R. N., and Davies, D. J. A. (1977). Polychlorinated biphenyl and organochlorine pesticide residues in adipose tissue of Canadians. *Bull. Environ. Contam. Toxicol.* **17**, 196–203.

Metcalf, C. L., Flint, W. P., and Metcalf, R. L. (1962). "Destructive and Useful Insects: Their Habits and Control," 4th ed. McGraw-Hill, New York.

Metcalf, R. L. (1971). Structure–activity relationships for insecticidal carbamates. *Bull. W.H.O.* **44**, 43–78.

Metcalf, R. L., Kapoor, I. P., and Hirwe, A. S. (1971). Biodegradable analogues of DDT. *Bull. W.H.O.* **44**, 363–374.

Miller, T. A., and Adams, M. E. (1982). Mode of action of pyrethroids. *In* "Insecticide Mode of Action" (J. R. Coats, ed.), pp. 3–27. Academic Press, New York.

Misawa, M., Doull, J., and Uyeki, E. M. (1982). Teratogenic effects of cholinergic insecticides in chick embryos. III. Development of cartilage and bone. *J. Toxicol. Environ. Health* **10**, 551–563.

Moriya, M., Ohta, T., Watanabe, K., Miyazawa, T., Kato, K., and Shirasu, Y. (1983). Further mutagenicity studies on pesticides in bacterial reversion assay systems. *Mutat. Res.* **116**, 185–216.

Mourot, D., Delépine, B., Boisseau, J., and Gayot, G. (1979). High-pressure liquid chromatography of a new pyrethroid insecticide, sumicidin. *J. Chromatogr.* **168**, 277–279.

Muralidhara, and Krishnakumari, M. K. (1980). Mammalian toxicity of aromex and xylene used in pesticidal formulations. *Indian J. Exp. Biol.* **18**, 1148–1151.

Murphy, S. D., and DuBois, K. P. (1957). Quantitative measurement of inhibition of the enzymatic detoxification of malathion by EPN (ethyl *p*-nitrophenyl thionobenzenephosphonate). *Proc. Soc. Exp. Biol. Med.* **96**, 813–818.

Nakatsugawa, T., and Morelli, M. A. (1976). Microsomal oxidation and insecticide metabolism. *In* "Insecticide, Biochemistry and Physiology" (C. F. Wilkinson, ed.), pp. 61–114. Plenum, New York.

Narahashi, T. (1976). Effects of insecticides on nervous conduction and synaptic transmission. *In* "Insecticide, Biochemistry and Physiology" (C. F. Wilkinson, ed.), pp. 327–352. Plenum, New York.

Narahashi, T. (1979). Nerve membrane ionic channels as the target site of insecticides. *In* "Neurotoxicology of Insecticides and Pheromones" (T. Narahashi, ed.), pp. 211–243. Plenum, New York.

Narahashi, T. (1982). Cellular and molecular mechanisms of action of insecticides: Neurophysiological approach. *Neurobehav. Toxicol. Teratol.* **4**, 753–758.

Nelson, J., MacKinnon, E. A., Mower, H. F., and Wong, L. (1981). Mutagenicity of *N*-nitroso derivatives of carbofuran and its toxic metabolites. *J. Toxicol. Environ. Health* **7**, 519–531.

Nelson, J. O., and Matsumura, F. (1975). Separation and comparative toxicity of toxaphene components. *J. Agric. Food Chem.* **23**, 984–990.

Newsome, W. H. (1986). Development of an enzyme-linked immunosorbent assay for triadimefon in foods. *Bull. Environ. Contam. Toxicol.* **36**, 9–14.

Newsome, W. H., and Shields, J. B. (1981). A radioimmunoassay for benomyl and methyl 2-benzimidazolecarbamate on food crops. *J. Agric. Food Chem.* **29**, 220–222.

Nigg, H. N., Metcalf, R. L., and Kapoor, I. P. (1976). DDT and selected analogues as microsomal oxidase inducers in the mouse. *Arch. Environ. Contam. Toxicol.* **3**, 426–436.

O'Brien, R. D. (1967). "Insecticides, Action and Metabolism." Academic Press, New York.

O'Brien, R. D. (1976). Acetylcholinesterase and its inhibition. *In* "Insecticide, Biochemistry and Physiology" (C. F. Wilkinson, ed.), pp. 271–296. Plenum, New York.

O'Brien, R. D., Hetnarski, B., Tripathi, R. K., and Hart, G. J. (1974). Recent studies on acetylcholinesterase inhibition. *In* "Mechanism of Pesticide Action" (G. K. Kohn, ed.), pp. 1–13. Am. Chem. Soc., Washington, D. C.

Olson, K. L., Boush, G. M., and Matsumura, F. (1980). Pre- and postnatal exposure to dieldrin: Persistent stimulatory and behavioral effects. *Pestic. Biochem. Physiol.* **13**, 20–33.

O'Reilly, R. A., Trager, W. F., Motley, C. H., and Howald, W. (1980). Interaction of ecobarbital with warfarin pseudoracemates. *Clin. Pharmacol. Ther.* **28**, 187–195.

Pardini, R. S., Heidker, J. C., Baker, T. A., and Payne, B. (1980). Toxicology of various pesticides and their decomposition products on mitochondrial electron transport. *Arch. Environ. Contam. Toxicol.* **9**, 87–97.

Pettersen, J. C., and Cohen, S. D. (1985). Antagonism of cyanide poisoning by chlorpromazine and sodium thiosulfate. *Toxicol. Appl. Pharmacol.* **81**, 265–273.

Pollack, J. D. (1979). Models of chemical and virus interaction and their relation to a multiple etiology of Reye's syndrome. *In* "Reye's Syndrome II" (J. F. S. Crocker, ed.), pp. 341–360. Grune & Stratton, New York.

Poulsen, E. (1978). Toxicological aspects of the food we eat. *In* "Proceedings of the First International Congress on Toxicology" (G. L. Plaa and W. A. M. Duncan, eds.), pp. 47–59. Academic Press, New York.

Pratt, I. S., Keeling, P. L., and Smith, L. L. (1980). The effect of high concentrations of oxygen on paraquat and diquat toxicity in rats. *Arch. Toxicol.* **4**, Suppl., 415–418.

Pritsos, C. A., Pisani, D. E., and Pardini, R. S. (1985). Inhibition of liver glycolysis in rats by dietary dichlone (2,3-dichloro-1,4-naphthoquinone). *Bull. Environ. Contam. Toxicol.* **35**, 23–28.

Rao, K. S., Burek, J. D., Murray, F. J., John, J. A., Schwetz, B. A., Bell, T. J., Potts, W. J., and Parker, C. M. (1983). Toxicologic and reproductive effects of inhaled 1,2-dibromo-3-chloropropane in rats. *Fundam. Appl. Toxicol.* **3**, 104–110.

Rattner, B. A., and Michael, S. D. (1985). Organophosphorus insecticide induced decrease in plasma luteinizing hormone concentration in white-footed mice. *Toxicol. Lett.* **24**, 65–69.

Reichel, W. L., Kolbe, E., and Stafford, C. J. (1981). Gas–liquid chromatographic and gas–liquid chromatographic–mass spectrometric determination of fenvalerate and permethrin residues in grasshoppers and duck tissue samples. *J. Assoc. Off. Anal. Chem.* **64**, 1196–1200.

Reiter, L., Kidd, K., Ledbetter, G., Gray, E. L., Jr., and Chernoff, N. (1977). Comparative behavioral toxicology of mirex and Kepone in the rat. *Toxicol. Appl. Pharmacol.* **41**, 143.

Reuber, M. D. (1979). Carcinogenicity of toxaphene: A review. *J. Toxicol. Environ. Health* **5**, 729–748.

Rohl, A. N., and Langer, A. M. (1974). Identification and quantitation of asbestos in talc. *Environ. Health Perspect.* **9**, 165–172.

Ross, R. D., Morrison, J., Rounbehler, D. P., Fan, S., and Fine, D. H. (1977). *N*-Nitroso compound impurities in herbicide formulations. *J. Agric. Food Chem.* **25,** 1416–1418.

Rumsey, T. S. (1979). Performance, ruminal measurements and blood plasma amino acids of steers fed ronnel. *J. Anim. Sci.* **49,** 1059–1065.

Rumsey, T. S., Williams, E. E., and Evans, A. D. (1975). Tissue residues, performance and ruminal and blood characteristics of steers fed ronnel and activated carbon. *J. Anim. Sci.* **40,** 743–749.

Sandifer, S. H., Wilkins, R. T., Loadhold, C. B., Lane, L. G., and Eldridge, J. C. (1979). Spermatogenesis in agricultural workers exposed to dibromochloropropane (DBCP). *Bull. Environ. Contam. Toxicol.* **23,** 703–710.

Seifert, J., and Casida, J. E. (1982). Possible role of microtubules and associated proteases in organophosphorus ester induced delayed neurotoxicity. *Biochem. Pharmacol.* **31,** 2065–2070.

Shankland, D. L. (1979). Action of dieldrin and related compounds on synaptic transmission. *In* "Neurotoxicology of Insecticides and Pheromones" (T. Narahashi, ed.), pp. 139–153. Plenum, New York.

Shankland, D. L. (1982). Neurotoxic action of chlorinated hydrocarbon insecticides. *Neurobehav. Toxicol. Teratol.* **4,** 805–811.

Shiau, S. Y., Huff, R. A., and Felkner, I. C. (1981). Pesticide mutagenicity in *Bacillus subtilis* and *Salmonella typhimurium* detectors. *J. Agric. Food Chem.* **29,** 268–271.

Singh, A., Valli, V. E. O., Ritter, L., and Villeneuve, D. C. (1981). Ultrastructural alterations in the liver of rats fed photomirex (8-monohydromirex). *Pathology* **13,** 487–496.

Singmaster, J. A., III (1980). Residue analysis of endosulfan in pigeon peas. *J. Agric. Univ. P. R.* **64,** 219–231.

Smith, D. C. (1971). Pesticide residues in the total diet in Canada. *Pestic. Sci.* **2,** 92–95.

Smith, D. C., Leduc, R., and Charbonneau, C. (1973). Pesticide residues in the total diet in Canada. III-1971. *Pestic. Sci.* **4,** 211–214.

Snow, R. L., and Hays, R. L. (1983). Phasic distribution of seminiferous tubules in rats treated with triphenyltin compounds. *Bull. Environ. Contam. Toxicol.* **31,** 658–665.

Spencer, E. Y. (1976). Organophosphorus insecticides. *In* "The Future for Insecticides: Needs and Prospects" (R. L. Metcalf and J. J. McKelvey, Jr., eds.), pp. 295–307. Wiley (Interscience), New York.

Steinhoff, D., Weber, H., Mohr, U., and Boehme, K. (1983). Evaluation of amitrole (aminotriazole) for potential carcinogenicity in orally dosed rats, mice, and golden hamsters. *Toxicol. Appl. Pharmacol. 69,* 161–169.

Street, J. (1981). Pesticides and the immune system. *In* "Immunologic Considerations in Toxicology" (R. P. Sharma, ed.). CRC Press, Boca Raton, Florida.

Taylor, J. R., Selhorst, J. B., Houff, S. A., and Martinez, A. J. (1978). Chlordecone intoxication in man. *Neurology* **28,** 626–631.

Toia, R. F., March, R. B., Umetsu, N., Mallipudi, N. M., Allahyari, R., and Fukuto, T. R. (1980). Identification and toxicological evaluation of impurities in technical malathion and fenthion. *J. Agric. Food Chem.* **28,** 599–604.

Trankina, M. L., Beitz, D. C., Griffith, D. R., and Ware, D. R. (1981). Effects of an organophosphate, ronnel, on growth in male rats. *Nutr. Rep. Int.* **23,** 37–42.

Trankina, M. L., Custer, K. G., Beitz, D. C., Griffith, D. R., and Ware, D. R. (1982). Effects of feeding on organophosphate, ronnel, on lactating rats and pup growth. *Nutr. Rep. Int.* **25,** 71–74.

Turner, W. V., Khalifa, S., and Casida, J. E. (1975). Toxaphene toxicant A. Mixture of 2,2,5-*endo*,6-*exo*,8,8,9,10-octachlorobornane and 2,2,5-*endo*,6-*exo*,8,9,9,10-octachlorobornane. *J. Agric. Food Chem.* **23,** 991–994.

Tyagi, S. R., Singh, Y., Srivastava, P. K., and Misra, U. K. (1984). Induction of hepatic mixed function oxidase system by endosulfan in rats. *Bull. Environ. Contam. Toxicol.* **32,** 550–556.

Uchida, M., Fujita, T., Kurihara, K., and Nakajima, M. (1978). Toxicities of γ-BHC and related compounds. *In* "Pesticide and Venom Neurotoxicity" (D. L. Shankland, R. M. Hollingworth, and T. Smyth, eds.), pp. 133–151. Plenum, New York.

Udall, J. A. (1975). Clinical implications of warfarin interactions with five sedatives. *Am. J. Cardiol.* **35**, 67–71.

Umetsu, N., Mallipudi, N. M., Toia, R. F., March, R. B., and Fukuto, T. R. (1981). Toxicological properties of phosphorothioate and related esters present as impurities in technical organophosphorus insecticides *J. Toxicol. Environ. Health* **7**, 481–497.

van den Bercken, J. (1980). Mode of action of pyrethroids. *Dev. Anim. Vet. Sci.* **6**, 242–248.

Wassermann, M., Tomatis, L., and Wassermann, D. (1974). Storage map of organo-chlorine compounds (OCC) in humans. Epidemiological deductions for further monitoring. *CED-EPA-WHO Int. Symp.—Environ. Health.*

Wilkinson, C. F. (1976a). Insecticide interactions. *In* "Insecticide, Biochemistry and Physiology" (C. F. Wilkinson, ed.), pp. 605–647. Plenum, New York.

Wilkinson, C. F. (1976b). Insecticide synergism. *In* "The Future for Insecticides: Needs and Prospects" (R. L. Metcalf and J. J. McKelvey, Jr., eds.), pp. 195–218. Wiley (Interscience), New York.

Wong, R., and Stevens, J. B. (1985). Paraquat toxicity in vitro. I. Pulmonary alveolar macrophages. *J. Toxicol. Environ. Health* **15**, 417–429.

Wood, R. W., Rees, D. C., and Laties, V. G. (1983). Behavioral effects of toluene are modulated by stimulus control. *Toxicol. Appl. Pharmacol.* **68**, 462–472.

Woolley, D. E., Chernobieff, J. R., and Reiter, L. W. (1979). Effects of parathion on the mammalian nervous system. *In* "Neurotoxicology of Insecticides and Pheromones" (T. Narahashi, ed.), pp. 155–181. Plenum, New York.

Wyrobek, A. J., Watchmaker, G., Gordon, L., Song, K., Moore, D., II, and Whorton, D. (1981). Sperm shape abnormalities in carbaryl-exposed employees. *Environ. Health Perspect.* **40**, 255–265.

Wysocka-Paruszewska, B., Osicka, A., Brzezinski, J., and Gradowska, I. (1980). An evaluation of the toxicity of thiuram in combination with other pesticides. *Arch. Toxicol.* **4**, Suppl., 449–451.

Yamaguchi, T., and Matsumura, F., and Kadous, A. A. (1979). Inhibition of synaptic ATPases by heptachlorepoxide in rat brain. *Pestic. Biochem. Physiol.* **11**, 285–293.

Yang, R. S. H. (1976). Enzymatic conjugation and insecticide metabolism. *In* "Insecticide, Biochemistry and Physiology" (C. F. Wilkinson, ed.), pp. 177–225. Plenum, New York.

Zoeteman, B. C. J., Harmsen, K., Linders, J. B. H. J., Morra, C. F. H., and Slooff, W. (1980). Persistent organic pollutants in river water and ground water of the Netherlands. *Chemosphere* **9**, 231–249.

11

Nutritional Importance of Pesticides

S. Berger and K. Cwiek

I. INTRODUCTION

There are at least three aspects to the nutritional importance of pesticides: (1) protection of agricultural crops and commodities from various pests and consequent contribution to the increase of total food production so badly needed for a growing and undernourished world population; (2) impact on nutritive values of various agricultural products; (3) alteration of several physiological metabolic processes related to quantitative nutritional requirements and responses.

This last point is linked not only to the biological processes involved in the utilization of food, but also to nutritional status and health of populations often covered by national or international legislation or standards for nutrient intakes and for pesticide residues [Food and Agriculture Organization/World Health Organization (FAO/WHO), 1978].

Previous reports on nutrition (Ernahrungsbericht, 1984) have addressed the pesticide residues in consumed foods. In the United States, the Environmental Protection Agency sets legal tolerances for the pesticide residues in various raw agricultural commodities. Also, in other countries, including Poland, similar official regulations are operational.

Often, such regulations influence food trade between countries and thereby restrict consumption of products from a country with higher maximum residue limits (MRL) for some commodities. Limited availability of particular foods may

281

Copyright © 1987 by Academic Press, Inc.
All rights of reproduction in any form reserved.

be especially important in relation to vulnerable groups in the population, such as pregnant women, infants, and children. These restrictions or limitations are of concern not only to food buyers but also to food processors, marketers, and others involved with special food products, such as baby foods or therapeutic food formulas for adults. The possible consequences of residues exceeding the MRL levels should be taken into account by these groups as well as by those who are responsible for good agricultural practice.

All these aspects are important because of the possibility of excessive human intake of pesticides; this could occur through various routes of exposure.

For the general population, residues in foods are the main source of exposure to pesticides. Some pesticides are very persistent in the environment and therefore can be present not only as residues in food but also as contaminants in water, air, and soil. Their movement and persistence in the environment can be influenced by many factors. All these factors can influence the impact of pesticides on the nutritional value and safety of foods.

II.   PESTICIDE EFFECTS ON NUTRIENTS IN FOODS

In general, the use of pesticides increases total food production and availability by protection of crops and produce from pests. Persistent residues in the soil, however, sometimes have adverse effects on crop yields (Karanth *et al.*, 1981). Pesticides influence not only quantity but also quality of yield of the raw or processed products; this often includes their nutritive values (Berger *et al.*, 1980; Srimanthi *et al.*, 1983) or flavors (Machoney, 1962). Pesticide residues are an important concern for public health, which is shown by the large numbers of international publications and recommendations (FAO/WHO,1978) on this topic. Pesticide residues in food products are of interest to agricultural workers, hygienists, sanitary inspectors, food chemists, nutritionists, food scientists, and toxicologists, as well as to regulatory decision makers.

Herbicides may affect the carbohydrate, protein, and free amino acid composition of plants, as well as their uptake of minerals from the soil (Ploszynski, 1972). Vitamin content is influenced by pesticides. In three varieties of cabbage, decreases in ascorbic acid and niacin content were observed after treatment with the insecticide carbotox (Maruszewska and Gertig, 1982). In studies on insecticides applied to tomatoes and spinach, however, ascorbic acid content was increased by dichlorphos treatment, and no changes were observed after malathion treatment (Zadrozinska, 1973).

On the other hand, while the use of several pesticides resulted in decreased amounts of various carbohydrates in apples (Engst *et al.*, 1969), ascorbic acid concentrations were not changed.

Somewhat different results have been obtained in black currants treated with some insecticides; no changes in reducing sugars occurred, but there were significant decreases in ascorbic acid content (Cwiertniewska, 1973). When application of pesticides (either heptachlor or simazine) is combined with mineral fertilizer in potato production, ascorbic acid, nonprotein nitrogen, starch, and disaccharides are decreased, while protein nitrogen or monosaccharides are increased.

Although combinations of pesticides with mineral fertilizers were investigated in relation to nutrients in foods by Persin and Krasner in 1966, further investigation is needed to sort out the various factors that influence the relationships.

Ziegler (1957) and Schuphan and Weinmann (1964) demonstrated that treatment of beans, peas, and spinach which parathion caused decreases in ascorbic acid but increases in sugar, total protein, and specific amino acids, as well as phosphatase, peroxidase, and respiratory activity. Monnberg (1960) reported that disaccharides were increased in yellow turnips and beets when treated with lindane and dieldrin. When parathion was applied, total protein in plants was increased while ascorbic acid diminished in oranges (Borys, 1964). Thiuram and ziram, synthetic fungicides, did not influence sugar and ascorbic acid content in apples (Schubert, 1970), but the herbicides simazine and atrazine mixed with amitrol diminished sugar content in these fruits (Schubert, 1974). Some insecticides used on tomatoes and cucumbers in greenhouses decreased carbohydrates and ascorbic acid levels along with catalase activity, but had no effect on protein levels or peroxidase (Wedzisz *et al.*, 1977b).

In several vegetables, sugars, proteins (except in celery), and carotene concentrations were decreased by tetrachlorofenvinphos (Wedzisz *et al.*, 1977a), confirming earlier observations (Engst *et al.*, 1967) that the application of lindane resulted in a decrease of carotene in carrots by 15–50%.

Szajkowski and Gertig (1978) found some decreases in vitamin levels in gooseberries and red currants after Karathane 25 application: vitamins with the greatest decreases were riboflavin (~30%) and ascorbic acid (20–30%). When fenitrothion is used on soil, large decreases (7–32%) of carotene in carrots have occurred (Mlodecki *et al.*, 1973).

In experiments with maneb and mancozeb, however, carotenoids and carotene were not affected in tomatoes, whereas maneb decreased ascorbic acid and reducing sugars in black currants (Zolnierz-Piotrowska, 1975). After soil was treated with insecticides, Walkowska *et al.* (1982) found that carrots underwent several metabolic changes and had a higher (≤16%) content of protein and a lower content of carotene and carotenoids.

In several studies on herbicides used in wheat production (Szymczak and Biernat, 1980; Szymczak and Grajeta, 1980; Sykut *et al.*, 1984), there were changes in contents of lipids, proteins, calcium, and iron. It was pointed out, however, that several factors, including variety, climatic, conditions, and vegetation periods, are important. It is not possible to predict any specific effect on nutrient content. More experimental work is needed to establish these effects.

Although the results are inconsistent (Table I), it is obvious that the applica-

TABLE I

Changes in Selected Nutrients in Plant Products as a Result of Pesticide Application

Nutrient	Increase[a]	Decrease[a]	No change[a]
Protein	6	2	6
Amino acids	—	1	—
Lipids	—	—	1
Starch	—	3	5
Sugars	2	2	1
Ascorbic acid	3	7	3
Carotene, carotenoids	—	5	—
Niacin	—	1	—
Thiamin	—	1	—
Riboflavin	—	1	—
Vitamin D activity	—	—	1
Calcium	1	1	5
Phosphorus	1	3	3
Iron	4	—	3

[a]Number of reports; summarized from the text.

tion of pesticides, substances with high biological activity, cause several disturbances in plant metabolism and commonly alter the nutritive values of plant products. These effects, along with the possible toxicity to animals or humans, is a legitimate concern related to the impact of pesticides on food value and safety. Therefore, studies to identify and diminish any negative effects of pesticides on human nutrition and health are very desirable. The choice of pesticide, dosage, formulation, method, and time of application deserve attention; also both home and industrial food processing plays an important role in this regard (Berger *et al.*, 1980).

Kubacki and Lipowska (1980) demonstrated that several different technological processes can eliminate or reduce organochlorine and organophosphorus pesticide residues in meat products, fruit products, and vegetable oils. Thermal or mechanical processes (e.g., straining and peeling) were the effective means of decreasing pesticide content of these food products.

Recent studies on chlorinated hydrocarbon residues in meals provided in student cafeterias in Poland (Amarowicz and Smoczynski, 1984) indicated that intake of lindane was 0.9% and DDT 13.8% of the acceptable daily intakes (ADIs). Most of these intakes (70%) originated in products of animal origin, especially milk.

Although results on particular pesticides usually show that they seldom reached the MRLs in food products or the ADI in the diet, we should remember that multiple pesticide interactions can occur and that other foreign substances are present in food and water. The proper regulatory response to the possible toxic potentiation is debatable.

Whenever possible, studies of pesticide effects on human and animal metabolism, including enzymatic or hormonal changes, should be done to provide further evaluation of food safety (Murré *et al.*, 1984: Ploszynski, 1972). Also modern methodologies for isolation, identification, and determination of pesticide residues, and their metabolites should be improved and further developed (Ludwicki, 1984; Miedwied, 1977; Nikonorow, 1980; Stijve, 1984; Bierska *et al.*, 1982).

III. GENERAL REMARKS AND CONCLUSIONS

Pesticides, among other factors, significantly contribute to the food supply and therefore help combat hunger. Also, their potential to influence nutritive value of food and human health cannot be ignored.

While other pest control methods, including nonchemical ones, should be further investigated, it is difficult to estimate the optimal level and kind of pesticides that will be needed in the future. In the United States, the current annual use (500 million kg) of pesticides will perhaps be doubled by the year 2000. Programs of integrated pest management are aimed at reducing this volume of use by including nonchemical pest controls (Pimentel and Pimentel, 1983). While the application of some pesticides decreased or disappeared from 1974 to 1982 (e.g., DDT and lindane), others increased (e.g., carbamates and herbicides) (Food and Agriculture Organization 1984).

It is argued that the returns on an investment in pesticide use for crop production and protection are about fourfold an increased production. Returns on some of the nonchemical controls, however, are about 150 times the investment. Although food economics are important, it is desirable that nutrition and health impact be important considerations in decisions on pesticide use.

In general, data on pesticide use are not complete and are often given in terms not readily comparable, such as active ingredients or complete formulations, including diluents or adjuvants. This makes it difficult to prepare and compare usage totals for the world or regions. Data on pesticide consumption should be standardized.

The deleterious effects of pesticides on wild birds and other animals in the ecosystem (Moore, 1980) suggest far-reaching consequences for food safety and human health.

As indicated by Corbett (1974), "... unless and until we understand the enzyme systems involved in vital processes and their vulnerability in different organisms, rational development of specific pesticides will be well-nigh impossible." This conclusion is equally valid for nutritional effects of pesticides.

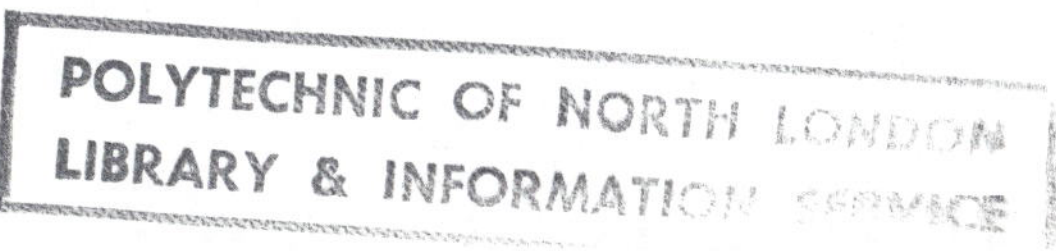

Because use of pesticides for agricultural, veterinary, domestic, and environmental purposes seems likely to be continued in the future, special attention should be given to the concept of ''good agricultural practice'' in the use of pesticides and similar restrictions in nonagricultural uses. This concept has been expressed as follows (FAO/WHO, 1978):

> Good Agricultural Practice in the use of pesticides is the officially recommended or authorized usage of pesticides under practical conditions at any stage of production, storage, transport, distribution and processing of food and other agricultural commodities, bearing in mind the variations in requirements within and between regions and taking into account the minimum quantities necessary to achieve adequate control, the pesticides being applied in such a manner as to leave residues that are smallest amounts practicable and that are toxicologically acceptable.

Analogous restriction should be applied to nonagricultural uses of pesticides.

There is an urgent need for efficient and updated monitoring systems that take into account conditions and practical possibilities in each country, food consumption patterns, economics, and technical development, especially in the case of new pesticides. Pesticide monitoring should be international and include all links in the food chain.

To assess the implications of pesticide residues in agricultural products, the food consumption pattern must be considered in relation to the MRL values (Hathcock *et al.*, 1983). The necessity of fairly uniform international residue standards to permit unobstructed trade is obvious. The simultaneous need to give adequate margins of safety with widely different national, regional, and ethnic dietary patterns means that MRL values must be set quite conservatively.

All nutritional and health effects of pesticides should be included in training of specialists (agriculturalists, food chemists, nutritionists, and medical personnel) engaged in various public education and extension services.

REFERENCES

Amarowicz, R., and Smoczynski, S. (1984). Badanie skazenia posilkow w stolowce akademickiej pozostalosciami chlorowanych weglowodorow. *Roczn. Panstw. Zakl. Hig.* **35,** 323–326.

Berger, S., Pardo, B., and Skorkowska-Zieleniewska, J. (1980). Nutritional implications of pesticides in food. Foreign substances and nutrition. *Bibl. ''Nutr. Dieta''* **29,** 1–10.

Bierska, J., Kaminski, J., and Skwarska, S. (1982). Badania zawartosci weglowodorow chlorowanych w mleku w proszku, w odzywkach i serach. *Roczn. Inst. Przem. Mlecz.* **24,** 13–19.

Borys, M. (1964). Wplyw fungicydow i insektycydow na procesy fizjologiczne traktowanych roslin. *Postepy Nauk Roln.* **11,** 57–64.

Corbett, J. R. (1974). ''The Biochemical Mode of Action of Pesticides.'' Academic Press, New York.

Cwiertniewska, E. (1973). Wplyw insektycydow fosforoorganicznych—dimetoatu, tiometonu i metylodemetonu-S na zawartosc witaminy C i cukrow redukujacych w owocach czarnej porzeczki. *Roczn. Panstw. Zakl. Hig.* **24,** 151–158.

Engst, R., Blazovich, M., and Knoll, R. (1967). Über das Vorkommen von Lindan in Möhren und seinen Einfluss auf dem Carotengehalt. *Nahrung* **11**, 389–399.

Engst, R., Noske, R., and Voigt, J. (1969). Zum Einfluss von Pflanzenschutz und Schädlingsbekämpfungsmitteln auf einige Inhaltstoffe von Obst und Gemüse. 1. Mitt. Beeinflussung von Äpfeln und Erdbeeren. *Nahrung* **13**, 249–255.

Ernahrungsbericht (1984). DGE, Frankfurt, Fed. Repub. Germany.

Food and Agriculture Organization (1984). "1983 FAO Production Year Book," Vol. 37. FAO, Rome.

Food and Agriculture Organization/World Health Organization (FAO/WHO) (1978). "Codex Alimentarius Commission. Guide to Codex Maximum Limits for Pesticide Residues," FAO/WHO Food Stand. Program. FAO WHO, Rome.

Hathcock, J. N., Vary, A. Z., Berger, S., and Brzozowska, A. (1983). Evaluation of FAO/WHO pesticide standards in relation to Polish and Honduras diets. *Regul. Toxicol. Pharmacol.* **3**, 216–223.

Karanth, N. G., Jayaram, M., and Majumder, I. (1981). Phytotoxicity of X-factor. *Pesticides* **15**, 7–10.

Kubacki, S. J., and Lipowska, T. (1980). The role of food processing in decreasing pesticide contamination of food. In "Food and Health Science and Technology" pp. 215—226. Applied Science Publishers, London.

Ludwicki, J. (1984). Oznaczanie pozostalosci insektycydow fosforoorganicznych w mleku. [Determination of residues of phosphoroorganic insecticides in milk.] *Roczn. Panstw. Zakl. Hig.* **35**, 243–246.

Machoney, C. H. (1962). Flavor and quality changes in fruits and vegetables in the United States caused by application of pesticides chemicals. *Residue Rev.* **1**, 11–23.

Maruszewska, M., and Gertig, H. (1982). Wplyw stosowania "Karbatoksu zawiesinowego 75" na poziom niektorych witamin w warzywach kapustnych. *Bromatol. Chem. Toksykol.* **15**, 19–22.

Miedwied, L. I. (1977). "Gigiena primienienija, toxikologie piesticidow i klinika otrawlenii." Moskwa.

Mlodecki, H., Lasota, W., and Dutkiewicz, J. (1973). Wplyw fenitrotionu na zawartosc β-karotenu i sumy karotenoidow w marchwi. *Bromatol. Chem. Toksykol.* **6**, 221–228.

Monnberg, B. (1960). Effect of certain chlorinated hydrocarbons on the sugar component in plant. *Chem. Abstr.* **54**, 16554c.

Moore, N. W. (1980). Pesticides and other man-made chemicals and the food chain. In "Food Chain and Human Nutrition" (K. Blaxter, ed.), pp. 401–410. Applied Science Publishers, London.

Murré, D. J., Gripshuyer, B., Monroe, A., and Murré, J. T. (1984). Phosphatidylinositol turnover in isolated soybean membranes stimulated by the synthetic growth hormone 2,4-dichlorophenoxyacetic acid. *J. Biol. Chem.* **259**, 15364–15368.

Nikonorow, M. (1980). Zanieczyszczenia chemiczne i biologiczne zywnosci. *Wydawn. Nauk Techn., Warszawa*, pp. 186–220.

Persin, S. A., and Krasner, B. A. (1966). Effect of the combined application of insecticides, herbicides and mineral fertilizers on the yield and quality of potato. *Chem. Abstr.* **65**, 1336g.

Pimentel, D., and Pimentel, M. (1983). The future of American agriculture. In "Sustainable Food Systems" (D. Knorr, ed.), pp. 3–47. Avi Publ. Co., Westport, Connecticut.

Ploszynski, M. (1972). Stymulacyjny wplyw herbicydow na rosliny i ich metabolizm. *Postepy Nauk Roln.* **1**, 5564.

Schubert, E. (1970). Einfluss organisch-synthetischer Fungizide auf die Fruchtqualität des Apfels. *Nahrung* **14**, 491–494.

Schubert, E. (1974). Einfluss ausgewählter Insektizide und Herbizide auf die Fruchtqualität des Apfels. *Nahrung* **18**, 557–560.

Schuphan, W., and Weinmann, W. (1964). Über die Wirkung einer Parathion Behandlung von

Spinat auf wertgebende Inhaltsstoffe und auf den ernahrungsphysiologischen Wert des Blatt-proteins. *Z. Pflanzenkr. Pflanzenschutz* **71**, 12–24.

Srimathi, M. S., Karanth, N. G. K., and Majumder, I. (1983). Insecticide-induced shift in the nutritive quality of vegetables grown in BHC-treated soil. *Indian J. Nutr. Diet.* **23**, 216–222.

Stijve, T. (1984). Determination and occurrence of organophosphorus pesticide residues in milk. *Spec. Publ., R. Soc. Chem.* **49**, 293–302.

Sykut, A., Ciszewska, R., Wojcik, W., and Szynal, J. (1984). Wplyw herbicydow stosowanych w uprawie pszenicy ozimej na zawartosc frakcji bialkowych i bialka ogolnego w ziarnic. *Bromatol. Chem. Toksykol.* **17**, 143–148.

Szajkowski, Z., and Gertig, H. (1978). Wplyw opryskiwania krzewow agrestu i porzeczek pre-paratem "Karathane 25" na poziom niektorych witamin w owocach. *Bromatol. Chem. Toksykol.* **11**, 297–300.

Szymczak, J., and Biernat, J. (1980). Wplyw herbicydow na zawartosc wapnia i zelaza w ziarnie roznych odmian pszenicy. *Bromatol. Chem. Toksykol.* **13**, 139–143.

Szymczak, J., and Grajeta, H. (1980). Wplyw herbicydow stosowanych w uprawie pszenicy na zawartosc lipidow w ziarnie. *Bromatol. Chem. Toksykol.* **13**, 135–138.

Walkowska, A., Olejnik, D., Urbanowicz, M., and Walkowski, A. (1982). Zawarotsc i trawalosc αiβ-karotenow oraz wybranych podstawowych skladnikow marchwi uprawianej na glebach skazonych in sketycydami. *Bromatol. Chem. Toksykol.* **15**, 23–34.

Wedzisz, A., Sloczynska, T., and Szwejda, J. (1977a). Wplyw preparatu Gardona na niektore skladniki warzyw. *Bromatol. Chem. Toksykol.* **10**, 29–34.

Wedzisz, A., Sloczynska, T., and Szwejda, J. (1977b). Dynamika zanikania naledu (Alvory-64,5) w warunkach upraw szklarniowych pomidorow i ogorkow oraz wplyw tego insektycydu na niektore ich skladniki. *Bromatol. Chem. Toksykol.* **10**, 123–128.

Zadrozinska, J. (1973). Wyplyw stosowania dichlorfosu i malationu na wartosc odzywcza niektorych warzyw. *Roczn. Panstw. Zakl. Hig.* **24**, 1–10.

Ziegler, H. (1957). Über die physiologischen Grundlagen der Wirkung des Insektizides E-605 auf den pflanzlicher Organizmus. *Biol. Zentralbl.* **76**, 43–69.

Zolnierz-Piotrowska, M. (1975). Wplyw wybranych fungicydow na zawartosc witaminy C i cukrow redukujacych w owocach czarnej porzeczki oraz na zawartosc β-karotenu i sumy karotenoidow w pomidorach. Ph.D. Thesis, Library of the National Institute of Hygiene, Warsaw, Poland (unpublished).

Index